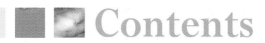 Contents

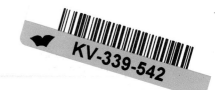
KV-339-542

Tables

Clinical Protocols

About the Executive Editors

Fred M. Wilson II, MD, is professor emeritus of ophthalmology, Indiana University School of Medicine, and consultant, Roudebush Veterans Administration Medical Center, Indianapolis. He trained at Indiana University, where he received his MD degree, and the Francis I. Proctor Foundation, San Francisco. He served for 15 years on the faculty of the Academy's *Basic and Clinical Science Course*, including 5 years as chair of the External Disease and Cornea Section.

Preston H. Blomquist, MD, is an associate professor of ophthalmology and ophthalmology residency program director at the University of Texas Southwestern Medical Center in Dallas, Texas. He serves as chief of the Ophthalmology Service at Parkland Memorial Hospital and medical director for ophthalmology for Parkland Health and Hospital System in Dallas.

Preface

Practical Ophthalmology: A Manual for Beginning Residents, sixth edition, is intended to help first-year ophthalmology residents function effectively as soon as possible during the first few months of their residencies. New residents usually have limited ophthalmologic knowledge and clinical capabilities yet are expected to work as clinicians almost immediately. In the hope of easing this abrupt and understandably stressful transition, this manual covers practical principles and techniques that are essential or useful for performing a variety of ophthalmologic examinations and tests and interpreting the results. Some clinical and background information is included to help residents understand the practical information presented.

The authors of this manual and the previous (fifth) edition are ophthalmologists who have much experience and interest in the training of ophthalmology residents: Preston H. Blomquist, MD (University of Texas Southwestern Medical Center, Dallas, Texas); Steven J. Gedde, MD (Bascom Palmer Eye Institute, University of Miami Miller School of Medicine, Miami, Florida), Karl C. Golnik, MD (University of Cincinnati and the Cincinnati Eye Institute, Cincinnati, Ohio); David K. Wallace, MD, MPH (Duke Eye Center, Durham, North Carolina); and Fred M. Wilson II, MD (Indiana University School of Medicine, Indianapolis, Indiana).

Text has been updated in this edition, particularly in the chapters on ophthalmic emergencies and common ocular medications. Tables, resources, and certain illustrations have been updated as well. In an effort to make the manual of maximal instructional value, we have incorporated several specific features, including:

- Chapters covering each element of a thorough ophthalmic examination, organized in the order in which each element is usually performed
- Clinical Protocols that include step-by-step instructions for some of the most important clinical procedures in various chapters
- Pitfalls and Pointers that present practical tips for avoiding or resolving common problems in certain subject areas
- Suggested Resources that list relevant and useful sources of more detailed information

This manual is obviously not intended to cover every procedural topic that needs to be learned by new ophthalmology residents. For example, residents should learn about diagnostic and procedural coding, managed care, electronic patient records and electronic prescribing, privacy concerns, evidence-based medicine, and outcomes/research data. Although these subjects are beyond the scope of this manual, the Academy publishes instructional materials concerning such matters. The reader should consult Suggested Resources at the end of each chapter for additional information.

We expect this manual to be of value mainly for the first 3–6 months of a new resident's experience. Beginning residents should also focus their attention on the

Academy's *Basic and Clinical Science Course* (BCSC) and on major ophthalmologic textbooks and journals, realizing that they will learn most and best from their fellow residents, departmental faculty members, and other teachers. We shall have fulfilled our goals if this manual eases the transition of new ophthalmology residents into a rewarding, exciting career in ophthalmology.

Acknowledgments

This manual is a revision of the fifth edition of *Practical Ophthalmology: A Manual for Beginning Residents*, which evolved from an earlier Academy publication titled *A Manual for the Beginning Ophthalmology Resident* (which was published in 3 editions).

The executive editors thank the authors of the fourth and fifth editions, whose work is still conspicuous in the current manual: Judith E. Gurland, MD; Latif M. Hamed, MD; Karla J. Johns, MD; and Kirk R. Wilhelmus, MD. The executive editors also thank the following members of the Ophthalmology Liaisons Committee who served as peer reviewers of the manuscript: Donna M. Applegate, COT; James W. Gigantelli, MD; Kate Goldblum, RN; Karla J. Johns, MD; David Sarraf, MD, FACS; Mary A. O'Hara, MD; Judy Petrunak, CO; Miriam T. Schteingart, MD; and Samuel P. Solish, MD.

The Academy wishes to thank Daniel F. Goodman, MD, San Francisco, California, for providing the photography staff with the use of his examination rooms. Dan McGarrah was the photographer for the following figures: 4.2, 4.5, 5.11(B), 5.12, 5.13, 7.3, CP 9.3 (1, 2), CP 9.11 (1), 13.6(A), 13.7(A), 13.15, and 13.16.

Introduction to the Practice of Ophthalmology

1

Like most important new endeavors, beginning an ophthalmology residency is both exciting and intimidating. This chapter offers some insights regarding what it means to become an ophthalmologist and to practice ophthalmology ethically, responsibly, and competently. It also describes ways in which this book can help you in your first few months of residency (and beyond if you wish) and offers practical tips on dealing with some of the challenges you will face. Here you will find some general guidelines about how to approach the task of assimilating the large body of knowledge, the skills, and the attitudes needed to practice ophthalmology, your chosen specialty. You successfully addressed similar challenges before when you embarked on your medical training, and you have undoubtedly developed your own system of acquisition and assimilation of knowledge along the way. The material in this chapter might be familiar to many beginning residents, but it is certainly fundamental enough to warrant emphasis.

■ Practicing Ophthalmology

Congratulations on your decision to study ophthalmology, a discipline with ancient roots dating back 2000 years. The remarkable success of ophthalmology as a discipline is based on 2 main intertwined elements: ophthalmology's intrinsic strength as a medical and surgical specialty, and its competitive appeal that ensures a perpetual flow of talented individuals into the field. The field has attracted some of the brightest minds throughout history. Several Nobel laureates have been named for their work in vision research. Ophthalmology can claim several firsts in medicine. For example, ophthalmology established the first medical specialty examining board in the world (1916). Originally called the American Board for Ophthalmic Examinations, it was renamed the American Board of Ophthalmology in 1935. Ophthalmology was the first medical discipline to perform randomized clinical trials, the first to use lasers, the first to use antiviral agents, and the first to perform successful allografts (corneal transplants).

Practicing ophthalmology is a privilege, and ophthalmologists are intimately familiar with the rewards and personal satisfaction their efforts bring. The broad scope of ophthalmology practice combines medicine and surgery, and treatment of pediatric as well as adult patients. The nature of ophthalmic practice permits the establishment of durable and satisfying doctor–patient relationships, often lasting a lifetime. The subject matter of ophthalmology is intellectually challenging and fulfilling, sufficiently broad to ensure that everyone can find an intellectual niche in its vast array of topics. The intrinsic strengths of our chosen specialty and the love that it inspires in its practitioners will ensure the continued progress of ophthalmology.

Ophthalmologic services are regarded with respect by patients. Sight is so valued among Americans that, according to a survey by the National Society to Prevent Blindness, blindness is feared second only to cancer. This fear emanates from the feeling that blindness has a catastrophic effect on one's social, economic, and personal life. It is particularly important for a new resident to understand this attitude, because ophthalmic practice involves the care of patients with vision-threatening disorders. Some such patients believe, correctly or otherwise, that they will go blind. The treatment of these patients draws not only on the technical skills of the physician but also on the physician's compassion, understanding, and counseling ability.

Much of the practice of medicine, including ophthalmology, involves communication as a key skill. Communication might be with the patient, with the family, with other health care providers, or with various sectors of society. Such communication should always be clear, forthright, timely, and free of jargon. Communication with patients in general, but especially with patients or parents of children found to harbor serious ophthalmic disease, is an art acquired over many years of experience. However, some general guidelines are helpful for the beginning resident. You might want to defer breaking the news of a serious ocular condition or the interpretation of a difficult clinical circumstance, leaving these tasks to the attending physician, who should have more experience in this area and possibly a different interpretation of the patient's condition. It is awkward to have to rescind your earlier message to the patient as well as confusing to the patient to hear 2 possibly conflicting messages with different implications. In situations in which you do break the news, approach the situation truthfully, with clarity, empathy, compassion, and professional kindness. The communication should be done in private, and should be conducted in an unrushed atmosphere. Try to strike a balance between being too exhaustive on the one hand and brief on the other. Finally, most children with blinding conditions still have some visual function, although it might be as poor as mere light perception. It is legally correct to label them as blind, but it might not be a suitable description when counseling parents who build hope on the scenario the physician describes. Most patients interpret the word "blindness" to mean no light perception. The terms *visual impairment*, *low vision*, or *limited vision* are usually preferable.

Consultation reports to other physicians should be written in clear language with few, if any, abbreviations. A poorly written consultation report, replete with abbreviations and jargon, carries little value if others cannot understand it; instead, it can create barriers between ophthalmology and other medical fields.

Responsibilities of the Resident

As a beginning resident, you will be a new member in an academic health care facility. Your goal is to acquire the knowledge, skills, attitudes, and behaviors needed to practice ophthalmology. It is helpful to be familiar with the general goals of the residency program and with the forces that affect the academic missions of medical schools and residency programs. Goals of the residency program are generally patient care, education, and research. Patient care is listed first because the primary goal of education and research is ultimately to enhance patient care.

Patient care is an excellent source of clinical education, but beginning residents must be able to recognize the limits of their abilities to ensure the continued delivery of high-quality care to all patients. Be willing to accept supervision freely, because it is the ethical and professional responsibility of the supervising ophthalmologist to ensure that the quality of medical care does not suffer as a consequence of resident education.

Ophthalmologists are physicians. Because of the close interrelationship between ophthalmic and systemic health and disease, the modern practice of ophthalmology requires a wide base of medical knowledge. You must maintain general medical knowledge and attitudes and thoughtfully integrate new ophthalmic knowledge into the general medical knowledge you have already acquired. Residents should strive to maintain a balance between their responsibilities to home and family on the one hand, and to the health care team of which they are members on the other. A well-developed support system should help in this respect, and you should not hesitate to convey to the appropriate supervisors any concerns you might have about situations or events that interfere with your effectiveness or well-being. Pace your activities as a resident for the duration of the residency and beyond. Display your spirit of cooperation and helpfulness with your fellow residents. Take the opportunity to build lasting relationships with faculty, fellow residents, and other coworkers. Such relationships are usually as rewarding as anything else you acquire during your residency.

Stress During Residency Training

The formal literature addressing the topic of stress during residency training has increased dramatically since the Libby Zion case, which involved the unexpected death in 1984 of an 18-year-old patient, allegedly caused in part by overworked and undersupervised medical trainees. The cost that stress during residency training can exact on society has since been analyzed, and various steps have been undertaken to reduce stress on trainees. Numerous factors can contribute to stress during residency training, only a few of which include:

- *Sleep deprivation.* Sleep deprivation is considered one of the most significant sources of stress during residency training. Night call might sometimes subject residents to a level of repetitive sleep loss unsurpassed by many other work groups. The Accreditation Council for Graduate Medical Education (ACGME) has established duty hour rules to minimize sleep deprivation. These include an 80-hour work week, at least 10 hours between shifts, 1 day in 7 without clinical duties and no more than 30 consecutive hours worked on call.
- *Role conflict and role ambiguity.* Role conflict arises when the resident's perceived image of the physician as a kind of superhero clashes with the reality of life as a resident. Role ambiguity is produced by the resident's status as both

practicing physician and student. The resident can occupy the important and dignified role of the primary physician for very ill patients, and at the same time be expected to perform less exalted work, such as transporting patients or materials, and have to answer to nurses and others whom the resident may perceive as lower in status and knowledge. Ambiguity of the job role creates an unfixed and expandable workload. This wide discrepancy between the various roles is often the basis of resident stress and discontent.

- *Newer stresses.* Most research to date has focused on the stresses arising from the residents' work environment. Other evolving factors may also be influencing residents' attitudes and feelings about their profession and their patients. The rapid evolution of health care, societal attitudes about physicians, the rising cost of training, and the uncertainties of job availability and future income are stress factors that are assuming increasing significance.

Recognizing Stress and Its Sources

The consequences of stress in residency adversely affect the resident, the resident's family, the patients, and society. Addictive behaviors (alcohol and drug abuse), divorce and broken relationships, psychopathologic behavior and disorders (anxiety, depression, and suicide), and professional dysfunction can result. The symptoms and signs can be subtle or overt. Residents and medical educators need to learn to identify the signals of stress and to establish effective methods to deal with it. These signals can be divided into 4 categories:

- Physical problems, including sleep and eating disorders, deteriorated personal hygiene and appearance, inability to concentrate, multiple physical complaints, and proneness to accidents
- Family problems, including disrupted spousal relationships (separation and divorce, impotence, and extramarital affairs)
- Social problems, including isolation from peers, withdrawal from nonmedical activities, unreliable and unpredictable behaviors at work, and inappropriate behavior at social functions
- Work-related problems, including tardiness, absence without explanation, loss of interest in work, giving inappropriate orders or responses to telephone calls regarding patient care, spending excessive time at the hospital, and demonstrating marked mood changes, such as moroseness, irritability, anger, hostility, and difficulty getting along with others

Given all the adverse effects of residency stress addressed above, it might come as a surprise that there is no unanimity among medical educators and trainees about the effect of stress. Some view stress as necessary and beneficial, and others see it as harmful. Most would agree, however, that stress becomes pathologic beyond a certain point.

Stress harms the doctor–patient relationship. Patients can be perceived as unwanted impositions during times of stress. The ability to empathize with patients is extremely important for delivery of health care with compassion. It can be argued that a stressed, sleep-deprived physician could be ill prepared to have or to show empathy, often finding the patient's complaints frivolous and minute in comparison to his or her own. Because of the sacrifices they make, trainees can become egocentric and feel that "the world owes us something."

Recognizing the potential sources of stress and its deleterious effects is essential when devising effective coping strategies. There may be circumstances beyond the ability of the individual resident to resolve, for which the resident should consider seeking external help. Residents occasionally fall victim to the common misconception that a physician must have an answer for everything and must be able to cope independently with every problem. This misconception is exemplified by the adage "Physician, heal thyself," which might imply to some that asking for help is an admission of unworthiness and might deter residents and trained physicians from seeking help, admitting fault, and accepting guidance. Although many perceive this aura of infallibility to be essential for the doctor–patient relationship and even to have a therapeutic value to patients, it should be clearly recognized that, like many other medical traditions and mythologies, this perception has not been subjected to scientific scrutiny and could very well be false.

■ Dealing With Early Discouragement

Discouragement early in residency is common. It stems largely from the psychologic impact of having to assimilate a novel body of knowledge dealing with unfamiliar regional anatomy and physiology and using special terminology, equipment, instrumentation, and procedures. The typically variable knowledge base among residents at the beginning of the residency can discourage those who feel they are starting behind their peers. Discouragement can be compounded by any of the types of stress described earlier. Throughout the history of medical education, residents have found that such discouragement is nearly always self-limited. It generally resolves within a few months as its sources are addressed and overcome.

The most effective method of dealing with early discouragement is a mature, methodical, long-term approach to the process of learning. Comparing and sharing experiences and feelings with colleagues at various levels of experience and training is helpful. The fact remains that the task of mastering ophthalmology can appear daunting to the beginning resident. There are no good substitutes for hard work combined with effective time management. A disciplined approach to knowledge acquisition, patient care, and ethical practice will lead to a professional life with continually increasing rewards.

■ Ethical Considerations

Ethics are reflections of our moral values. Your ethical standing is a reflection of your actions and attitudes. The ethical practice of ophthalmology must at all times be borne in mind by the physician-in-training. It safeguards the healthy foundations of the doctor–patient relationship. The principles involved, formalized in the Code of Ethics of the American Academy of Ophthalmology, are designed to ensure that the best interest of the patient is paramount. These principles can be summarized as the following:

- Provide care with compassion, honesty, integrity, and respect for human dignity.
- Do not refer to a patient as *the retinal detachment*. Instead, always refer to patients by their names, except in public situations where patient confidentiality must be maintained.
- Seek a healthy personal lifestyle. An ill, problem-ridden physician is less likely to empathize genuinely with the minor ailments of patients.
- Understand the psychology of illness. Patients or family members might appear frightened, angry, or hostile. Learn to recognize and to deal effectively with these emotions without ever becoming defensive or hostile yourself.
- Maintain clinical and moral competence to avoid doing harm (Hippocrates: *primum non nocere*) and to ensure provision of excellent care. Clinical competence is accomplished by continued study and by appropriate consultation. Moral competence calls upon the physician to practice moral discernment (understand and resolve the ethical implications of clinical encounters), moral agency (act faithfully and respectfully on behalf of the patient), and caring in the doctor–patient relationship.
- Communicate openly and honestly with patients. Never misrepresent your status. Introduce yourself by name and identify yourself as a resident. Provide complete and accurate information about treatment options.
- Safeguard the patient's right to privacy within the constraints of the law, and maintain patient confidentiality in accordance with the policies of the Health Insurance Portability and Accountability Act (HIPAA) of 1996.
- Do not allow fees for ophthalmologic services to exploit patients or third-party payers.
- Always strive to preserve, to protect, and to advance the best interests of the patient. Reflect this in your own actions and attitude by placing your patient's welfare ahead of your personal ambitions and desires.
- Take thoughtful measures to effect corrective action if colleagues deviate from professionally or ethically accepted standards.

■ Education and Training

The physician-in-training must strive to achieve a balance between education and training. Training connotes learning to perform specific tasks, such as examination steps and surgical procedures. The meaning of education is much broader, entailing the thoughtful integration of new knowledge into one's own personal experiences, insights, and actions. Residency training must be supplemented by individually driven education. It can be argued that the single most important factor that determines an excellent residency training outcome is the individual's own input into the education and training. A well-balanced education can be obtained by diversifying sources of learning to encompass a thoughtful mixture of reading books and journals, attending lectures and conferences, and participating in informal discussions. One time-honored approach to continuing education is to read about the disorders you find in your own patients as you encounter them. Your knowledge will be tested annually with the Academy's Ophthalmic Knowledge Assessment Program (OKAP) examination. This will help you identify areas of strength and areas requiring further study. All residents should strive to obtain certification by the American Board of Ophthalmology. Such certification is based on continuing education, licensure, verification of credentials by the chairperson of the residency program, the Written Qualifying Examination, and the Oral Examination. To ensure continued learning after residency, the American Board of Ophthalmology began a process of maintenance of certification (MOC). The MOC process requires proof of state licensure, documentation of continued medical education, office record review, open book practice examinations, and a closed book examination. The process is repeated every 10 years.

Active pursuit of education and training must continue beyond residency. The beginning resident must make a commitment to sharpen medical skills and knowledge through continual study, instruction, and experience. Maintaining competence is essential to the ethical practice of ophthalmology and to the promotion of intellectual and professional growth. Keeping up with medical and surgical discoveries and inventions, which seem to change the practice of medicine almost daily, is necessary to remain competitive in a marketplace that demands excellent outcomes.

The demands of health care reform will affect the challenge of becoming an excellent ophthalmologist. Increasing constraints on the time and economic resources available for education are further strained by the need to remain current and fully competent in an ever-evolving field. The American Academy of Ophthalmology offers a framework of Academy resources that can help members accomplish their continuing educational goals in the face of new challenges and imperatives. For a listing of products and services from the Academy, visit the web site at www.aao.org.

Pitfalls and Pointers

- Avoid cutting corners or taking shortcuts in your practice as a new resident. Learn it right the first time.
- Do not compromise patient care for the sake of training or any other personal benefit. Always consult a more knowledgeable or experienced physician if you are uncertain about how to proceed in a clinical situation.
- Do not be embarrassed to use this (or any) introductory manual. Adopt a lifelong approach to learning.
- Do not hide your own limitations in skill and knowledge as you begin your residency. Strive to improve upon them and be receptive to criticism.
- Remember that professional success involves more than learning the medical facts and the surgical techniques. The art of practicing medicine is best achieved by a well-rounded, mature, and compassionate physician who also knows the medical facts well.

- Do not publicly denounce or belittle the care given by previous practitioners by saying, "Your doctor did not know what he or she was doing," or "That was malpractice." Avail yourself of the facts before passing any judgments, but remember that you are a medical resident, not a judge.

Suggested Resources

Appropriate Examination and Treatment Procedures [Advisory Opinion]. San Francisco: American Academy of Ophthalmology; 2003.

Basic and Clinical Science Course. American Academy of Ophthalmology web site. http://one.aao.org/CE/EducationalProducts/BCSC.aspx. Accessed June 15, 2009.

Code of Ethics. American Academy of Ophthalmology web site. http://www.aao.org/about/ethics/code_ethics.cfm. Accessed June 15, 2009.

Duty hours language. Accreditation Council for Graduate Medical Education web site. http://www.acgme.org/acWebsite/dutyHours/dh_Lang703.pdf. Accessed June 15, 2009.

Ethical Obligations in a Managed Care Environment [Advisory Opinion]. San Francisco: American Academy of Ophthalmology; 1997.

Learning New Techniques Following Residency [Advisory Opinion]. San Francisco: American Academy of Ophthalmology; 2003.

OKAP exam. American Academy of Ophthalmology web site. http://one.aao.org/CE/EducationalContent/oKAP.aspx. Accessed June 15, 2009.

Parke II DW, ed. *The Profession of Ophthalmology: Practice Management, Ethics, and Advocacy.* San Francisco: American Academy of Ophthalmology; 2005.

The Ethical Ophthalmologist: A Primer. San Francisco: American Academy of Ophthalmology; 1999.

The Moral and Technical Competence of the Ophthalmologist [Information Statement]. San Francisco: American Academy of Ophthalmology; 1999.

Overview of the Ophthalmic Evaluation

2

The purpose of the ophthalmic evaluation is to document objective and subjective measurements of visual function and ocular health. The specific objectives of the comprehensive ophthalmic evaluation include the following:

- Obtain an ocular and a systemic history.
- Determine the optical and health status of the eye, visual system, and related structures.
- Identify risk factors for ocular and systemic disease.
- Detect and diagnose ocular abnormalities and disease.
- Establish and document the presence or absence of ocular signs or symptoms of systemic disease.
- Discuss with the patient the nature of the findings and the implications.
- Initiate an appropriate response, such as diagnostic tests, treatment, or referral when indicated. Often the patient needs only explanation and reassurance, which is best offered after the examination has been completed; otherwise, the reassurance will not be credible.

The physician accomplishes these objectives by obtaining the patient's history and performing the necessary examinations, using specific equipment as needed. A successful encounter also requires that the physician approach the patient with a professional demeanor. Finally, timely and accurate documentation is important.

■ History

Obtaining a thorough history from the patient is the important first step in an ophthalmic evaluation (see Chapter 3). In general, the history includes the following information:

- Demographic data, including name, date of birth, sex, race/ethnicity, and occupation
- The identity of other pertinent health care providers utilized by the patient, including the name of the physician requesting consultation, if applicable
- Chief complaint, or the main problem that prompted the visit
- History of present illness, which is a more detailed description of the chief complaint(s)
- Present status of vision, including the patient's perception of his or her own visual status, visual needs, and any ocular symptoms

- Past ocular history, including prior eye diseases, injuries, diagnoses, treatments, surgeries, ocular medications, and use of glasses
- Past systemic history, including allergies, adverse reactions to medications, medication use (including prescription and nonprescription medications and herbal and nutritional supplements), and pertinent medical problems and hospitalizations
- Family history, including poor vision (and cause, if known), and other pertinent familial ocular and systemic diseases

■ Examination

The comprehensive ophthalmic evaluation includes an analysis of the physiologic function and anatomic status of the eye, visual system, and related structures. Components of the evaluation and chapters in this book in which they are discussed are noted here:

- Visual acuity examination (visual acuity is determined with and without the present correction, if any, at distance and at near; see Chapter 4)
- Determination of best-corrected visual acuity utilizing retinoscopy and refraction (see Chapter 5)
- Ocular alignment and motility examination (see Chapter 6)
- Pupillary examination (see Chapter 7)
- Visual field examination (see Chapter 8)
- Examination of the external eye and ocular adnexa (see Chapter 9)
- Examination of the anterior segment (see Chapters 10 and 11)
- Tonometry to determine intraocular pressure (see Chapter 12)
- Posterior segment examination (see Chapter 13)

■ Ophthalmic Equipment

The ophthalmic examination room and its equipment are sometimes referred to as a lane. Although the equipment in examining rooms varies widely, the components typically include the following:

- *Snellen acuity chart.* This printed hanging chart, projected chart, or video display is used in determining visual acuity and in refraction (see Chapter 4).
- *Near visual acuity chart.* This printed handheld chart is used to determine near visual acuity and as an aid in refraction (see Chapter 4).
- *Penlight or Finnoff transilluminator (muscle light).* These instruments are used to check pupillary light reflexes and the corneal light reflex. Auxiliary uses include illumination for the external examination and transillumination of the globe (see Chapters 6, 7, and 9).
- *Slit-lamp biomicroscope.* This optical magnifying instrument is primarily used to perform anterior segment examinations. When combined with an auxiliary lens such as a Hruby lens, a +90 diopter lens, a +78 diopter lens, or

a Goldmann 3-mirror lens, it can be used to examine the posterior segment. It is also used in conjunction with a gonioscopy lens to examine the anterior chamber angle (see Chapters 10, 11, and 13).

- *Goldmann applanation tonometer.* This device attaches to the slit-lamp biomicroscope and is used to measure intraocular pressure. A handheld device (Tonopen) can also be used to measure intraocular pressure (see Chapter 12).
- *Streak retinoscope.* This handheld instrument is used to perform retinoscopy, an objective measurement of a patient's refractive state (see Chapter 5).
- *Phoroptor.* This device (also called a refractor) stores a range of trial lenses and is used when performing retinoscopy and refraction (see Chapter 5).
- *Trial frame and loose trial lenses.* This equipment is used when performing retinoscopy and refraction and to confirm refractive findings (see Chapter 5). It is also useful when performing tests evaluating ocular alignment when a patient is without his or her glasses.
- *Distometer.* This handheld device is used to measure vertex distance, which is the distance between a patient's eye and the back surface of a spectacle lens (see Chapter 5).
- *Direct ophthalmoscope.* This handheld instrument is used for posterior segment examinations and also to assess the red reflex (see Chapter 13).
- *Indirect ophthalmoscope.* This device, worn on the head, is used for the posterior segment examination in conjunction with auxiliary handheld diagnostic condensing lenses (see Chapter 13).
- *Keratometer.* This device measures corneal curvature and is typically used when fitting contact lenses and to diagnose disorders such as keratoconus.
- *Prisms.* These optical devices, available individually or held together in a prism bar, are used to measure strabismus (see Chapter 6).
- *Sensory testing equipment.* The Worth 4-dot testing equipment consists of red-green eyeglasses and a flashlight that illuminates 4 colored dots. The Titmus test utilizes a stereoscopic test booklet and a pair of polarized spectacles. Both of these tests are used to assess binocular vision as a part of the motility examination (see Chapter 6).
- *Color vision testing equipment.* Standardized books of colored plates, such as the Ishihara pseudoisochromatic color tests, are used when congenital or acquired color vision defects are suspected (see Chapter 4).
- *Exophthalmometer.* This instrument is used to assess the anterior-posterior position of the globes by measuring the distance from the lateral orbital rim to the corneal apex (see Chapter 9).

Ancillary Equipment

Other equipment is commonly used to measure visual function or to assess ocular structures:

- *Visual field analyzer (perimeter).* This device is usually automated, but it may be manual. It is used for assessing the central and peripheral field of vision (see Chapter 8).

- *Corneal topography system.* This automated system is used for measuring corneal curvature. It is most useful in refractive surgery, after corneal transplant surgery, and in evaluating patients with keratoconus.
- *Optical coherence tomography (OCT).* This system provides a high-resolution cross-sectional image of the optic nerve and retina. It is useful in evaluating retinal disease such as macular edema and in monitoring glaucomatous nerve disc changes. OCT can also be used to visualize anterior segment structures.
- *Ultrasonography.* This imaging modality provides 1- or 2-dimensional cross-sectional views of the eye. It is often used to evaluate retinal structure when the view of the posterior segment is obscured by opacities in the cornea, lens, and/or vitreous (see Chapter 13).
- *Specular microscope.* This device is used to evaluate the corneal endothelium. It demonstrates cell morphology and calculates endothelial cell density (see Chapter 11).
- *Pachymeter.* This instrument is used to measure corneal thickness. It may be found as a slit-lamp attachment or as a handheld device.

■ Physician Demeanor and Approach to the Patient

When performing the ophthalmic evaluation, the ophthalmologist's approach to the patient should be compassionate and professional. He or she should listen to patients' concerns carefully and with undivided attention. Patients' descriptions of ocular problems, in their own words, are of vital importance. After completing the ophthalmic evaluation and counseling the patient, it is advisable to ask if the patient has any additional questions or concerns and to address them at that time. As in any medical setting, it is important to maintain the confidentiality of all patient information and interactions.

Certain situations can create barriers to effective patient–physician communication. When the patient and the ophthalmologist do not speak the same language, bilingual family members or staff can often bridge the communication gap by translating for the patient and physician. If a translator is needed to obtain informed consent for a procedure, it is advisable to consult hospital administration regarding institutional policies. In these situations, family members might not be permitted to be the sole translators, particularly if they are minors.

In some situations, the mental status of the patient limits the extent of first-person history taking. In these cases, the family members, guardians, or attendants of the patient can usually provide additional important information. Some patients have a deep-seated fear of the health care environment that inhibits their ability to communicate, while other patients have an unspoken fear of blindness that can cause them to minimize or exaggerate ocular complaints. By creating an atmosphere of trust, respect, and openness, the ophthalmologist can encourage the patient to communicate freely, and effective patient–physician communication can be achieved.

Pediatric Patients

Pediatric patients warrant special consideration. The parent or caretaker will be the primary source of information for preverbal children. Older children should be involved as much as possible in history taking and in discussions of the findings and treatment plans, depending on the child's age and ability to communicate and comprehend.

Elderly Patients

Ophthalmologists typically interact with patients of all age groups, many of whom are elderly. With advancing age comes an increased prevalence of major causes of visual impairment (eg, diabetic retinopathy, glaucoma, cataract, and age-related macular degeneration). The ophthalmologist-in-training needs to give specific consideration to the special needs and impact of visual loss in aged patients.

The word "senile," as in *senile cataract*, is well established in medical terminology; but this word has unpleasant connotations and should not be used in the presence of patients. *Involutional* or *age-related* are far preferable if an equivalent adjective is needed.

Loss of visual function increases the incidence and severity of falls and fractures. Falls occur in a substantial number of older people (up to 35% per year), and poor vision is an obvious risk factor for falls, which are associated with considerable morbidity and even mortality. Preventing falls is a much more effective strategy than treating them. Possible interventions for reducing the risk of falling include the following:

- Increasing lighting and decreasing glare
- Increasing contrast at dangerous areas such as steps and corners
- Removing obstacles and clutter from floors
- Anchoring loose rugs and eliminating uneven surfaces
- Installing well-designed hand rails and other safety features such as nonskid flooring
- Using appropriate aids for walking (walkers and canes)
- Avoiding footwear such as high heels

Visual loss and hearing impairment often coexist, and the presence of both sensory deficits is worse than either one alone. Ophthalmologists should recognize hearing-impaired patients and refer them as needed for management.

Visual loss is also commonly associated with depression, especially in elderly patients. Depression should not be overlooked or ignored, as it is a debilitating, yet treatable, condition. Patients rarely tell their ophthalmologists that they are depressed, and they often do not recognize their own depression. The ophthalmologist may simply ask, "Do you feel sad or depressed?" If the answer suggests possible depression, appropriate referral should be considered and discussed with the patient.

Loss of visual cues can worsen symptoms of dementia, and visual impairment is associated with Alzheimer's disease. Patients who have dementia might report visual complaints such as "I have trouble reading," "I get lost easily," or "I can see but I can't read." Rapid screening techniques can help the ophthalmologist identify patients who might have dementia. One such test is the "clock draw." The patient is asked to draw a clock face including the numbers of the hours (1 to 12) and to draw the hands to show a time of 10 minutes past 11 o'clock. Patients who fail the test should have evaluation for possible dementia.

Visual loss can have profound effects on many activities of daily living, such as walking, going outside, getting in and out of bed, grocery shopping, paying bills, cleaning house, answering the telephone, cooking, and driving. Visual impairment increases the risk of a driving accident, especially in the elderly patient. Many of these problems can be helped by low-vision evaluation and treatment using optical and nonoptical rehabilitative aids. One of the most simple, common, and useful aids is a high-plus reading prescription that serves to magnify reading material. Social, family, community, and other support services often improve the visually impaired patient's quality of life.

Medical Record Keeping

Timely, legible, and thorough documentation of the ophthalmic evaluation allows the ophthalmologist and other caregivers to refer to the data in the future and is thus of tremendous importance to patient care and continuity of care. Many ophthalmologists now use an electronic (computerized) medical record, and advantages of such a system include improved legibility, accessibility from multiple sites, and reduced space requirements for storage. Although some abbreviations are widely used, ophthalmologic medical records should be written using terminology that will be understandable to other health care providers who will access the medical records. Excessive use of jargon should be avoided. As a medicolegal document, the medical record must present sufficiently detailed findings and treatment recommendations. The record must be sufficiently complete to justify coding levels for charges and reimbursement.

Communication with referring physicians and other health care providers, whether written or verbal, is crucial in providing the patient with continuity and co-ordination of care. Such communication should be clear, timely, and informative.

Some ocular conditions occur as manifestations of systemic diseases that constitute a threat to public health, such as gonococcal conjunctivitis and HIV-related ocular infections. Some such diseases, by statutory guidelines, must be reported to the state health department. States also often want reports about patients who have recently become legally blind. Reporting guidelines vary from state to state; the ophthalmologist should contact the state health department for appropriate guidelines.

Pitfalls and Pointers

- The beginning resident should strive to learn a systematic, comprehensive approach to the history and examination of each patient. In this way, key historic points or examination findings are much less likely to be omitted.

- New residents in ophthalmology might at first feel overwhelmed by unfamiliar diagnostic techniques, equipment, and nomenclature. This reaction is normal. With hard work, perseverance, and diligent study, what is unfamiliar now will seem like second nature in a relatively short time.
- As the beginning resident strives to master new ophthalmologic techniques and skills, he or she should not lose sight of the fact that a patient sits behind the refractor.

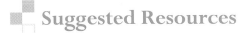

Suggested Resources

Comprehensive Adult Medical Eye Evaluation [Preferred Practice Pattern]. San Francisco: American Academy of Ophthalmology; 2005.

Miller AM. *Clinical Pearls for Pediatric Ophthalmology.* American Academy of Ophthalmology YO Info Newsletter, July 2008.

Movaghar M, Lawrence MG. Eye Exam: The Essentials. In *The Eye Exam and Basic Ophthalmic Instruments* [DVD]. San Francisco: American Academy of Ophthalmology; 2001. Reviewed for currency 2007.

Parke II DW, ed. *The Profession of Ophthalmology: Practice Management, Ethics, and Advocacy.* San Francisco: American Academy of Ophthalmology; 2005.

Pediatric Ophthalmology and Strabismus. Basic and Clinical Science Course, Section 6. San Francisco: American Academy of Ophthalmology; published annually.

Screening and comprehensive ophthalmic evaluation. In: *Pediatric Eye Evaluations: Screening and Comprehensive Ophthalmic Evaluation.* [Preferred Practice Pattern] San Francisco: American Academy of Ophthalmology; 2007.

3 History Taking

Although similar to the general medical history that you learned in medical school, the ophthalmic history naturally emphasizes symptoms of ocular disease, present and past ocular problems, and ocular medications. The history is intended to elicit any information that might be useful in evaluating and managing the patient; it may be as brief, or extensive, as required by the patient's particular problems. This chapter provides an overview of the ophthalmic history, its goals, recording methods, and components.

■ Goals of the History

The history should allow for the recording of important information that could affect the patient's diagnosis and treatment. The 5 most important objectives include the following:

1. *Identify the patient.* If not already collected, record demographic information about the patient such as name, address, date of birth, sex, race, and medical record number. Strict confidentiality of this information should be maintained according to HIPAA standards.

2. *Identify other practitioners who have cared for the patient or who may care for the patient in the future.* Such individuals might need to be contacted for additional information or be given information about the patient, especially if the patient was referred for consultation, in which case a written report is required. Reports also are often needed following referrals from attorneys, insurance companies, or governmental agencies.

3. *Obtain a diagnosis.* The likely diagnosis, or at least a reasonable differential diagnosis, can often be suspected merely on the basis of a good history. This, in turn, allows for the planning and tailoring of a more useful and efficient examination.

4. *Select therapy.* Knowledge of treatments that have already been tried, and whether or not (and in what ways) they were helpful, is invaluable in planning therapy for the future. An awkward situation can arise if a physician recommends therapy, only to learn that the same therapy has already been tried and has failed. Insufficient knowledge of the results of prior therapeutic efforts can also lead to misdiagnosis.

   Where therapy is concerned, it is important also to try to ascertain what the patient wants and expects from the physician. This can be done directly by questioning the patient or, in many cases, indirectly by listening attentively to, and interpreting, what the patient says. Some patients require definitive therapy, whereas others need only explanation and reassurance, documentation of a problem, or periodic observation.

5. *Consider socioeconomic and medicolegal factors.* Insurance payments, worker's compensations, disability payments, and the like (on the patient's behalf), as well as legal proceedings, often depend on detailed, accurate reports (or even testimony) from the physician. Such reports can be inadequate, and sometimes even humiliating for the physician, if a thorough history has not been obtained. In addition, a well-taken history can save time and expense by obviating needless tests and examination procedures. Such efficiency and cost containment is important in the current environment of managed care. Also, the components and thoroughness of the history are considered, and may be audited, by Medicare to determine the appropriateness of coding and charges for services.

■ Methods of Recording the History

The precise method of recording the history is unimportant unless a practice or institution has specific requirements. The history may be handwritten on blank paper or on a preprinted form, dictated for later transcription, or entered into a computerized database. Figure 3.1 displays one type of preprinted history chart that some physicians find useful.

Figure 3.1 One type of pre-printed history chart.

Patient Data
Name _____
Address _____
_____
Telephone (work) _____ (home) _____
Date of Birth __/__/__   Sex □M □F   Race _____
Referred by _____
Referrer's address _____
Medical Record Number _____
Insurance carrier _____

Patient History   Date _____

1. Chief complaint

2. Present illness

3. Past ocular history

4. Ocular medications

5. General medical/surgical history

6. Systemic medications

7. Allergies

8. Social history

9. Family history

■ Components of the History

As described below, the components of the ophthalmic history are essentially the same as the components of any general medical history, except that ophthalmic aspects are, of course, emphasized. The components of the history are:

- Chief complaint
- Present illness
- Past ocular history
- Ocular medications
- General medical and surgical history
- Systemic medications
- Allergies
- Social history
- Family history

Chief Complaint

The patient's main complaint(s) should be recorded *in the patient's own words* or in a nontechnical paraphrasing of the patient's words. It is not advisable in this early phase of the history for the ophthalmologist to draw hasty conclusions by employing medical terms that suggest premature diagnoses. For example, chief complaints should be listed as *redness, burning, and mattering* or *light flashes* instead of *conjunctivitis* or *photopsias*. The patient's own words are important for knowing, and being able to document, the patient's point of view, as distinct from that of the physician. The physician's impression is appropriate only later, after a proper history has been taken and a suitably thorough examination has been performed.

Of course, patients are sometimes troubled by more than 1 symptom or problem and so might have more than 1 chief complaint. Even problems that are of lesser importance should be cited along with the chief complaint. Here are some examples of kinds of questions that can help to elicit the patient's main complaints:

- What are the main problems that you are having with your eyes?
- What other problems are you having with your eyes?
- Why did you come (or why were you sent) here?
- In what way are you hoping that you might be helped?
- What is it about your eyes that worries or concerns you? (This type of question sometimes reveals entirely unfounded fears, such as blindness or cancer.)
- What is the main problem that you would like me to address?

Present Illness

Evaluation of the patient's present illness consists mainly of an effort to record additional information and details about the chief complaint(s). The patient's own words may be used here when desired, although the physician's words, including medical terminology and abbreviations, are more often used to represent what the patient said. Information elicited about the present illness allows the ophthalmologist to begin developing a preliminary diagnostic impression.

The following general areas of inquiry are given as suggestions for developing information about the present illness.

- *Time and manner of onset.* Was it sudden or gradual?
- *Severity.* Has the problem improved, worsened, or remained the same?
- *Influences.* What might have precipitated the condition, made it better or worse, or made no difference? Asking about prior therapeutic efforts is especially important, and it is helpful to know when the patient's refractive prescription was last changed.
- *Constancy and temporal variations.* Has the problem been intermittent or seasonal, or does it worsen at a particular time of day? If so, were there any influences that seemed to precipitate exacerbations or remissions?
- *Laterality.* Is the problem unilateral or bilateral?
- *Clarification.* It is sometimes necessary to clarify what the patient means by certain complaints. For example, does mattering of the eye mean sealing of the eyelids by sticky discharge, the mere presence of strands of mucus at times, or simply the noting of tiny granules on the eyelids (as from dried mucus or the drying and crystallization of eyedrops)? Countless other situations exist in which it is important to clarify just what the patient means, so it is vital to question the patient thoroughly.
- *Documentation.* Old records, or even old photographs, can be of value in documenting the presence or absence of particular problems in the past (eg, ptosis, abnormal ocular motility, proptosis, facial nerve palsy, anisocoria).

Specific complaints that might be recorded under "Present Illness" are too numerous to list here in their entirety. Nevertheless, one needs to keep in mind certain general categories of complaints, which are listed below together with examples of accompanying specific complaints.

Disturbances of vision

- Blurred or decreased central vision (distance, near, or both)
- Decreased peripheral vision
- Altered image size (micropsia, macropsia, metamorphopsia—the last referring to distorted images)
- Diplopia (monocular, binocular, horizontal, vertical, oblique)
- Floaters (moving lines or specks in the field of vision)
- Photopsias (flashes of light)
- Iridescent vision (halos, rainbows)
- Dark adaptation problems
- Dyslexia (medical inability to read understandingly)
- Color vision abnormalities
- Blindness (ocular, cortical, perceptual)
- Oscillopsia (apparent movement or shaking of images)

Ocular pain or discomfort

- Foreign-body sensation (a feeling of scratchiness, as though a particle were present on the surface of the eye)
- Ciliary (deep) pain (an aching, often severe, pain within and around the eye, sometimes radiating to the ipsilateral temple, forehead, malar area, and even the occiput, secondary to spasm of the ciliary muscles)
- Photophobia (a less severe form of ciliary pain that is present only upon exposure to light)
- Headache (not attributable to ciliary pain)
- Burning
- Dryness
- Itching; true itching, which compels the patient to rub the eye(s) vigorously (and which usually indicates allergy), must be differentiated from burning, dryness, and foreign-body sensation
- Asthenopia (eyestrain)

Abnormal ocular secretions

- Lacrimation (tearing—welling up of tears on the ocular surface)
- Epiphora (actual spilling of tears over the margin of the eyelid onto the face)
- Dryness (also considered discomfort, as listed above)
- Discharge (purulent, mucopurulent, mucoid, serous, or watery; the first 2 kinds of discharge are associated with neutrophils and cause true sealing of the eyelids in the mornings)

Abnormal appearances

- Ptosis (drooping of the eyelid)
- Proptosis or exophthalmos (protrusion of the eye or eyes)
- Enophthalmos (the opposite of proptosis)
- Blepharitis (sometimes referred to by patients as *granulated eyelids*)
- Misalignment of the eyes
- Redness, other discolorations, opacities, masses
- Anisocoria (inequality of the pupils)

Other complaints

- "Something my doctor wanted to be checked"
- The need for a second opinion regarding diagnosis, surgery, or other management

Trauma

Cases of ocular trauma, especially, can require very detailed reports based on a thorough history (and examination). For medical, medicolegal, and compensation purposes, it is important to obtain the following information:

- The date, time, and place (including the precise address) of the injury
- What happened, in the patient's own words (particularly in the case of trauma, the patient's words are useful in the present illness, as well as in the chief complaint)

- What safety precautions were taken, if any, including the wearing of safety glasses
- What measures were taken for emergency treatment, because treatment takes priority over obtaining a history in a true emergency (see Chapter 14), although the history remains important
- The type and roughly estimated speed of any foreign body
- Whether or not the vision has been affected

Past Ocular History

Prior ocular problems can have a bearing on a patient's current status. The existence of any such problems should be discovered so that their possible role in the present illness can be evaluated, and so that they can be managed if necessary.

To begin with, the patient is usually asked simply if there have been any eye problems in the past, but it is often useful for eliciting additional information to ask about the following:

- Use of eyeglasses or contact lenses (the date of the most recent prescription may be recorded here or with the present illness)
- Use of ocular medications in the past
- Ocular surgery (including laser surgery)
- Ocular trauma
- History of amblyopia (lazy eye) or of ocular patching in childhood

If the patient responds positively to any of the above, it might be valuable to ask why, when, how, where, and by whom, as applicable.

Ocular Medications

Knowledge of the patient's use of ocular medications is essential for 2 reasons. First, it is necessary to know how the patient responded to prior therapy. In addition, recent therapy (within the past 6 weeks, approximately) can affect the patient's present status, because toxic and allergic reactions to topical medications and pre-servatives sometimes resolve slowly.

All current and prior ocular medications used for the present illness should be recorded, including dosages, frequency, and duration of use. Also ask about the use of any over-the-counter (nonprescription) medications, home remedies, herbal medicines, and dietary supplements.

Patients sometimes do not know the names of their medications. In such cases the physician might learn the general classes of medications being used by asking the color of the cap on the container, because containers for eyedrops have caps of different colors to facilitate identification:

- Green: cholinergic (miotic) drugs such as pilocarpine, carbachol, echothiophate iodide (Phospholine Iodide)
- Red: anticholinergic (dilating cycloplegic or mydriatic) drugs such as atropine, homatropine, scopolamine, cyclopentolate, tropicamide, phenylephrine
- Yellow: beta-adrenergic blocking agents (timolol 0.5%, levobunolol 0.5%, metipranolol)

- Blue: timolol 0.25%, betaxolol (a β_1 blocking agent), levobunolol 0.25%, Combigan (timolol /brimonidine combination)
- White: many medications, including certain antibiotics, artificial tears, corticosteroids, and anti-allergy drops
- Purple: alpha agonists such as brimonidine
- Teal: prostaglandins (latanoprost, travoprost, bimatoprost)
- Orange: tropical carbonic anhydrase inhibitors (dorzolamide, brinzolamide)
- Tan: fluoroquinolone antibiotics (ciprofloxacin, levofloxacin, gatifloxacin, moxifloxacin)
- Gray: nonsteroidal anti-inflammatory medications (ketorolac, nepafenac, diclofenac)
- Pink: loteprednol corticosteroid drops

General Medical and Surgical History

The patient's present and past general medical history is important for 2 reasons. First, many ocular diseases are manifestations of, or are associated with, systemic diseases. In addition, the general medical status must be known to perform a proper preoperative evaluation.

All medical and surgical problems should be recorded, along with the approximate dates of onset, medical treatments, or surgeries when possible. A pertinent review of systems, tailored to the patient's complaints, should be conducted, including questions about diabetes mellitus and hypertension, and malignancy, as well as dermatologic, cardiac, renal, hepatic, pulmonary, gastrointestinal, central nervous system, and autoimmune collagen vascular (including arthritic) diseases. Diabetes mellitus should be identified as insulin dependent or non–insulin dependent, and the duration of diabetes and hypertension should be determined. The adequacy of glycemic control is important information to acquire. The patient's sexual history, including previous sexually transmitted diseases, can be pertinent in selected situations.

The evaluation of a pediatric patient might call for historic information from the mother about pregnancy (prenatal care, drugs used, complications in labor, prematurity, delivery, birth weight, and the neonatal period). The family history can also be important but is usually recorded separately, as described later in this chapter.

Systemic Medications

Systemic medications can cause ocular, preoperative, intraoperative, and postoperative problems and can provide clues to systemic disorders the patient might have. In questioning the patient, give particular attention to the use of aspirin and other anticoagulant agents, as they can cause intraoperative and postoperative bleeding. The patient's use of systemic medications (eg, acetazolamide, vitamins) that are taken for ocular problems may be recorded here or, preferably, under "Ocular Medications."

It is sometimes sufficient merely to ask what systemic (general) medications the patient takes, but it can be useful in selected cases to inquire specifically about antibiotics, tranquilizers, narcotics, sleeping pills, anticonvulsants, anti-inflammatory agents, oral contraceptives, or vitamins, especially when the patient seems to be unsure about medications being used. Certain medicines such as hydroxychloro-quine sulfate (Plaquenil), phenothiazines, amiodarone, tamoxifen, and systemic steroids can have ocular toxicity. Patients may also be taking alternative medications, herbal compounds, and vitamins that should be noted here.

Allergies

The patient's history of allergies to medications is important for avoiding drugs to which a patient is allergic. However, patients often cannot differentiate true allergic reactions from side effects or other nonallergenic adverse effects of medications, so it is important to ask about (and to record) the nature of any claimed reaction. Itching, hives, rashes, wheezing, or frank cardiorespiratory collapse clearly suggest true allergy, whereas statements such as "the drops burned" or "the pills upset my stomach" do not.

In addition to inquiries about allergic reactions to topical and systemic medications, the physician should ask about allergies to environmental agents (atopy), resulting in any of the following:

- Atopic dermatitis
- Allergic asthma
- Allergic rhinitis, conjunctivitis (hay fever)
- Urticaria (hives)
- Vernal conjunctivitis

In some instances the presence of these kinds of disorders might already have been elicited in the taking of the present illness, past medical history, or review of systems, in which case it need not be again recorded under "Allergies."

Before injecting dye for fluorescein or other angiography, establish whether the patient has previously been given such an injection and whether any kind of adverse reaction occurred.

Social History

A social history is not always necessary, although Medicare requires this information for certain levels of coding for reimbursement. When relevant, a social history should be taken, including information on such matters as tobacco and alcohol use, drug abuse, sexual history (including sexually transmitted diseases and, perhaps, HIV status), tattoos, body-piercing, environmental factors, and occupation. The questioning should be pursued in a nonjudgmental way, with sensitivity and due respect for privacy. Except as might be required by law, or with the patient's permission, such information should not usually be revealed to third parties.

Family History

The family history of ocular, or nonocular, diseases is important when genetically transmitted disorders are under consideration. The physician might begin by asking a general question such as, "Are there any eye problems, other than just needing glasses, in your family background?" before asking specifically about corneal disease, glaucoma, cataract, retinal disease, or other heritable ocular conditions.

Knowledge of familial systemic diseases can be helpful in ophthalmic evaluation and diagnosis. Examples include atopy, thyroid disease, diabetes mellitus, certain malignancies, various hereditary syndromes, and many others. Inability of the patient to provide information about the family medical background should not be construed or recorded as a negative family history. Rather, the chart should reflect the fact that the patient's knowledge was incomplete or lacking. Examination of family members is occasionally useful when patients present with possibly heritable disorders.

Pitfalls and Pointers

- Avoid taking an insufficiently detailed history. The history need not be of great length, but it should contain all the details that are pertinent to the patient's complaints and problems.
- Although sufficient detail in a history is important, it is important not to emphasize minutiae to the detriment of the main sources of concern (ie, why is the patient here and what does he or she need and want from the ophthalmologist?).
- Parents, guardians, other relatives, or friends are sometimes needed to give histories for patients who are unable to speak for themselves because of age or other reasons. An interpreter can be invaluable for any patient who does not speak the physician's language.
- A good history may be brief or lengthy, so long as it is thorough relative to the ultimate goal of helping the patient. The ability to take an essentially complete, yet efficient, history is an important aspect of the art of medicine. Nevertheless, the beginning ophthalmology resident whose histories fall short of being ideal should not be dismayed; the skill improves greatly, and almost automatically, with experience.
- When taking a prenatal and gestational history, avoid phrasing your questions in a way that would elicit guilt feelings or imply causal relationship between a child's ocular disorder and anything the mother might have done or not done.

Suggested Resources

Fundamentals and Principles of Ophthalmology. Basic and Clinical Science Course, Section 2. San Francisco: American Academy of Ophthalmology; published annually.

Intraocular Inflammation and Uveitis. Basic and Clinical Science Course, Section 9. San Francisco: American Academy of Ophthalmology; published annually.

Pediatric Ophthalmology and Strabismus. Basic and Clinical Science Course, Section 6. San Francisco: American Academy of Ophthalmology; published annually.

Trobe JD. *The Physician's Guide to Eye Care.* 3rd ed. San Francisco: American Academy of Ophthalmology; 2006.

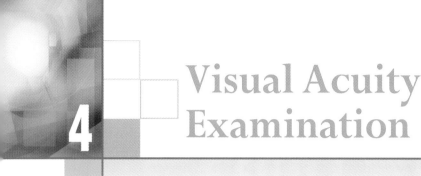

Visual Acuity Examination

Vision is a complex human sense with many facets that cannot be measured. Ophthalmologists rely on a variety of psychophysical assessments and express vision as a measure of visual acuity, although acuity is only 1 component of vision. Vision consists of, but is not limited to, visual acuity, peripheral vision, visual field, and contrast sensitivity. This chapter deals mainly with measuring distance and near visual acuity, near points of accommodation and convergence, and stereopsis.

Testing Conventions and Materials

The term visual acuity refers to an angular measurement relating testing distance to the minimal object size resolvable at that distance. Ophthalmologists typically use Snellen acuity as a measure of the resolving ability of the eye. The traditional measurement of distance acuity refers to a visual test in which a target subtends a visual angle on the retina of 5 minutes of arc when a subject is 20 feet (6 m) away from that target. The distance to the test target may be arbitrary, but the visual angle subtended for the standard 20/20 test object must be 5 minutes of arc. Thus, the 20/20 size test object may vary in height, depending on the distance between it and the eye, so that the size of the retinal image will be the same for any object that covers the same 5 minutes of arc. The expression that relates the test target size and the distance at which it is seen is the Snellen acuity notation, which is described below.

A variety of measurement and notation methods, test targets, and abbreviations have been developed for the purpose of performing visual acuity and visual function testing and for documenting the results. This section presents an overview of the standard conventions and steps used in performing these tests.

Measurement Notation

The Snellen notation is the most common method of expressing visual acuity measurement. By convention, this expression is written as a fraction, but it is not a mathematical fraction or expression. The number in the numerator position is the equivalent of the testing distance from the eye to the chart being used, in either feet or meters. The number in the denominator position is the distance at which a subject with unimpaired vision can read the same figure. This notation quantifies visual discrimination of fine detail.

Other types of visual acuity notations are used besides the Snellen notation. A decimal notation converts the Snellen fraction to a decimal; for example, Snellen 20/20 equals decimal 1.0, Snellen 20/30 equals decimal 0.7, Snellen 20/40 equals decimal 0.5, and so forth. Other expressions of acuity are the M, or metric, and the logMAR notations. The latter expresses visual acuity as the logarithm of the minimum angle of resolution (logMAR). The minimum angle of resolution is the inverse of the Snellen fraction. Acuity of 20/20 has a logMAR value of 0 ($\log_{10} 1=0$), 20/50 a value of 0.4 ($\log_{10} 2.5=0.4$), and 20/200 a value of 1.0 ($\log_{10} 10=1.0$). The Jaeger (J) notation, which assigns arbitrary numbers to Snellen equivalent figures, is used by many practitioners to express near visual acuity. Methods of calculating these acuities and detailed comparisons with Snellen acuity can be found in more comprehensive textbooks.

Test Targets

Various test targets are used in visual acuity testing (Figure 4.1). Each individual letter, number, or picture on a testing chart is referred to as an optotype. Charts with such optotypes have achieved almost universal acceptance in the United States. Some optotypes are more difficult to recognize than others. For example, B (a relatively complex letter form) is the hardest for patients to recognize and can easily be interpreted as an E or the number 8. The letters C, D, and O are often confused because their shapes are similar. The easiest letter to recognize is L, which can be mistaken for few letters other than the letter I. This means that the examiner can consider a patient's misinterpreting a B during visual acuity testing to be less significant than missing an L.

Most letter and number charts available require some degree of literacy and some verbalization skills. The tumbling E and Landolt C tests can be done by matching, but both involve some degree of laterality and therefore test psychophysical components other than vision. Picture charts are nonthreatening for young children but can result in overestimation of visual acuity because, as with certain letters, the optotypes are not equally recognizable. Children easily learn the limited number of optotypes used, which can result in inaccurate acuity measurements due to educated guessing. A test involving a chart and matching cards employing the 4 letters H, O, T, and V is particularly useful with young children. These letters

Figure 4.1 Charts for distance visual acuity testing. **(A)** Snellen letter chart. **(B)** Allen picture chart.

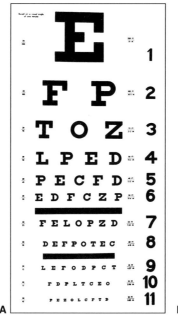

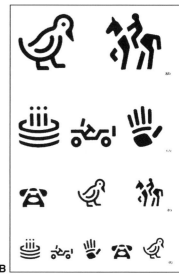

A
B

were chosen because they are symmetric, can be used for matching, and are useful with nonverbal or illiterate patients. A newer procedure for testing visual acuity using isolated, surrounded HOTV optotypes is the Amblyopia Treatment Study (ATS) visual acuity testing protocol, and it is gaining widespread acceptance for use with young children. Studies have demonstrated that this protocol has a high level of testability in 3- to 7-year-olds and excellent test-retest reliability.

Most charts have a notation either to the side or below each line of optotypes. This notation compares the size of the optotype with that of the standard 20/20 line. When the patient can read at least one-half of the letters correctly in any given line, the size of that optotype becomes the denominator of the Snellen acuity expression for that patient. The distance at which the patient is placed in reference to the chart is the numerator of the Snellen expression. For example, if a patient is 20 feet from the test chart and reads one-half of the optotypes on the 20/40 line correctly, the vision may be recorded as 20/40, but if the patient is only 15 feet from the chart and reads the same line, the vision should be recorded as 15/40. The examiner should also record whether the patient missed some letters on that line by adding the number of letters missed as a superscript notation to the acuity measurement. For example, if 2 letters are missed on the 20/40 line, the acuity may be expressed $20/40^{-2}$. If the patient misses 2 letters on that same line but was only 15 feet away from the chart, the expression is modified to $15/40^{-2}$. If the patient reads several letters on the next smallest line, the examiner may modify the superscript notation with a plus sign instead of a minus sign and denote the number of letters read correctly.

Standard Abbreviations

In addition to Snellen or other numeric notation, certain conventional abbreviations and notations are used in the patient record to indicate the type, circumstances, and results of visual acuity or visual function testing. The most common of these are shown in Table 4.1. The use of these abbreviations in recording the results of patient testing is described throughout this chapter where individual tests are detailed. Other abbreviations such as C, S, M (central, steady, maintained fixation) and F & F (fixes and follows) are used for preverbal or nonverbal children.

Table 4.1   Visual Acuity Notations and Abbreviations

Abbreviation	Stands for	Abbreviation	Stands for
VA	Visual acuity	CF or FC	Count fingers or finger counting
$\overline{cc}$	With correction	HM	Hand motion
$\overline{sc}$	Without correction	LP $\overline{c}$ proj	Light perception with projection (specify quadrants)
N	Near	LP $\overline{s}$ proj	Light perception without projection
D	Distance	NLP	No light perception
PH	Pinhole	C	Central
OD or RE	Right eye	S	Steady
OS or LE	Left eye	M	Maintained
OU	Both eyes (together)	F/F	Fixes/follows
J	Jaeger notation	NPA	Near point of accommodation
HOTV	HOTV chart	$20/40^{-2}$	Missed 2 letters on 20/40 line
E	Tumbling E chart or E game	$20/50^{+2}$	Read 2 letters on the line following the 20/50 line

■ Testing Procedures

The most basic types of vision testing are the distance and near visual acuity tests. Even though they test 2 different aspects of fine-detail central vision, these tests share some conventions, such as the use of corrective lenses and an established order for testing each eye. This section presents general background and specific steps for performing distance, pinhole, and near visual acuity testing and for measuring near points of accommodation and convergence.

Distance Acuity Test

On an initial visit, a patient should be tested both with and without corrective lenses. When recording visual acuity test results in the patient's record, the abbreviation cc indicates that corrective lenses were worn for the test.

When vision is measured without the use of corrective lenses, the abbreviation sc is used. On subsequent tests, a patient who habitually wears eyeglasses or contact lenses should wear them for the test, and it should be documented in the record. Distance correction should be used to test distance vision. To avoid confusion in recording information, a testing routine should be established. The right eye is tested first by convention. Clinical Protocol 4.1 presents instructions for performing a distance visual acuity test.

A variety of occluders, held by either the patient or the examiner, can be used to cover the eye that is not being tested. These include a tissue, a paddle, or an eye patch. The palm of the patient's or the examiner's hand can also be used to occlude the eye not being tested. If a standard occluder is not used, it is important to ensure that the patient cannot see through or around it. Any occluder that is used for more than 1 patient should be cleaned before reuse.

Before the test begins, determine if the patient is familiar with the optotypes being used. This is particularly important for children. If a patient is comfortable with letters, use that chart, if it is available. If the patient prefers numbers, use that chart. Because people tend to memorize the sequence of images that they have seen numerous times, present different charts or optotype sequences whenever possible. If only 1 type of chart is available, a patient can quickly memorize the order of the optotypes, whether intentionally or not. In this case, it is useful to ask the patient to read the letters in reverse order with the second eye. The type of chart and the method of presentation used should be noted in the patient's record; for example, "isolated numbers," "linear letters," or "pictures."

Pinhole Acuity Test

A below-normal visual acuity can be the result of a refractive error. This possibility can be inferred by having the patient read the testing chart through a pinhole occluder. The pinhole admits only central rays of light, which do not require refraction by the cornea or the lens. If the pinhole improves the patient's acuity by 2 lines or more, it is likely that the patient has a refractive error. If poor uncorrected visual acuity is not improved with the pinhole, the patient's reduced visual acuity is likely due either to an extreme refractive error or to nonrefractive causes (eg, cataract).

A pinhole no more than 2.4 mm in diameter should be used, and a single or multiple pinhole design is acceptable. One commonly used multiple pinhole design has a central opening surrounded by 2 rings of small perforations.

Clinical Protocol 4.2 describes the pinhole acuity test. Patients should be positioned as for the distance acuity test, and they should wear their habitual optical correction. The test is done for each eye separately and is not repeated under binocular viewing conditions.

Near Acuity Test

Near acuity testing assesses the ability of a patient to see clearly at a normal reading distance. The examiner should determine whether or not the patient uses near spectacles and, if so, the patient should use them during near vision testing. Occasionally, as with patients who are bedridden or who are examined in the emergency room, near vision testing might be the only available method of measuring visual acuity.

The test is usually performed at 16 inches (40 cm) with a printed, handheld card (Figure 4.2). If the distance is not accurate, the near visual acuity measurements will not be equivalent to the distance acuity. Most test cards specify in writing the distance at which they are to be held to correlate properly the measurements with those obtained for distance acuity. Some near reading cards come equipped with a chain that is 40 cm long to facilitate obtaining an accurate testing distance.

A Rosenbaum pocket vision screener, a Lebensohn chart, or the equivalent should be used to test near visual acuity. Clinical Protocol 4.3 presents instructions for testing near vision in adults. For children, near visual acuity can be tested with Allen reduced picture cards, the Lighthouse picture card, the HOTV equivalent cards, or the Lea figure set.

As with the Snellen chart, the near test card shows numeric notations alongside each line of optotypes. Most cards should have an equivalent Snellen acuity fraction next to each line. Other notations might also be present, the most common being the Jaeger notation, also referred to as *J (number)* acuity.

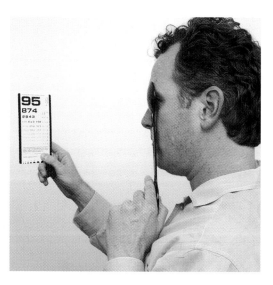

Figure 4.2 For near vision testing, the patient can hold the small near vision card at a normal reading distance.

Other Tests of Near Vision

Near vision depends not only on the eye's focusing ability, but on the near point of accommodation (NPA), a monocular attribute, and the near point of convergence (NPC), a binocular characteristic. The NPA is the nearest point at which the eye can focus so that a clear image is formed on the retina. With increasing age, the NPA recedes, a condition referred to as *presbyopia*. Clinical Protocol 4.4 describes the procedures for measuring the near points of accommodation and convergence. The distance noted when measuring the NPA, if expressed in meters, can be converted into diopters. A Prince or RAF (Royal Air Force) rule that has distance and diopters noted on the side is attached between the eyepieces of some phoropters and can be used for the conversion. This information is useful in determining the add power that will be needed for corrective lenses, or in assessing residual accommodative capacity. The NPC is the nearest point to which both eyes can move nasally (converge) and still maintain a single image. The normal NPC is between 6 cm and 10 cm, irrespective of age.

■ Acuity Tests for Special Patients

Patients with extremely low vision need special testing. Infants and toddlers, as well as illiterate adults and nonverbal patients, also need special testing methods and attention.

Low-Vision Testing

If a patient is unable to read the largest line of the visual acuity testing chart at the standard distance, repeat the acuity test at successively shorter distances. For example, repeatedly halve the distance between the patient and the chart. In this situation, note the distance at which the acuity measurement is successfully taken. This distance is used as the numerator of the Snellen fraction. For example, the notation 5/200 indicates that the patient read the 20/200 line successfully while standing 5 feet in front of the chart.

If the patient is unable to read the standard chart even at extremely close distances, the examiner can hold up fingers and ask the patient to count them. The patient with extremely low vision can also be asked to recognize the examiner's hand movements or identify the position of a penlight. Accepted abbreviations for recording low-vision test results are noted in Table 4.1. Clinical Protocol 4.5 describes the specific steps in a visual acuity examination for patients with low vision.

Testing Children and Special Adults

Many young toddlers are uncomfortable with strangers, and most do not want to be touched by someone they do not know. For these reasons, the examiner should allow these children to sit with a parent or other familiar caretaker and approach them slowly to avoid frightening them. Ask the parents questions regarding their child's visual behavior, such as whether their child recognizes their faces from a distance, responds to their smiles, or uses visual or auditory clues to identify objects or people.

In infants and preverbal children, an estimation of visual function can be made based on the ability to look directly at (fixate) a visual object, follow the object, and maintain steady fixation. Infants with normal visual function are able to manifest steady fixation and to follow an object by approximately 2 or 3 months of age.

Newborns should show a consistent blink response to a bright light, even through closed eyelids while they are sleeping. Teller acuity cards (discussed later in this chapter) can be used to obtain a more formal measurement of infant visual acuity. Clinical Protocol 4.6 describes standard procedures for testing an infant's vision.

Compare the infant's visual following responses, testing each eye separately with the other eye covered with a hand or a patch. If 1 eye fixes or follows better than the other eye, amblyopia or an alternate cause of reduced vision is suspected. If the infant objects only when 1 eye is covered, a difference in vision between the 2 eyes is strongly suspected. Fixation preference testing, usually using the induced tropia test, is a useful adjunct for detecting amblyopia in preverbal children. Clinical Protocols 4.7 and 4.8 describe the induced tropia test.

Teller acuity cards, if available, can be used to estimate acuity (Figure 4.3). These cards are large photographic plates (approximately 3 feet × 1 foot) with line gratings printed at 1 end. Cards are presented to the infant with progressively smaller line gratings. The examiner looks through a central pinhole to determine the baby's direction of gaze. The baby will look preferentially toward the side of the card that has a discernible image. Once the resolving ability of the eye has been surpassed, the baby's gaze will be random. These cards are reliable until a child is approximately 1 year of age. The examiner must be experienced to obtain reliable acuity measurements, lighting must be good, and the cards must be kept meticulously clean. Detailed testing and interpretation instructions are included with the test kits.

As an alternative testing method, optokinetic nystagmus (OKN) can be elicited using any regularly striped object. This can be as simple as lines drawn on paper or a standard tape measure, or as formal as a commercially produced OKN drum (Figure 4.4). In all cases, the stripes are passed slowly and steadily in front of the baby while the examiner observes the movement of the baby's eyes. Fine oscillatory movements, with the slow phase going in the direction that the stripes rotate, indicate that the baby has a potential for discriminating detail of at least the width of the stripe. Neurologic implications in the interpretation of the OKN response are covered in greater detail in more advanced texts. Horizontal OKN should be present before 3 months of age, whereas vertical optokinetic nystagmus might not be elicited until a child is approximately 6 months of age.

Toddlers and preliterate children as well as illiterate or nonverbal adult patients might be tested using a picture chart, the Landolt ring test, the tumbling E chart, or the HOTV chart and cards. When the HOTV chart and cards are used, the patient may be given a card with the 4 letters marked in large print. The patient is asked to point to each letter in turn as the examiner presents them on a separate screen or chart from a specified distance. The appropriate equivalent Snellen notation is then made, with an addendum that the optotypes were H, O, T, and V.

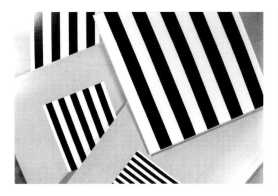

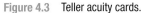

Figure 4.3   Teller acuity cards.

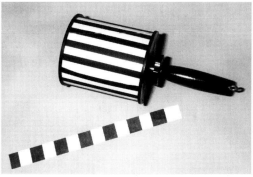

Figure 4.4   An OKN drum (top) and a homemade striped OKN target used to test nonverbal or preverbal patients.

The ATS visual acuity testing protocol is available on computerized visual acuity testers such as the electronic visual acuity (EVA) tester and M & S Technologies Smart System II PC-Plus. The protocol is automated on these instruments, so that the examiner only needs to indicate correct or incorrect. The surround bars are used to induce the crowding phenomenon, which makes the test more sensitive for amblyopia.

In the screening phase of the ATS visual acuity protocol, single letters are presented in descending logMAR sizes until one is missed. In the testing phase, letters are shown, starting 2 logMAR levels above the missed level in the screening phase, to determine the lowest level at which 3 of 4 letters are correctly identified. In the reinforcement phase, the child is shown 3 larger letters starting 2 levels above the lowest correct level in the testing phase to get the child, whose attention might be drifting, back on track. In the retest phase, the child is given a second chance on the last level missed in the test phase; if 3 of 4 levels are correctly identified, the test continues at the next smallest line until a level is failed. The visual acuity score is the lowest level at which 3 of 4 letters are correctly identified in the testing or retesting phase.

To help determine the most appropriate test, the examiner should ask whether the patient knows letters of the alphabet or numbers, because many patients can identify specific letters or numbers even though they cannot read. Some of the pictures are more readily recognizable than others, and there are only a limited number of pictures. Therefore, the use of picture charts generally leads to an overestimation of the child's visual ability and is a less sensitive method of detecting mild amblyopia.

Young children often become bored very quickly with vision testing. Some children do better with numbers, whereas others prefer letters. If a child seems bored or hesitant with 1 kind of chart, try another. If you are using the tumbling E chart, position yourself on 1 side of the chart and the parent on the other and ask the child, "Which direction are the legs pointing—to the ceiling, to the floor, to me, or to Mommy?" Alternatively, you can ask the child to point a hand or finger in the same direction that the legs of the letter form point. When using the Landolt ring you can position yourself and the parent as with the tumbling E chart and ask the child to indicate, for example, which side of the "cookie" has a bite in it. Some very shy children will not talk but can be coaxed into whispering the answer to a parent. Positive reinforcement, such as cheering for correct answers, can encourage a child to complete the test.

■ Variables in Acuity Measurements

Falsely high or low acuity measurements can be obtained under a variety of circumstances. In general, the near and distance acuities should be comparable unless myopia is present. Possible causes of near acuity being poorer than distance acuity include the following:

- Presbyopia/premature presbyopia
- Undercorrected or high hyperopia
- Overcorrected myopia
- Small, centrally located cataracts
- Accommodative insufficiency
- Systemic or topical drugs with anticholinergic effect
- Convergence insufficiency (applies to binocular visual acuity)
- Adie's pupil
- Functional visual loss

Other conditions can cause variability in acuity measurements for both near and distance. Examples of external variables include the following:

- Lighting conditions must remain equivalent for acuity tests to be comparable.
- Charts with higher contrast will be seen more easily than those with lower contrast.
- If a chart is not kept clean, smaller letters become more difficult to identify. When a projector chart is used, the cleanliness of the projector bulb and lens and the condition of the projecting screen will affect the contrast of the letters viewed by the patient.
- The distance between the projector and the chart will affect the size of the letters. The sharpness of the focus of a projected chart and the incidental glare on the screen can also influence the patient's ability to read the optotypes.
- Charts that have the letters crowded together might be more difficult to read.
- Patient fatigue or boredom are difficult variables to assess but will also affect acuity measurements and may be noted in the chart at the examiner's discretion.

Optical considerations also influence the ability of the patient to discern detail. They include the following:

- If a patient is wearing eyeglasses, the lenses need to be clean. Dirty lenses of any kind, whether trial lenses, phoropter lenses, eyeglass lenses, or contact lenses, will decrease acuity, and the measurements obtained will be falsely low.

- Effects of tear film abnormalities, such as dry eye syndromes, can be minimized by the generous use of artificial tear preparations.
- Corneal surface abnormalities can produce distortions.
- Corneal or lenticular astigmatism might necessitate the use of special spectacle or contact lenses. Discussions regarding the prescribing of these lenses can be found in specialized clinical texts.
- Other interferences from media opacities might have to be addressed either medically or surgically.

Patients with neurologic impairments might have motility problems or central nervous system abnormalities that can influence the measurement of acuity, as described here:

- A visual or an expressive agnosia will usually be identified while obtaining the history by the way questions are, or are not, answered.
- Motility defects such as nystagmus (the presence of spontaneous oscillatory movements of the eyes) or any other movement disorder that interferes with the ability to align the fovea on the object of regard will lower the acuity measurement.
- Nystagmus might be difficult to determine when the amplitude of the nystagmus is small. In latent nystagmus, a condition that occurs only when 1 eye is occluded, the unoccluded eye develops nystagmus and the measured visual acuity will be lower than expected and significantly lower than the binocular acuity.
- Other neurologic considerations include the following:
- Visual field defects
- Optic nerve lesions
- Pupillary abnormalities
- Impairment by drugs, legal or illicit

If latent nystagmus is suspected or diagnosed, the fellow eye may be blurred using a +10.00 to +20.00 diopter lens instead of a standard occluder. "Fogging" the fellow eye in this manner does not induce latent nystagmus because it allows light to enter both eyes; therefore, the best possible monocular visual acuity is obtained. As an alternative, the vectographic projection slides can be used to conduct visual acuity examinations using polarized images, with a different polarized image presented to each eye.

When nystagmus is present, the patient might have a null position. In this situation, the patient maintains a head position to decrease the amplitude of the nystagmus. Visual acuity will improve when the head is held in that position. If the patient assumes a head position when looking at objects, determine if this improves acuity by allowing the patient to maintain that head position while you measure binocular visual acuity for distance and near. The anomalous head position may also be allowed for monocular visual acuity testing, as long as it does not cause the patient to see around the occluder or fogging lens. Frequently patients with congenital nystagmus will have significantly better visual acuity for near than for distance. This occurs if the nystagmus dampens with convergence.

Psychologic factors, whether conscious or unconscious, affect visual acuity measurement results. In an attempt to please the examiner or parent(s) or to "score" better on the test, children might try to peek around the occluder. Familiarity with the test can also lead to inadvertent memorization of the lines by the patient. External variables such as patient distraction, fatigue, and age should be considered when an unexplained, poor acuity measurement is obtained.

■ Uncorrectable Visual Acuity

The Snellen standard of 20/20 is considered normal vision. Sometimes, this acuity cannot be achieved with optical correction such as eyeglasses or contact lenses. The terms visual impairment or visual acuity impairment are used to describe this situation. Visual impairment is not the same as a visual disability, which implies a subjective judgment by the examiner. The World Health Organization divides low vision into 3 categories based on visual acuity (VA) and visual field. The criteria for the categories based on visual acuity are as follows:

- Moderate visual impairment: best corrected VA is less than 20/60 (including 20/70 to 20/160).
- Severe visual impairment: best corrected VA is less than 20/160 (including 20/200 to 20/400).
- Profound visual impairment: best corrected VA is less than 20/400 (including 20/500 to 20/1000).

The visual acuity is an important factor that the examiner may use to make estimates regarding a patient's potential disability. The acuity level is considered when determining reading aids and reading distances. These factors are summarized in Table 4.2. Severe visual impairment in both eyes is required for inclusion in the category "legal blindness" and is the criterion usually used to determine eligibility for disability benefits.

The disabling effect, if any, of a visual impairment depends upon the individual and might or might not be perceived by the patient as a disability. Table 4.2 also summarizes levels of visual impairment and visual disability, which are important for evaluating legal or physical limitations for a patient. Definitions of legal blindness differ from state to state, especially regarding eligibility for a driver's license. In most states, the visual acuity must be correctable to 20/40 or better for an unrestricted license, which was the level of acuity proposed by the Low Vision Rehabilitation Committee of the American Academy of Ophthalmology in a Policy Statement regarding vision requirements for driving. The guidelines for issuing noncommercial driving licenses also include the recommendation that an uninterrupted visual field of 140° horizontal diameter be present for individuals with 20/40 or better visual acuity.

Table 4.2 Visual Impairment and Estimates of Visual Disability

Visual Impairment	Visual Disability	Comment	Reading Distance: Reading Aids
20/12 to 20/25	Normal vision at normal reading distance	Healthy young adults average better than 20/20.	*> 33 cm:* Regular bifocals (up to 3 D)
20/80 to 20/160	Moderate low vision; (near) normal performance with magnifiers	Strong reading glasses or vision magnifiers usually provide adequate reading ability; this level is usually insufficient for a driving license.	*16–10 cm:* Half-eye glasses (6–10 D), with prisms for binocularity Stronger magnifiers (> 8 D)
20/200 to 20/400	Severe low vision: legal blindness by US definition	Gross orientation and mobility generally adequate, but difficulty with traffic signs, bus numbers, etc. Reading requires high-power magnifiers; reading speed is reduced, even with reading aids.	*8–5 cm (cannot be binocular):* High-power reading lenses (12–20 D) High-power magnifiers (> 16 D)
20/500 to 20/1000	Profound visual impairment	Limited spot reading with visual aids.	*4–2 cm (cannot be binocular):* High-power reading lenses (24–28 D) High-power magnifiers (> 28 D) Video magnifier Talking devices and vision substitutes
CF 8 ft to 4 ft	Unreliable vision	Increasing problems with visual orientation and mobility. Long cane is useful to explore environment. Talking devices and vision substitutes are useful.	
Less than CF 4 ft	Nearly total blindness	Vision unreliable, except under ideal circumstances; must rely on nonvisual devices.	
NLP	Total blindness	No light perception; must rely on talking devices and vision substitutes.	

Amblyopia

Amblyopia, when unilateral, is a visual disorder defined as a difference in optically correctable acuity of more than 2 lines between the 2 eyes that results from abnormal visual input in early childhood. The lay term for amblyopia is *lazy eye*. Normal development of vision occurs early in life through ongoing stimulation of vision-receptive cells in the brain. Amblyopia results when there is an interruption of this process. A patient with amblyopia demonstrates impaired vision not explained by organic damage to the eye because the problem is primarily in the brain, which does not receive proper visual input from the affected eye.

Causes of unilateral amblyopia include anisometropia, strabismus, and unilateral media opacities such as monocular congenital cataracts. Amblyopia can also be bilateral and can be associated with a variety of other conditions, including long-standing uncorrected refractive errors and nystagmus. Causes of amblyopia are dealt with in greater detail in other textbooks of clinical ophthalmology. In general, the younger the patient, the more successful is the amblyopia treatment. Many patients with amblyopia exhibit the crowding phenomenon, in which smaller optotypes can be correctly identified when they are viewed singly rather than in a line with figures on both sides. As a result, many amblyopic patients correctly identify the first and last letters of a line more easily than those in the middle. If visual acuity is checked using isolated figures, it should be recorded in the medical record. The crowding phenomenon is not specific to amblyopia.

Although many practitioners end treatment when a patient is 8 to 10 years of age, evidence indicates that some improvement in vision can be achieved in older children and teenagers. Therefore, a trial of amblyopia therapy may be attempted in an older child after a thorough discussion with the parents and the child of the benefits and drawbacks of such treatment.

Other Tests of Sensory Visual Function

The ability to use both eyes together is referred to as *fusion* or *single binocular vision*. Single binocular vision results from simultaneous stimulation of corresponding retinal elements that have the same visual direction. For example, an object to a person's left stimulates a spot on the temporal retina of the right eye and a corresponding spot on the nasal retina of the left eye. The brain then perceives the object as a single image in space. Many tests have been devised to assess different aspects of binocular vision, and they are discussed in detail in most strabismus textbooks.

Stereopsis is the perception of depth or 3 dimensions that occurs when slightly disparate (noncorresponding) retinal elements are stimulated at the same time. To achieve stereopsis, both eyes must be used simultaneously. The tests used to measure stereopsis consist of either polarized images or random-dot stereograms that may be nonpolarized or polarized. Figure 4.5 illustrates the Titmus (fly) test, which is the most common test for near stereopsis. Clinical Protocol 4.9 summarizes the procedure for the Titmus stereoacuity test. Random-dot stereogram tests also are used to test near stereoacuity. Vectographic polarized projection slides can be used to test distance stereopsis. Stereoscopic acuity is expressed in seconds of arc, but

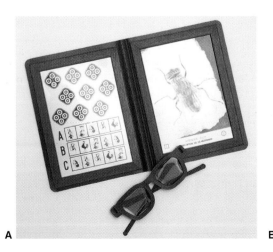

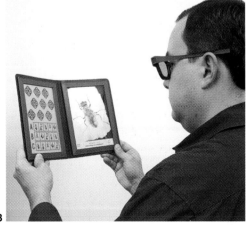

A   B

Figure 4.5   The Titmus stereopsis test. **(A)** Light-polarizing eyeglasses and targets. **(B)** The patient views the target through polarizing filters and reports perception of depth.

there are no standards for stereoacuity tests as there are for Snellen acuity charts to allow comparison among different tests.

Entoptic phenomena include the visualization of images of one's internal retinal blood vessels and corpuscles after a light has been applied. Although the presence of these images implies that the retina is functioning, it is not a measure of acuity and is rarely used to characterize vision. Eliciting this phenomenon can be helpful in determining a reasonable level of function behind very opaque media.

Contrast Sensitivity, Glare, and Color Vision Tests

Contrast sensitivity refers to the ability to discern relative darkness and brightness and the ability to see details, edges, or borders of images. Contrast sensitivity can be impaired even in the presence of excellent Snellen acuity. Alterations in contrast sensitivity imply abnormalities in the anterior visual receptive systems, from the tear film to the optic nerve. Specific patterns of alteration of contrast sensitivity function are discussed in more advanced textbooks.

In the simplest contrast sensitivity tests, patients are shown printed charts with contrasting lines, referred to as *gratings*, which are presented in varying orientations. The difference in the intensity between the background of the chart and the printed lines is gradually decreased, and the patient is asked to identify the direction of the lines. The endpoint is reached when the patient can no longer correctly identify either the presence of any lines or the direction of their orientation. Testing methods that are more technical involve presenting grating patterns or letters on an oscilloscope screen. The endpoints and reporting methods are similar in the 2 techniques.

Glare occurs when light from a single bright source scatters across the visual field, reducing the quality of the visual image. The perception of troublesome glare, which causes distorted vision and, in some cases, mild pain, can be a symptom of cataract. As with contrast sensitivity testing, glare testing (by exposing the patient to bright light under controlled circumstances) can suggest the presence of cataract or other opacity.

The most commonly recognized color vision abnormalities are the sex-linked congenital red-green deficiencies, but many other color vision anomalies exist. Optic nerve or retinal disease can result in color vision defects that can be acquired or asymmetric. Most patients with inherited color vision defects see red as less bright than nonaffected individuals and, according to a standard established by testing nonaffected individuals, fail to identify color mixtures that include red. Although not disabling, color vision anomalies can impair performance in some careers or activities. However, colors can often be altered to accommodate those who have difficulty discriminating certain shades, as is available in some computer graphics applications.

Evaluation of color vision is often performed with a book that displays circles in multicolored patterns, called *pseudoisochromatic color plates*. Patients with normal color vision easily detect specific numbers and figures composed of and embedded in the dot pattern, but patients with impaired color vision do not detect the same numbers. Various combinations of colors are used to identify the nature of the color vision deficit.

Another test of color vision, the 15-hue test (Farnsworth-Munsell D-15 test), consists of 15 pastel-colored chips, which the patient must arrange in a related color sequence. The sequence is obvious to patients with normal color vision, but patients with color deficits arrange the chips differently.

Principles and performance of contrast sensitivity, glare, and color vision testing are covered more thoroughly in other, more detailed textbooks and in manufacturers' instructions that accompany testing materials.

Pitfalls and Pointers

- Be aware of the variables possible in visual acuity measurement. Ensure that all lenses, projectors, and charts are clean.
- Avoid glare on the viewing chart or screen.
- Avoid glare in patients' eyes from overhead lights or outside windows.
- Learn appropriate ways of interacting with patients who have low vision or are blind. Warn the patient of your movement, particularly if there is severe visual impairment. Offer an arm to the patient, but do not attempt to grab his or her hand or arm.
- Ensure that you are using the appropriate tests for the patient's abilities.
- Refrain from using the term *blindness* when counseling patients or parents of children with severe visual impairment. Most of these patients have some useful vision, and many of them will amaze you with their resourcefulness.
- Use a demeanor and a test of visual function that is appropriate for the patient's age. Infants and young toddlers will respond best to a gentle, gradual approach and to the use of interesting toys to assess their fixing and following behaviors.

Suggested Resources

Amblyopia [Preferred Practice Pattern]. San Francisco: American Academy of Ophthalmology; 2008.

Frisen L. *Clinical Tests of Vision.* New York: Raven Press; 1990.

Clinical Optics. Basic and Clinical Science Course, Section 3. San Francisco: American Academy of Ophthalmology; published annually.

Pediatric Ophthalmology and Strabismus. Basic and Clinical Science Course, Section 6. San Francisco: American Academy of Ophthalmology; updated annually.

Visual Rehabilitation for Adults [Preferred Practice Pattern]. San Francisco: American Academy of Ophthalmology; 2007.

Clinical Protocol 4.1 — Testing Distance Visual Acuity

1. Ask the patient to stand or sit at a designated testing distance (20 feet from a well-illuminated wall chart is ideal). If a projected chart is used, distance may vary; the projected optotype size must be focused and adjusted to be equivalent to the corresponding Snellen acuity for the distance used.

2. Occlude the left eye. Be sure that the occluder is not touching or pressing against the eye. Observe the patient during the test to make sure there is no conscious or inadvertent peeking.

3. Ask the patient to say aloud each letter or number, or name the picture object on the lines of successively smaller optotypes, from left to right or, alternatively, as you point to each character in any order, until the patient correctly identifies at least one-half of the optotypes on a line. If a patient is hesitant (at times for fear of being wrong), tell him or her that it is all right to guess.

4. Note the corresponding acuity measurement shown at that line of the chart. Record the acuity value for each eye separately, with correction and without correction, as illustrated below. If the patient misses half or fewer than half the letters on the smallest readable line, record how many letters were missed; for example, $20/40^{-2}$. If acuity is worse than 20/20, recheck with a 2.4 mm pinhole (see Clinical Protocol 4.2).

5. Repeat steps 1 through 4 for the left eye, with the right eye covered.

6. If desired, retest acuity with the patient using both eyes simultaneously and record acuity OU (see the following example).

$$ \mathrm{D} \, \mathrm{V} \, \overline{\mathrm{sc}} \quad \begin{matrix} \text{OD } 20/200 \\ \text{OS } 20/100 \end{matrix} \quad \text{OU } 20/80 $$

$$ \mathrm{D} \, \mathrm{V} \, \overline{\mathrm{cc}} \quad \begin{matrix} \text{OD } 20/20 \\ \text{OS } 20/25 \end{matrix} \quad \text{OU } 20/20 $$

7. Record the power of the corrective lenses worn for the distance acuity determination (see Clinical Protocol 5.1).

Clinical Protocol 4.2 — Testing Pinhole Visual Acuity

1. Position the patient and occlude the eye not being tested, as done for the distance acuity test.

2. Ask the patient to hold the pinhole occluder in front of the eye that is to be tested. The patient's habitual correction may be worn for the test.

3. Instruct the patient to look at the distance chart through the single pinhole or through any one of the multiple pinholes.

4. Instruct the patient to use small hand or eye movements to align the pinhole to resolve the sharpest image on the chart.

5. Ask the patient to begin to read the line with the smallest letters that are legible as determined on the previous vision test without the use of the pinhole.

6. Record the Snellen acuity obtained and precede or follow it with the abbreviation *PH*.

Clinical Protocol 4.3 — Testing Near Visual Acuity

1. With the patient wearing the habitual corrective lens for near and the near card evenly illuminated, instruct the patient to hold the test card at the distance specified on the card.
2. Ask the patient to occlude the left eye.
3. Ask the patient to say each letter or read each word on the line of smallest characters that are legible on the card.
4. Record the acuity value for each eye separately in the patient's chart according to the notation method accepted (see the example below).
5. Repeat the procedure with the right eye occluded and the left eye viewing the test chart.
6. Repeat the procedure with both eyes viewing the test card.
7. Record the binocular acuity achieved (see the following example).

$$N \bigvee \overline{sc} \quad \begin{array}{l} \text{OD } 20/200 \\ \text{OS } 20/100 \end{array} \quad \text{OU } 20/80$$

$$N \bigvee \overline{cc} \quad \begin{array}{l} \text{OD } 20/20 \\ \text{OS } 20/25 \end{array} \quad \text{OU } 20/20$$

Clinical Protocol 4.4 — Testing for NPA and NPC

Testing for Near Point of Accommodation (NPA)

1. With the patient wearing full distance correction and with the left eye occluded, place the near testing card at a distance of 16 inches (40 cm) from the patient and ask the patient to read the 20/40 line with the unoccluded eye.
2. Move the test card slowly toward the patient as you ask the patient to state when the letters have become blurred.
3. Record this distance in centimeters or inches (whichever you are using).
4. Repeat steps 1 to 3 for the other eye and record as described above.
5. The NPA is that point (in centimeters or inches) where the patient can no longer bring the image into clear focus.

Testing for Near Point of Convergence (NPC)

1. With the patient wearing appropriate correction and with neither eye occluded, hold a target, such as a pencil tip, at a distance of approximately 16 inches (40 cm) from the patient and ask the patient to fixate on it.
2. Move the object slowly forward and ask the patient to tell you when the object doubles.
3. Observe whether both eyes are converging.
4. Note the position at which the image doubles or 1 eye deviates away from the fixation target. The NPC is that point where a single image can no longer be maintained. Record the distance (in centimeters or inches) between that point and the upper bridge of the nose at the midpoint between the eyes.

Clinical Protocol 4.5

Testing Acuity for Patients With Low Vision

1. If the patient is unable to resolve the largest optotype on the distance acuity chart from the standard testing distance, ask the patient to stand or sit 10 feet from the well-illuminated test chart. A projected chart is less desirable to use in this situation than a printed wall chart. A low-vision test chart, if available, is preferable for these patients.

2. Occlude the eye not being tested.

3. Repeatedly halve the testing distance (up to 2.5 feet) and retest the distance visual acuity at each stage until the patient successfully identifies half the optotypes on a line.

4. Note the corresponding acuity measurement shown at that line of the chart. Record the acuity value for each eye separately, with correction and without correction, as would be done for standard distance acuity testing, recording the distance at which the patient successfully reads the chart as the numerator of the Snellen acuity designation; for example, *5/80*.

5. If the patient is unable to resolve the largest optotypes on the chart from a distance of 2.5 feet, display 2 or more fingers of 1 hand and ask the patient to count the number of fingers displayed. Record the longest distance at which counting is done accurately; for example, *CF at 2 ft.*

6. If the patient cannot count fingers, move your hand horizontally or vertically before the patient at a distance of approximately 2 feet. Record the distance at which the patient reported seeing your hand movement; for example, *HM at 2 ft.*

7. If the patient cannot detect your hand motion, shine a penlight toward the patient's face from approximately 1 foot and turn it on and off to determine if light perception is present. If the patient cannot see the light, dim the room lights and shine the brightest light available (usually the indirect ophthalmoscope) toward the patient's eye again. If the patient cannot see even the brightest light, record the response as *NLP* (no light perception). If the patient can see the light, record the response as *LP* (light perception). No record of distance is required.

8. If light is perceived from straight ahead, move the light sequentially into each of the 4 quadrants of the visual field. Turn the penlight on and off in each field, and ask if the patient can see the light.

9. If the patient correctly identifies the direction from which the light is coming, record the response as *LP with projection*. Specify the quadrant(s) in which light projection is present. If the patient is unable to identify any direction but is able to discern light in the straight-ahead position, record the response as *LP without projection*.

10. If the light can be seen from straight ahead, colored filters can be placed in front of the light and the patient is asked to identify the color of the light. Record whether or not color perception is present.

11. Repeat steps 1 to 10 for the fellow eye, as appropriate.

Clinical Protocol 4.6 — Testing an Infant's Fixing and Following Behavior

1. Seat the infant on a familiar adult's lap, so that the infant is comfortable.

2. Select a small toy or other attention-attracting object that stimulates sight only; do not use a sound-producing object. Hold the object about 1 to 2 feet from the infant's face and move it horizontally to either side.

3. Watch the infant's eyes for fixation and following movements.

4. Cover 1 eye and repeat the test. Cover the other eye and repeat again. Observe for any difference between the eyes in the quality of fixation and smooth pursuit or in the amount of objection to occlusion. If you suspect a difference but are unsure, repeat these tests, using a different toy if available to maintain the infant's interest.

5. When tested monocularly, very young infants will respond with better following movements for objects moved from temporal to nasal field; this preference decreases after an infant is approximately 6 months old.

Clinical Protocol 4.7 — Performing the Induced Tropia Test in Nonstrabismic Infants

1. This test is used to detect a fixation preference (and amblyopia) in an infant without strabismus or with a very small strabismic angle. Position the infant and select a toy as you would to elicit fixing and following, and present an interesting target at near fixation.

2. Place a 15 or 20 PD base-down prism in front of the right eye. Determine if the infant looks upward through the prism to view the target (maintains right eye fixation), views the target without an upward shift of fixation (maintains left eye fixation), or shifts fixation upward and downward spontaneously (alternates fixation).

3. Repeat the test with the prism placed before the left eye.

4. Combine the results from the 2 eyes, and record as:

   a. Alternates fixation (amblyopia unlikely)

   b. Alternates, but prefers fixation with OD / OS (amblyopia suspected)

   c. Fixes only with OD / OS (amblyopia likely)

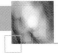

Clinical Protocol 4.8 — Testing Fixation Preference in Strabismic Patients

1. This test is used to detect a fixation preference (and amblyopia) in an infant with strabismus. Position the infant and select a toy as you would to elicit fixing and following, and present an interesting target at near fixation.

2. Determine which eye is fixing on the target (preferred eye).

3. Cover the preferred eye. Observe the shift of the fellow eye (nonpreferred eye) to assume fixation on the target.

4. Uncover the preferred eye. Determine if fixation is maintained by the previously nonpreferred eye or switches back to the preferred eye, noting the timing of the fixation switch. Observe the presence or absence of a blink preceding a fixation switch.

(continued)

Clinical Protocol 4.8 *(continued)*

5. Record the results as:

   a. Alternates fixation (amblyopia unlikely)

   b. Prefers OD / OS, holds OS / OD through a blink (amblyopia unlikely)

   c. Prefers OD / OS, holds OS / OD to a blink (amblyopia suspected)

   d. Prefers OD / OS, holds OS / OD briefly (amblyopia suspected)

   e. Prefers OD / OS, will not hold OS / OD (amblyopia likely)

Clinical Protocol 4.9      Testing for Stereoacuity

1. Check the polarization of the glasses being used to ensure that each eye sees a different image; the left eye should see only the L on the lower left of the Titmus fly, and the right eye should see only the R.

2. Place the polarizing glasses on the patient. If glasses are usually worn, place the polarizing glasses over them.

3. Hold the fly image facing the patient approximately 16 inches (40 cm) away, with the surface of the page parallel to the surface of the glasses.

4. Ask the patient to touch or to pinch the wings of the fly. Reassure young children who might respond with surprise or fright if the image appears too real to them. If the image is perceived as having height, the patient will be observed to attempt to touch the wings as if they were above the page surface.

5. If the fly test is positive, show the patient the 3 rows of animal figures. Ask which figure in each row is coming forward or is above the page.

6. After noting the responses to the animals, direct the patient's attention to the squares with the 4 circles in each. Ask the patient to tell you which circle is coming forward in each square. Alternatively, you may ask the patient to point to the appropriate circle or, particularly with children, to push the button that is popping up.

7. Score the response as the last correctly identified before 2 consecutive circles are missed.

8. Record the stereopsis as seconds of arc as designated in the instruction booklet that is included with each test. It is advisable to copy the scoring chart for each test and attach it to the back of the test chart for ready reference; you will probably not remember the numbers for each target, and if the test that you are using is not the standard one, the scoring could vary.

9. Be sure that the patient has both eyes open while doing the test. Some patients are so accustomed to being tested monocularly that they automatically close 1 eye.

10. You might suspect that some patients are using monocular clues to choose the correct responses. If so, turn the book upside down and ask them to describe the images. If they do not describe the images as going behind or sinking into the page, then you have confirmed your suspicion that they were relying on monocular clues instead of stereopsis.

5 Refraction

Refraction is the process by which the patient is guided through the use of a variety of lenses so as to achieve the best possible acuity on distance and near vision tests. Refraction involves both objective and subjective measurements. The objective portion of the process of refraction is called *retinoscopy* and can be accomplished by manual or automated methods. The measurements obtained by retinoscopy can be refined by subjective methods to achieve a final prescription for eyeglasses or other optical aids. This chapter offers instruction in these basic techniques of refraction, including guidelines for spectacle lens prescription. Because refraction requires an understanding of basic refractive states of the eye and the basic characteristics of lenses used for optical correction, this chapter briefly reviews those topics and provides instruction in determining the prescription of existing corrective lenses.

■ Overview of Refraction

The physicist defines refraction as the bending of light rays as they encounter interfaces between materials with differing refractive indices. In clinical ophthalmology, the term *refraction* is employed to describe the process to measure a patient's refractive error, determine the optical correction needed to focus light rays from distant and near objects onto the retina, and provide the patient with clear and comfortable vision. The clinical process of refraction comprises several activities, which are discussed in greater detail later in this chapter.

1. *Retinoscopy* (or objective refraction) is a clinical test used to determine the approximate nature and extent of a patient's refractive error (ie, nearsightedness, farsightedness, or astigmatism). It is sometimes called *objective refraction* because it does not require subjective responses from the patient. Retinoscopy is performed primarily with a retinoscope, a handheld instrument consisting of a light source and a viewing component. Sometimes an automated machine is used for retinoscopy.

2. *Refinement* (or *subjective refraction*) provides a precise measurement of refractive error and appropriate lens correction. Refinement utilizes patient participation and reaction ("I can see better with this lens than with that one") to obtain the refractive correction that gives the best visual acuity. Tools used in refinement include the refractor (also called a *Phoroptor*) or trial lenses and trial frame and a visual acuity chart. Because refinement requires subjective participation from the patient, it is not possible to

perform this part of refraction with infants, most toddlers, and other patients who are unable to communicate adequately.

Both retinoscopy and refinement can be done in the presence or absence of *cycloplegia*. Cycloplegia is the use of eyedrop medication to paralyze accommodation temporarily, enabling the refractionist to determine the patient's baseline nonaccommodative refractive error. If cycloplegic drops are not used, then the refraction is said to be manifest (or "dry").

3. *Binocular balancing* is the final step in refraction that determines whether accommodation has been equally relaxed in the 2 eyes.

4. *Prescription of spectacle lenses* is the outcome of the clinical process of refraction. The patient is given an optical prescription (a written description of the optical requirements for correction of the patient's refractive error) based on the results of the steps 1 to 3.

Overview of Ophthalmic Optics

Performing accurate retinoscopy and refinement and prescribing appropriate optical correction require a fundamental understanding of the properties of light rays, of the types and properties of optical lenses, and of the interaction between the two. This chapter touches on the principles of ophthalmic optics only briefly; more detailed information is available in Section 3, *Clinical Optics*, of the Basic and Clinical Science Course, published by the American Academy of Ophthalmology.

Principles of Vergence

As applied to light rays, the term *vergence* describes the direction of a ray as it passes between some luminous point to a lens in question. Vergence is the reciprocal of the distance from the lens to the point of convergence of the light. Light rays that are moving away from each other are termed *divergent*. Light rays that are moving toward each other are termed *convergent*. Parallel light rays have zero vergence; ie, they do not move toward or away from each other. Figure 5.1 illustrates these 3 types of rays. Light rays emanating from a point source of light are divergent. Convergent light rays do not usually occur in nature but are the result of the action

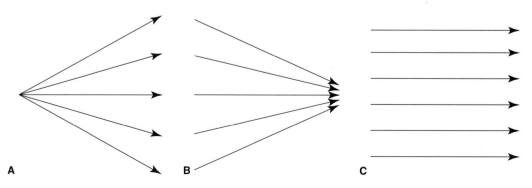

Figure 5.1   Light rays can be divergent **(A)**, convergent **(B)**, or parallel (zero vergence) **(C)**.

of an optical system (eg, a lens). Light rays emanating from the sun are essentially parallel and have zero vergence.

Power (or *vergence power*) describes the ability of a curved lens to converge or diverge light rays. By convention, divergence is expressed in minus power; convergence is expressed in plus power. A *diopter* (abbreviated D) is the unit of measurement of the refractive power of a lens. The *focal length* of a lens is the distance between the lens and the image formed by an object at infinity:

$$f = 1/D$$

where f = focal length (in meters) and D = lens power (in diopters).

Types of Lenses

Lenses may be spheres, cylinders, or spherocylinders. A *spherical lens* has the same curvature over its entire surface, and thus the same refractive power in all meridians. Convex spherical lenses converge light rays and are called *plus lenses*; concave spherical lenses diverge light rays and are called *minus lenses* (Figure 5.2). The *focal point of a plus lens* is that position where parallel light rays that have passed through the lens converge to form an image. The *focal point of a minus lens* is the point from which parallel light rays entering the lens appear to diverge. Examples of plus and minus lenses illustrating the relationship of lens power to focal length are shown in Figure 5.3. In the case of convex, or plus, lenses, using the mathematical formula D = 1/f, 1 diopter of plus power converges parallel rays of light to focus at 1 m from the lens. A ι0.25 D lens focuses parallel light rays 1/0.25 m, or 4 m, from the lens. A +4.00 D lens converges parallel light rays to a focus at 1/4.00 m, or 0.25 m from the lens. In the case of concave, or minus, lenses, parallel light rays entering the lens diverge; a virtual image is considered to appear at a focal point in front of the lens.

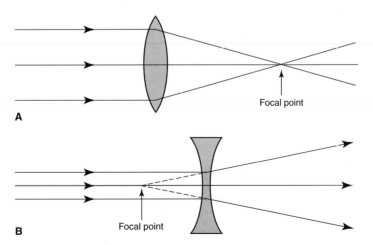

Figure 5.2 Types of lenses include **(A)** converging (convex or plus) lenses, and **(B)** diverging (concave or minus) lenses. The focal point of a plus lens occurs where parallel light rays that have passed through the lens converge to form an image. The focal point of a minus lens occurs where parallel light rays entering the lens appear to diverge.

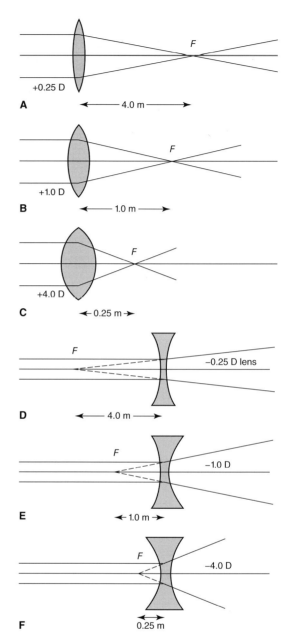

Figure 5.3 Relationship of lens power to focal length for plus lenses **(A, B, C)** and minus lenses **(D, E, F)**. *F* = focal point.

A minus lens with a focal length of 1 m has a power of –1.00 D; a minus lens with a focal length of –0.25 m has a power of 1/(–0.25) D or –4.00 D.

Cylindrical lenses have vergence power in only 1 meridian, the one perpendicular to the axis of the cylinder. They have no power in the meridian parallel to the axis (Figure 5.4). Cylindrical lenses focus light rays to a line (Figure 5.5). The orientation of the axis of cylindrical lenses is assigned by convention, when looking at a patient, as noted in Figure 5.6. The orientation of corrective cylindrical lenses is the same for the right and left eyes; ie, 0° to 90° is to the patient's left, whereas 90° to 180° is to the patient's right.

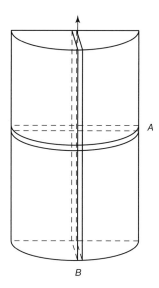

Figure 5.4   Refracting (vergence) power of a cylindrical lens. Maximum refractive power occurs in the meridian perpendicular to the axis of the cylinder (curved undotted line *A*). The cylinder has no refractive power in the meridian that corresponds to the axis of the cylinder (vertical undotted lines *B*).

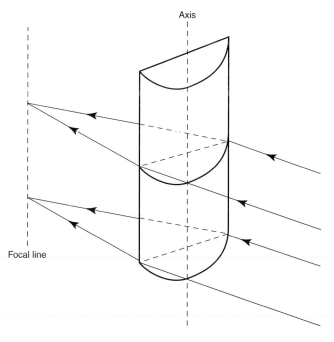

Figure 5.5   Because a cylindrical lens has refracting power in only 1 meridian (which is perpendicular to its axis), it focuses light rays to a focal line.

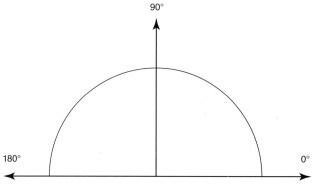

Figure 5.6   Conventional assignment of the orientation of the axis of cylindrical lenses, when looking at a patient.

Spherical and cylindrical lenses can be combined in 1 lens to form a *spherocylindrical lens*, also known as a *compound lens* or *toric lens*. A spherocylindrical lens focuses the light in 2-line foci. The shape of the light rays as they are focused by the spherocylindrical lens is called the *conoid of Sturm* (Figure 5.7). Between the 2-line foci produced by the conoid of Sturm is a point called the *circle of least confusion*, which represents the point of best overall focus for a spherocylindrical lens.

Prisms are technically not lenses, but prismatic effects are inherent characteristics of lenses. A *prism* is a wedge of refracting material with a triangular cross section that deviates light toward its base. Objects viewed through a prism appear to be displaced toward the apex of the prism (Figure 5.8). Spherical lenses can be thought of as paired prisms, with convergent (plus) lenses made of prisms that are base to base, and divergent (minus) lenses made of prisms that are apex to apex. Thus, a spherical lens has prismatic power at every point on its surface except at the optical center of the lens.

The power of a prism to deviate light rays is expressed in *prism diopters* (abbreviated PD or with a superscript delta $^\Delta$). A prism measuring 1 PD (1^Δ) deviates parallel rays of light 1 cm when measured at a distance of 1 m from the prism (Figure 5.9). A prism that deviates light rays 1 cm at a distance of 2 m measures 0.5 PD; a prism that deviates light rays 1 cm at a distance of 1/2 meter (0.5 m) measures 2 PD.

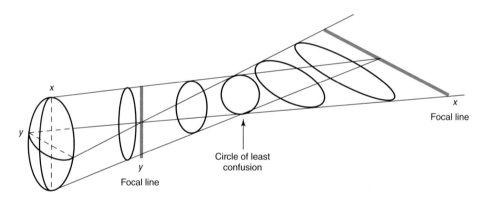

Figure 5.7 Because its 2 radii of curvature (*x, y*) are not equal, a spherocylinder does not focus light to a point, but to 2 lines (*y* focal line, *x* focal line) in different places. The clearest image is formed between the two, at the circle of least confusion. The conoid of Sturm is the name given to the shape the light rays take as they are focused by a spherocylindrical lens.

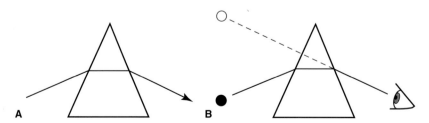

Figure 5.8 **(A)** Because of its shape, a prism refracts light rays toward its base. **(B)** If an object is viewed through a prism, the object appears in space as if it were displaced toward the prism apex.

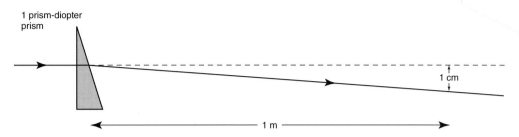

Figure 5.9 Measurement of prism power. A prism measuring 1 PD deflects a light ray 1 cm at a distance of 1 m.

■ Refractive States of the Eye

In the normal eye, parallel light rays are focused sharply on the retina, a condition known as *emmetropia*. When the relaxed, or *nonaccommodating*, eye is unable to bring parallel light rays from a distant object into focus, the condition is referred to as *ametropia*. The 3 basic conditions that may produce ametropia are:

- Myopia (nearsightedness)
- Hyperopia (farsightedness, also called *hypermetropia*)
- Astigmatism

A *myopic* (nearsighted) eye has excessive convergent power; the light rays focus anterior to the retina. A minus (divergent) lens is used to correct myopia (Figure 5.10 A, B). A *hyperopic* (farsighted) eye has insufficient convergence power to focus light rays on the retina; the rays focus posterior to the retina. A plus (convergent) lens is used to correct hyperopia (Figure 5.10 C, D).

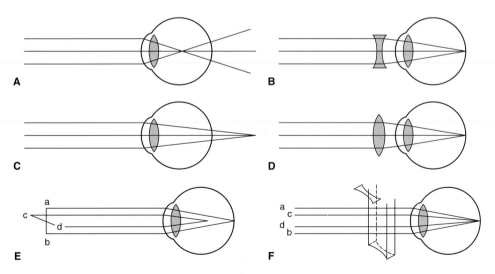

Figure 5.10 **(A, B)** A concave (minus) lens is used to correct myopia, in which parallel rays are focused anterior to the macula. **(C, D)** A convex (plus) lens is used to correct hyperopia, in which parallel rays are focused posterior to the macula. **(E, F)** A cylindrical (or spherocylindrical) lens is used to correct astigmatism, in which parallel rays are not focused uniformly in all meridians.

The cornea (and sometimes the eye's crystalline lens) might not have the same radius of curvature in all meridians. Aberration of the corneal or lenticular surfaces that produces differing radii of curvature is called *astigmatism*. A cylindrical lens is used to neutralize astigmatism (Figure 5.10 E, F). In most patients, the axis of plus cylinder needed to correct the astigmatism is either close to 90° (with-the-rule astigmatism) or close to 180° (against-the-rule astigmatism). In clinical practice, many myopic patients and hyperopic patients also have astigmatism. A sphero-cylindrical lens is used to correct myopic and hyperopic astigmatism.

Accommodation is the mechanism by which the eye changes refractive power by altering the shape of its crystalline lens. The point of focus moves forward in the eye during accommodation and allows one to focus on objects at near. *Presbyopia* is a progressive loss of accommodative ability of the crystalline lens caused by the natural process of aging. It generally manifests itself as difficulty with near visual work, such as reading. Presbyopia occurs in the presence of myopia, hyperopia, and astigmatism. It can be remedied optically with plus lenses.

■ Lens Notation

A written spectacle lens prescription follows a standard format. The power of the sphere (abbreviated sph) is recorded first, along with its sign (+ or –). This is followed by the power of the cylinder, if a cylinder is required, with its sign and axis. Sometimes the cylinder designation is preceded by the symbol ⌒, which means "combined with." The axis of the cylinder is designated by ×, followed by the degree of the orientation of the cylinder axis. The degree symbol is commonly omitted and only the numbers written. A prescription is recorded for each eye, using the abbreviations OD (*oculus dexter*) for the right eye and OS (*oculus sinister*) for the left eye. Table 5.1 displays examples of typical spectacle prescriptions. In writing spectacle prescriptions, many practitioners omit the "combined with" sign.

Lens Transposition

In a written spectacle lens prescription, cylinder power can be recorded in either plus form or minus form. Many ophthalmologists customarily record cylinder with

Table 5.1   Typical Spectacle Prescription Notations

Hyperopia	OD	+2.00 sph
	OS	+2.25 sph
Myopia	OD	−2.50 sph
	OS	−3.00 sph
Hyperopic astigmatism	OD +1.00 ⌒ +1.00 × 90 *or* +2.00 ⌒ −1.00 × 180	
	OS plano ⌒ +1.50 × 180 *or* +1.50 ⌒ −1.50 × 90	
Myopic astigmatism	OD −0.75 ⌒ +0.50 × 150 *or* −0.25: ⌒ −0.50 × 60	
	OS −1.00 ⌒ +0.50 × 120 *or* −0.50: ⌒ −0.50 × 30	

In writing spectacle prescriptions, some practitioners omit the "combined with" ⌒ sign. The myopic astigmatism example then might be recorded as follows:

OD −0.75 +0.50 × 150 *or* −0.25 −0.50 × 60
OS −1.00 + 0.50 × 120 *or* −0.50 −0.50 × 30

plus notation, except for contact lenses, whereas opticians and optometrists generally use minus notation. A plus cylinder is ground onto the anterior surface of a lens, and the minus cylinder is ground onto the posterior surface of the lens. Unless specifically stated by the practitioner, the lenses will be filled as minus cylinders. This generally allows for a more cosmetically acceptable lens, because plus cylinders produce more magnification than the equivalent minus-cylinder form. A conversion of a prescription from 1 form to the other is called *lens transposition* and is achieved in 3 steps:

1. Add algebraically the cylinder power to the sphere power.
2. Reverse the sign of the cylinder.
3. Add 90° to the cylinder axis. If the resulting number exceeds 180°, then subtract 180.

Examples of lens transposition:

−1.00 ⌒ +1.50 × 95	*is equivalent to*	+0.50 ⌒ −1.50 × 05
+3.00 ⌒ +2.00 × 20	*is equivalent to*	+5.00 ⌒ −2.00 × 110
−2.00 ⌒ +1.00 × 160	*is equivalent to*	−1.00 ⌒ −1.00 × 70

Spherical Equivalent

The average power of a spherocylindrical lens is called the *spherical equivalent*. It represents the dioptric position of the circle of least confusion of the conoid of Sturm. Spherical equivalent is useful when comparing or trying to balance the 2 eyes, or when trying to reduce an excessive cylindrical correction. The spherical equivalent is frequently used in the prescription of contact lenses. It is calculated as follows:

Spherical equivalent = power of the sphere + (cylinder power/2)

■ Lensmeter

The *lensmeter* is an instrument used to measure the power of a patient's present spectacle lenses. Both manual and automated lensmeters are available (Figure 5.11). The lensmeter measures 4 principal properties of spectacle lenses:

- Spherical and cylindrical *power*
- Cylindrical *axis* if cylinder is present
- Presence and orientation of *prism*
- Optical *centration*

Clinical Protocol 5.1 describes the steps in using a standard manual lensmeter for single-vision spectacles. Clinical Protocol 5.2 describes measurement of multifocal spectacles. Clinical Protocol 5.3 lists steps in measuring prism power and orientation, and Clinical Protocol 5.4 describes how to determine optical centration of lenses.

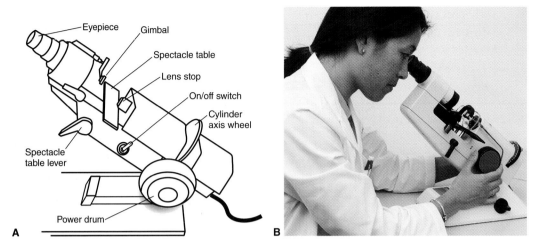

Figure 5.11 **(A)** Parts of the manual lensmeter. **(B)** Lensmeter in use.

■ Retinoscopy and Refinement

The goal of retinoscopy (objective refraction) is to determine the nature of the patient's refractive error (if any) and the approximate lens power that will diminish (neutralize) that error and approach clear vision. In the process of refinement (subjective refraction), the examiner further and exactly determines the patient's final refractive correction by presenting various lenses to the patient until the patient responds that a best—and balanced (if the patient has binocular vision)—Snellen visual acuity has been reached.

Retinoscopy and refinement, perhaps more than most other ophthalmologic examination techniques, require artistry and experience to perform successfully. They demand fine motor skills, ambidextrousness, clinical observation skills, knowledge of optical principles and subjective judgment. Retinoscopy and refinement are best learned through hands-on, guided training with an experienced practitioner. This text can only present an overview of the instrumentation and steps in these processes. A list of recommended books and videotapes that treat these topics in greater detail appears at the end of this chapter.

Instrumentation

The examiner must become familiar with and skilled in the use of the variety of specialized instruments that are used in retinoscopy and refinement, namely, the retinoscope, trial lenses and frames, refractor, Jackson cross cylinder, and distometer. Other instruments occasionally used in refraction include a single or multiple pinhole occluder and a lensmeter. Automated refractors are available that combine many of the individual refraction instruments or duplicate their functions automatically.

Retinoscope

The handheld streak retinoscope comprises a viewer (peephole), a mirror assembly, and a light bulb with a delicate filament that can be rotated and focused by

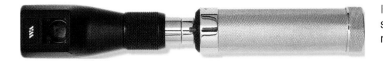

Figure 5.12 A standard streak retinoscope.

manipulating a sleeve on the instrument's handle (Figure 5.12). It produces a streak of light, as differentiated from the round dot of light produced by a spot retino-scope, which is used less frequently. The vergence of the slit (that is, the focus of the beam) on the streak retinoscope is adjusted by moving the sleeve up or down on the instrument's handle. To perform retinoscopy, the examiner looks through the retinoscope peephole viewer and aligns the retinoscope streak with the patient's visual axis. By shifting the position of the instrument, manipulating its light characteristics in specific ways, and observing the reaction of a light reflex from the patient's eye, the examiner can determine the patient's refractive state and estimate the corrective needs.

Trial lenses and frames

During retinoscopy (and subsequent refinement), the examiner has the patient look through a variety of lenses until an appropriate optical correction is determined. One way to do this is with the use of trial frames—eyeglasses that can hold a variety of lenses from a trial set of spheres, cylinders, and prisms (Figure 5.13). Trial frames have adjustable eyepieces, temple pieces, and nose pieces, and the examiner should become proficient in adjusting these elements to align the frame properly on the patient's face.

Halberg clips, which can be affixed onto the patient's own eyeglasses, also hold trial lenses and can be used to allow for modification of the patient's glasses with them in place, a procedure referred to as *overrefraction*. This term is also used to refer to the refraction, with a trial frame or refractor, of a patient who is wearing contact lenses.

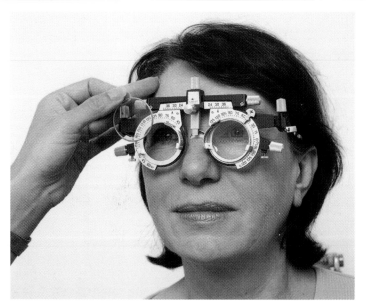

Figure 5.13 A trial frame can be adjusted to conform to the patient's anatomy and allows manual insertion of multiple lenses selected from a trial set.

Phoroptor

The Phoroptor, or refractor, provides an alternative to a trial frame and loose lenses. It consists of a face plate that can be suspended before the patient's eyes. The plate contains a wide range of spherical and cylindrical lenses that the examiner can dial into position (Figure 5.14). Most refractors have a variable setting for the interpupillary distance and have a tilt feature to allow the eyes to converge for determining near vision correction. Other accessories vary widely among makes and models. Table 5.2 lists the major Phoroptor controls and their uses.

Jackson cross cylinder

This instrument is a special lens used as part of the refinement process to confirm first the axis and then the power of a correcting cylindrical lens for astigmatism (Figure 5.15). The handheld device consists of a handle attached to a lens containing 2 cylinders of equal power, 1 minus and 1 plus, set at right angles to each other. A cross cylinder usually is built into the refractor.

Distometer

A distometer is a small handheld device used for determining vertex distance (that is, the distance between the patient's eye and the back of the corrective lens). A distometer is illustrated in Figure 5.16. A vertex distance of 13.5 mm is considered average but can vary among patients. It is important to keep the vertex distance for the patient's eyeglasses constant during refractometry. If the vertex distances

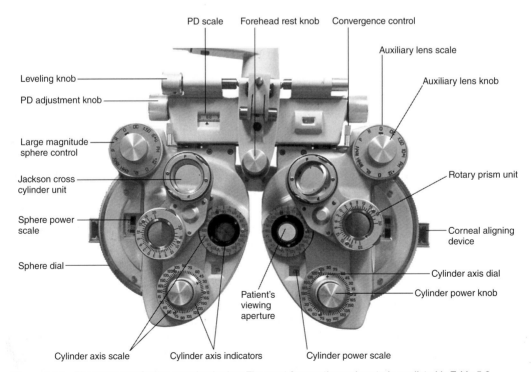

Figure 5.14   Phoroptor, or refractor, examiner's view. The most frequently used controls are listed in Table 5.2.

Table 5.2 Frequently Used Refractor Controls

Control	Purpose
PD adjustment	Adjusts viewing apertures to fit patient's interpupillary distance
Leveling knob	Tilts front face plate if eyes are not at same level
Forehead rest knob	Maintains constant distance from back surface of refractor lenses
Convergence levers	Adjusts angle of viewing apertures to about 150° for near vision measurements (not present on all models)
Sphere dial	Adjusts sphere in 0.25 D increments
Sphere power scale	Displays power of sphere
Cylinder dial	Adjusts power of cylinder in 0.25 D increments
Cylinder power scale	Displays power of cylinder
Cylinder axis dial	Adjusts axis of cylinder
Cylinder axis scale	Displays axis of cylinder
Large magnitude sphere control	Adjusts sphere in 3.00 D increments
Auxiliary lens knob and scale	**O** = Open (to test the eye) **OC** = Occlude (to occlude the eye) **R** = Refracting lens (usually +1.50 D sph)

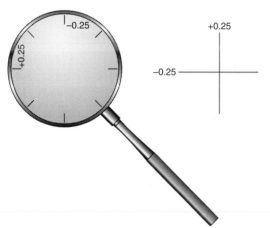

Figure 5.15 The Jackson cross cylinder with axes marked on the lens, and the corresponding power cross representation. The handle of the cross cylinder is attached 45° to the principal meridians, allowing quick twirling from 1 orientation of the cross cylinder to the exact opposite orientation.

used for the 2 eyes differ, the effective power of the patient's corrective lenses will be different and, probably, unacceptable. When the prescription is filled, unless the optician has been informed of a specific measurement, a distance of 13.5 mm is assumed for each eye. Vertex distance is especially critical in patients with high refractive errors (more than 5.00 D of plus or minus sphere). Clinical Protocol 5.5 details the method of using the distometer to measure vertex distance.

Retinoscopy Technique

For retinoscopy, the room lights are dimmed. The relative positions of the patient and the examiner are very important. With the patient in the examining chair and instructed to gaze past the examiner's ear at a fixation light located at effective optical infinity (20 feet or more), the examiner sits facing, eyes on the same level as the

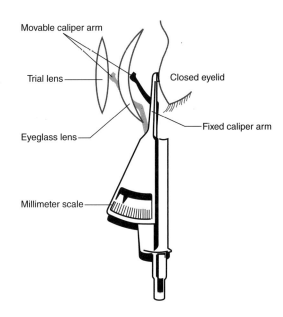

Figure 5.16 A distometer is used to measure vertex distance accurately. The separation distance between the patient's eye and the back surface of the refracting lens is the vertex distance. The distometer scale takes into account the thickness of the average eyelid.

Movable caliper arm

Trial lens

Closed eyelid

Fixed caliper arm

Eyeglass lens

Millimeter scale

patient, at a standard distance, usually about arm's length. In most cases, situate yourself as follows:

- *To examine the right eye:* Seat yourself slightly to the patient's right; hold the retinoscope in your right hand and look through it with your right eye. Use your left hand to manipulate the phoropter or trial lenses.
- *To examine the left eye:* Seat yourself slightly to the patient's left, in front of the patient's left shoulder; hold the retinoscope in your left hand and look through it with your left eye. Use your right hand to manipulate the phoropter or trial lenses.

It is critical to know that the eye being examined is the fixating eye, especially if the patient has strabismus. When the patient is unable to control alignment, as in the case of manifest exotropia, the retinoscopic reflex will not be in the visual axis but rather in the axis of the deviation. The measurement of the eye's refractive error made in this axis will not be accurate. If the eye is not aligned with the retinoscopic reflex, the examiner may sit more directly in front of the patient and can occlude the eye not being examined, either with a hand or an occluding device. If cycloplegia has been used, the patient is instructed to look directly into the light.

Working distance

The distance between the examiner and the patient's eye must be measured and converted into diopters. For the examination, the patient may be given a "working lens," the power of which equals the dioptric distance between examiner and patient. The power of this lens is then subtracted from the final dioptric amount that is measured. If a working lens is not used, simply subtract the dioptric equivalent of the working distance from the neutralization point reached in retinoscopy.

For convenience in changing lenses in the refractor or trial frame, most examiners use a working distance of arm's length, usually about 66 cm (approximately

2/3 m or 26 inches), and assign the patient a corresponding working lens of +1.50 D. A working distance of 1/2 m would require a +2.00 D working lens, and a working distance of 1 m would require a working lens of +1.00 D. The working distance must remain constant throughout the examination, although the examiner does move forward and backward slightly from this position to evaluate the movement of the patient's light reflex.

Neutralization With a Retinoscope

The term *neutralization* refers to the achievement of the point at which a lens placed before the patient's eye effectively "neutralizes" the retinoscopic reflex and the patient's pupil fills with reflected light. Because of its subtleties and complexities, retinoscopy is best learned by hands-on instruction. Nevertheless, the basic steps in retinoscopic neutralization are outlined next.

1. Set the retinoscope so that the light rays emanating are parallel. This can be ensured if the streak cannot be focused on a surface of any sort, such as the wall or the palm of your hand.
2. Adjust the patient and yourself for comfort and appropriate testing positions and distance (as discussed earlier in this section). Position the trial frame or refractor as necessary.
3. Direct the patient to look at a specific distance target, such as an optotype on a vision test chart. If cycloplegia has been used, you may direct the patient to look into your light.
4. Look through the examiner's eyepiece of the retinoscope and direct the light into the patient's pupil. Remember to seat yourself in front of the patient (as summarized earlier in this section). If the reflection from the patient's pupil is not easy to see, consider the following possible reasons:
   a. The retinoscope bulb is dim, dirty, or turned off.
   b. The patient has a very high refractive error.
   c. The room lights are not sufficiently dimmed.
   d. The patient has a cataract or other media opacity.

   If you see several reflections, the "extra" ones may be coming from other surfaces, such as the cornea or the trial lens that you are using. Try moving slightly to either side, tilting the trial lens slightly, ascertaining that the trial lens surface is clean, or checking that you are not seeing reflections of lights in the examining room.
5. Orient the streak of the retinoscope horizontally and then move it up and down. Alternatively, you may start by orienting the streak vertically and then moving it right and left. Whichever direction you first orient the streak, your hand movement, and that of the retinoscope, is always perpendicular to that direction.
6. Note if the motion of the reflex is the same as ("with") or opposite ("against") the direction of your sweeping movement. If the light reflex moves in the direction opposite your movement, add minus lenses in front of the eye in

half-diopter increments until you no longer see "against" movement. If the movement of the light reflex is in the same direction that you are sweeping the retinoscope light, the exiting rays are too divergent, so plus lenses must be added. Increments of 0.50 D are added until it becomes difficult to tell if the movement of the reflex is "with" or "against," at which time increments of 0.25 D are more helpful. Figure 5.17 illustrates the reflexes produced by the streak of the retinoscope.

7. Smaller sweeps are useful as the reflex band appears to widen. When the movement of the reflex fills the pupil and cannot be ascertained, the reflected light rays coming from the eye are parallel, and the lens combination that you have used to reach this point (with the dioptric equivalent of your working distance) is the objective measurement of the refractive error of the eye. This is referred to as *neutrality*.

8. To confirm that you have achieved neutrality, you can move your eye/ retinoscope several inches closer to the patient. At this point, "with" movement of the reflex band should occur as you continue to sweep. Return to your original working distance, while continuing the sweeping motion, and note that the reflex again fills the pupil and has no apparent motion. Additional confirmation of neutrality can be made by moving several inches farther away from the eye, repeating the sweeping movements, and noting that the reflex is now "against" your direction of movement.

9. Note the power of the lens or lenses that you have used to reach neutrality. Subtract the dioptric equivalent of your working distance. This gives you the refractive error in the axis that you were sweeping. For example, if you were sitting 66 cm in front of a patient and needed a –1.00 D lens

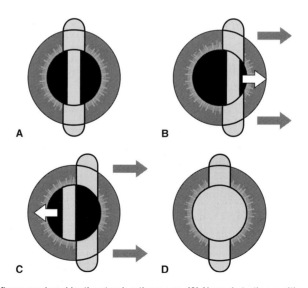

Figure 5.17 Reflexes produced by the streak retinoscope. (A) Normal starting position, before be-ginning sweeping movements. (B) "With" motion: The reflex moves in the same direction as the streak of light, indicating the need for a stronger converging (plus) lens. The eye is relatively more hyperopic than the lenses are correcting. (C) "Against" motion: The reflex moves in the direction opposite that of the streak, indicating the need for a stronger diverging (minus) lens. The eye is relatively more myopic than the lenses are correcting. (D) Neutralization point: There is no apparent movement of the reflex, and the pupil is filled with a red glow.

to obtain a neutral reflex with your streak in either the horizontal or the vertical direction, the patient's refractive error is –2.50 sphere. If you obtained different reflexes from the horizontal and the vertical orientation of the streak, an astigmatic refractive error is present, which will need to be neutralized with cylinders in the final eyeglass prescription.

Determining Cylinder

The following steps are taken to determine the presence of astigmatism:

1. Position yourself and the patient and illuminate the patient's pupil with the retinoscope as outlined in steps 1 to 4 above. Orient the streak horizontally and sweep it up and down. Change the orientation to vertical, and sweep it right and left.
2. Compare the intensity and the direction of the reflex. If both are comparable in intensity and direction, an insignificant astigmatism is present.
3. If the streak is brighter in 1 direction than it is in the other, or if the reflexes move in opposite directions, a cylindrical, or astigmatic, refractive error is present.
   a. Neutralize the reflex with your retinoscope streak oriented in the horizontal or vertical position as described in steps 1 to 8 of "Neutralization With a Retinoscope." If you are using minus cylinders, first neutralize the reflex that is moving more slowly, or more "with" your streak. Then neutralize the reflex that is perpendicular to it.
   b. If you are using plus cylinders, first neutralize the reflex that is more "against" your streak and then neutralize the one perpendicular to it.
4. Rotate the sleeve of the retinoscope so that the streak is oriented perpendicular to the direction of the initial orientation. In other words, if you first achieved neutrality with the streak oriented horizontally, now orient it vertically.
   a. If you are using only spheres for retinoscopy, neutralize the reflex in 1 orientation and note the power of the sphere used in that axis. Change the orientation of the streak by 90°, repeat the neutralization procedure as outlined above, note the power of the sphere used in this orientation, and then add the 2 sphere powers as outlined below.
5. If you cannot achieve neutrality with the streak oriented horizontally and vertically, an oblique astigmatism might be present. The 2 axes can be determined by rotating the sleeve of the retinoscope to change the orientation of the streak. They will be perpendicular to each other. Methods of neutralization for oblique astigmatism, which take more time and practice to acquire than the usual techniques, are detailed in textbooks and video presentations on retinoscopy and not here.
6. Note the power of the lens combination(s) that you used at each axis. If you are writing the eyeglass prescription in plus-cylinder form, write the power and the axis of the least-plus lens that you used to neutralize the reflex. For example, if you were sitting 66 cm in front of a patient and needed a –1.00 D lens to obtain a neutral reflex with your streak in the horizontal direction (ie, as you moved it up and down), the patient's refractive error at

180° is –2.50 D. If you needed a –0.50 D lens instead of the –1.00 D lens to neutralize the reflex when your streak was oriented vertically, the patient's refractive error at 90° is –2.00 D. You have a –1.00 D sphere together with a 0.50 D cylinder with the axis line oriented vertically. The resultant prescription is written –2.50 ⌒ +0.50 × 90.

As inferred from the preceding sentences, another method for determining the power of the astigmatism is first to determine the power of the sphere in 1 orientation. If you are using plus cylinders, you should achieve neutrality in 1 direction and still note "with" movement when the streak of the retinoscope is rotated 90°. If you are working with minus cylinders, "against" movement will be noted after you have neutralized all the "with" movement and then rotated the streak 90°. The axis of the cylinder should be placed so that it is aligned with the direction that you are moving the retinoscope reflex. The direction of the sweeping movement is the *meridian*, and it is at right angles to the axis of the cylinder.

Summary of Retinoscopy Steps

1. Establish alignment in front of the patient's pupil.
2. Shine the retinoscope light into the patient's eye while maintaining a constant distance between yourself and the patient.
3. Rotate the streak to determine the meridian that you wish to neutralize first. This will depend on whether you are using plus cylinders, minus cylinders, or spheres only. As you move the streak up and down, you are neutralizing the vertical meridian *with the axis at or close to 180°*. As you move the streak to the right and the left, you are neutralizing the horizontal meridian, for which the axis is 90°.
4. Neutralize the reflex at the chosen axis.
5. Orient the streak 90° to the original orientation and neutralize the reflex at that axis.
6. Note the power of the lenses needed to achieve neutrality at both orientations.
7. Calculate the power of the resultant eyeglass prescription.

Residents should review videotapes about retinoscopy, read more detailed textbooks, and gain hands-on training in order to master the finer details of neutralization, estimating cylinder axis and power, and interpretation of aberrations.

Refinement

Refinement, or subjective (acceptance) refraction, can be performed either with or without the use of cycloplegic drops. Refinement performed without the use of cycloplegic drops is often referred to as the "manifest" refraction or "dry" refraction. A cycloplegic (or "wet") refraction may be performed in addition to (or instead of) a manifest refraction. Because cycloplegia suspends accommodation, the examiner can make an accurate measurement of the nonaccommodative refractive state of the eye during the time that the cycloplegic drops have full effect. Some of the indications for performing a cycloplegic refraction are discussed later in this chapter in the sections on "Cycloplegic Refraction" and "Guidelines for Prescribing Glasses."

Several methods are used for performing subjective refraction. Some of them, such as the Lancaster astigmatic clock and the stenopeic slit, are rarely used. One of the more common methods involves the use of the refractor and the Jackson cross cylinder to adjust and refine the sphere and refine cylinder axis and power. The refinement instructions that follow apply to the use of a refractor, but refinement can be performed with the trial frame and trial lenses as well. As with retinoscopy, this text can only provide a basic outline of the procedure; residents should consult more detailed textbooks and videotapes and gain sufficient hands-on training with an experienced practitioner.

Adjust sphere

1. Place 1 of the following lens prescriptions in the refractor:
   a. Retinoscopic findings
   b. Previous eyeglass prescription
   c. Previous manifest refraction (useful for patients who have undergone cataract surgery or penetrating keratoplasty, especially if multiple refractions have been done but glasses have not been prescribed)
2. Occlude the eye not being tested by dialing in *OC* (occluding lens) on the auxiliary dial of the refractor. Adjust the auxiliary lens knob to position *O* (open) for the eye being tested.
3. Measure visual acuity for the eye to be tested, using the standard Snellen chart and technique. Use test figures 1 or 2 lines larger than the patient's best visual acuity for testing, because introduction of the cross cylinder produces blur, and the patient will be more aware of changes at this already slightly blurred level of acuity.
4. Adjust the sphere dial on the refractor to the most plus or the least minus that gives the patient the best visual acuity. Ask the patient, "Which lens makes the letters clearer, number 1 or number 2, or are they the same?" and dial 2 "clicks," or +0.50 D sphere. The patient is presented with 2 choices and will select either the original lens (choice number 1) or an addition of +0.50 D sphere (choice number 2).
   a. If the patient prefers choice number 2, repeat the process, adding another 2 clicks of plus (+0.50 D) and ask the patient, "Which is better, 3 or 4, or are they the same?" Continue adding increments of +0.50 D sphere until the patient notes that the 2 choices are equivalent.
   b. If the patient prefers choice number 1, subtract 2 clicks of sphere (that is, subtract −0.50 D sphere) and ask, "Which is clearer, number 3 or number 4, or are they the same?" Continue subtracting in increments of −0.50 D sphere until the patient notes that the 2 choices are equivalent. You might need to advise many myopic patients to choose the lens that lets them actually see the letters more clearly, not the one that just makes the letters smaller and darker. If the patient describes the change in the letters as just smaller and darker, too much minus power has been added.
   c. Avoid confusion with previous choices by giving the patient different numbers for subsequent choices, such as, "Which is better, 1 or 2, 3 or

4," and so on. If the patient persists in always choosing either the first or the second lens presented, reverse the order of presentation to check for consistency. Present the 2 choices quickly; give the patient adequate time to view the testing letters, then briskly present the second lens choice.

    d. If cycloplegia is not in effect and the patient tends to accommodate (as is the case with young patients or hyperopic patients), it can be helpful to start with more plus power than is needed and then slowly to decrease plus power until the best sphere is found. This technique, called *fogging*, encourages the patient to relax accommodation.

Refine cylinder axis

1. Position the Jackson cross cylinder in front of the eye to be tested, with the axis 45° to the principal meridians of the cylinder axis (this is referred to as *straddling the axis*). In the example in Figure 5.18A, the 90° axis is straddled.
2. Flip the cross cylinder (turn it over and then back) and ask the patient, "Which is better, number 1 or number 2, or are they the same?"
3. Rotate the cross cylinder 5° to 10° toward the plus axis (white dot) of the preferred choice.
4. Continue the process until the patient reports that the 2 choices look the same and are equally blurred.

Refine cylinder power

1. Align the cylinder axis with the Jackson cross cylinder axis. This is sometimes referred to as on axis. In Figure 5.18 B and C, the cross cylinder axis is aligned "on axis" with the 90° axis of the refracting lens.
2. Flip the cross cylinder and ask the patient, "Which is better, choice 1 or choice 2, or are they the same?"
3. If the patient prefers the plus cylinder (white-dot axis), add 1 click of cylinder power (+0.25 D). If the patient prefers the minus cylinder (red-dot axis), subtract *1* click of cylinder power (–0.25 D).
4. For each *2* clicks (+0.50 D) of cylinder power added, subtract 1 click (–0.25 D) of sphere power, using the sphere dial on the refractor to maintain the same

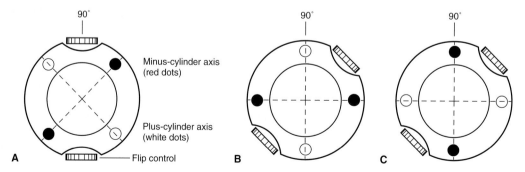

Figure 5.18 **(A)** The refractor's Jackson cross cylinder "straddling" the 90° axis. An imaginary line is drawn on the cross cylinder to indicate the position of the minus-cylinder and plus-cylinder axes. **(B)** The cross cylinder "on axis" with the 90° axis, showing the white dots of the plus-cylinder axis aligned with the 90° axis and **(C)** the red dots of the minus-cylinder axis aligned with the 90° axis.

spherical equivalent. Adding cylinder requires modifying the sphere so as to avoid final inaccuracy.

5. The end point has been reached when the patient notes that the choices presented appear equal. When the patient is asked whether choice 1 or 2 is better or whether they are the same, the patient may say that it is impossible to choose. Encourage a preference until the patient states that the 2 choices are equal. Patients sometimes think that they have performed poorly because they often could not decide which lenses were preferable. Explain that you were specifically looking for the point at which they could see no difference and that, therefore, they actually had done very well.

If the patient does not have a cylinder in the current spectacles or in the retinoscopic findings, it is a good idea to check for the presence of astigmatism during the refinement to see if visual acuity can be improved by adding cylinder. The Jackson cross cylinder is placed arbitrarily at 90° and 180°, the cylinder is flipped, and the patient is asked to make a choice. If a preferred flipped position is found, cylinder is added with the axis parallel to the respective plus or minus axis of the cross cylinder until the 2 flip choices are equal. If no preference is found with cross cylinder axes at 90° and 180°, check again with axes at 45° and 135° before assuming that no astigmatism is present. If cylinder power is found, refinement of both power and axis is performed in the usual manner. The axis of astigmatism is defined first, followed by power. After the power of the cylinder has been determined, the axis should be rechecked and readjusted if necessary.

Refine sphere

After refining the axis and power of the cylinder, a further refinement of sphere is performed.

1. Ask the patient, "Which lens makes the letters clearer, number 1 or number 2, or are they the same?" and dial 1 to 2 clicks, or +0.25 to +0.50 D sphere, on the sphere dial of the refractor. The patient is presented with 2 choices and will select either the original lens (choice 1) or an additional spherical power (choice 2).
2. If the patient prefers choice number 2, repeat the process, adding another 1 to 2 clicks of plus (+0.25 to +0.50 D), and ask the patient, "Which is better, 2 or 1, or are they the same?" Continue adding increments of +0.25 to +0.50 D sphere until the patient notes that the 2 choices are equivalent.
3. If the patient prefers choice number 1, subtract 1 to 2 clicks of sphere (that is, subtract –0.25 to –0.50 D sphere) and ask, "Which is clearer, 1 or 2, or are they the same?" Continue subtracting in increments of –0.25 to –0.50 D sphere until the patient notes that the 2 choices are equivalent.

Summary of refinement

1. Adjust sphere.
2. Refine cylinder axis.
3. Refine cylinder power.
4. Refine sphere.

Cycloplegic Refraction

Cycloplegia can be useful as an adjunct to refraction for almost any patient, but it is especially helpful for a patient who has active accommodation. A cycloplegic refraction should be done at least once for every patient, preferably during an initial evaluation. Cycloplegia achieved at the time of dilation for retinal examination can be used to verify noncycloplegic refraction measurements in adults, and it is the ideal time to do retinoscopy for children.

Cycloplegic refraction is indicated:

- In any patient under 15 years old before prescribing glasses (manifest refraction should rarely be relied upon under 10 years old and usually does not need to be done)
- In hyperopic patients up to 35 years old, especially if symptomatic
- In pre- and early presbyopia, especially when glasses have never previously been worn
- Whenever refraction yields variable results, especially under 50 years old
- Whenever the patient's symptoms are disproportionate to the manifest refractive error, or if symptoms suggest an accommodative problem
- For patients who tend to accommodate during refraction
- For obvious or suspected extraocular muscle imbalance
- Whenever the refractionist is forced to rely on retinoscopy to provide all of the refractive information
- In bilateral refractive asymmetry, or whenever a good binocular balance cannot be achieved

As with the use of any medication, the patient should be asked about allergies before cycloplegic drugs are given. Ascertaining the use of other medications and the existence of other medical conditions is also important because the side effects of cycloplegic drugs, especially cyclopentolate (Cyclogyl), can include exacerbation of seizures, cardiac arrhythmias, and precipitation of angle-closure glaucoma. Table 5.3 outlines the systemic effects of common cycloplegic drugs. Cycloplegics in common use include tropicamide (Mydriacyl), cyclopentolate (Cyclogyl), atropine (either as drops or as ointment), and a combination drop marketed as Cyclomydril.

Duochrome Test

The duochrome test (Figure 5.19) is a quick method of determining if the patient has too much minus or too much plus in the spectacle correction. The test uses a projected red bar and green bar of light, which are superimposed over the visual acuity test targets. The patient is asked, "Which are sharper (or darker), the letters on the green side or the letters on the red side, or are they the same?" If the patient answers that the letters on the green side are blacker, too much minus power has probably been added, so add plus sphere. If the answer is that the red side is blacker or sharper, then the overall power is probably too plus, and minus sphere should be added.

Table 5.3 Systemic Effects of Cycloplegic Drugs

Drug Name	Symptoms and Signs
Atropine	Dryness of mouth and skin Fever Delirium Urinary retention Tachycardia Flushed face Respiratory depression **Note**: If ingested, induce emesis and treat as emergency.
Cyclopentolate	CNS disturbance (particularly hypersensitivity) reported in infants, young children, and children with spastic paralysis or brain damage Psychotic reaction (particularly with 2%), ataxia, incoherent speech, restlessness, seizures, hallucinations, hyperactivity Disorientation; failure to recognize familiar people Feeding intolerance (vomiting is more frequent for several hours after administration in neonates) Abdominal distention in infants from paralytic ileus Other similar to atropine
Tropicamide	Similar to cyclopentolate but less frequent and less severe
Phenylephrine	Do not use within 21 days of MAO inhibitor use because phenylephrine can potentiate response of tricyclic antidepressants Tachycardia Rebound miosis Hypertension, systemic vasopressor response (especially 10% solution)

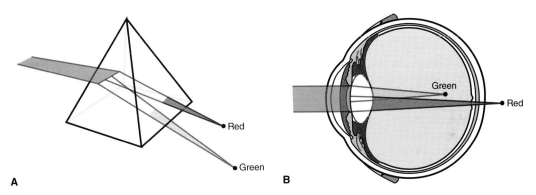

Figure 5.19 Duochrome test. **(A)** Green light is refracted more than red light as both enter optically dense media. **(B)** The endpoint of the duochrome test is achieved when the letters on the red background and the letters on the green background are imaged equidistant from the macula. (Illustration by Mark M. Miller.)

This test is based on the principle that shorter wavelengths of light are refracted more than longer wavelengths as both enter more optically dense media, as would be the case for light traveling through the cornea to retina. Therefore, relative to the macula, the letters seen in the green light are refracted more and, hence, are more anterior than the letters on the red side. If one sees the black letters on the green background as being darker, these letters are focused closer to the macula than are the letters on the red background, which in this case are actually imaged posterior to the macula. In this situation, plus lenses are needed to better focus the image on the macula. The end point of the duochrome test is achieved when the red and the green letters are equidistant from the macula.

Because this test is based on chromatic aberration and not color discrimination, it can be used even with colorblind patients. A drawback of the duochrome test is that accommodation can reduce the reliability of the results. The duochrome test is most reliable when conducted after the patient has been given cycloplegic eyedrops.

Binocular Balancing

The final steps in subjective refraction, known as binocular balancing, ensure that accommodation has been relaxed equally in the 2 eyes. Fogging, prism dissociation, and cycloplegia are but 3 of many methods commonly used; most balancing methods require that correctable vision be essentially equal in the 2 eyes.

Fogging

By fogging (blurring) the end point refraction using +2.00 D spheres for each eye, the visual acuity should be reduced to approximately 20/100. Placing a –0.25 D sphere first before 1 eye then the other and rapidly alternating occlusion of the eyes will enable the patient to identify clearly the eye with the –0.25 D sphere as having the clearer image. If the eyes are not in balance, sphere should be added or subtracted in steps of 0.25 D until balance is achieved.

Prism dissociation

The most sensitive method of binocular balance is achieved by fogging the refractive end point using +1.00 D spheres and then placing vertical prism of 4^{Δ} or 5^{Δ} before 1 eye. A single line, usually 20/40, is projected on the chart. The patient is then able to view a single line with both eyes simultaneously but with the 2 images vertically displaced, 1 above the other. The 2 images should be comparable in size and clarity. Differences between the fogged images in the 2 eyes of 0.25 D sphere or even less can be identified readily by the patient. A +0.25 D sphere is placed before 1 eye and then before the other. In each instance, if the eyes are balanced, the patient will report that the image corresponding to the eye having the additional +0.25 D sphere will be more blurred. Once a balance between the 2 eyes has been established, the prism is removed. The fogging lenses are then gradually reduced simultaneously from the 2 eyes, in 0.25 D increments. The desired end point is reached when the patient achieves maximum vision with the *lowest* minus or the *highest* plus spheres.

Cycloplegia

Binocular balance is achieved simply by the monocular findings when full cycloplegia has been used. It is important to ascertain that cycloplegia is complete in both eyes if this method is to be used. Residual accommodation can be determined by asking the patient to look at a distance target while you neutralize the reflex (the standard way of performing retinoscopy), and then asking the patient to look directly at the retinoscope light while you note if the reflex is moving more "with" your sweep. If additional "with" movement is noted, accommodation has not been fully reduced.

Near Point and Reading Add

As fine print is moved closer and closer to the patient, the print becomes blurred at a certain point. This point is called the *near point of accommodation* (NPA). Because of presbyopia, patients over the age of 40 or 45 typically require a plus-lens "reading add" in addition to their distance spectacle prescription to see near objects well. The binocular near point is usually closer than the monocular near point and can be estimated in a simple, practical way by asking the patient to fixate on small print and to state when the print blurs as it is moved closer to the eye.

To measure the NPA, place the patient's distance prescription in the refractor. Most refractors have a convergence control lever on the front that allows you to adjust the front tilt so that the eyes are converging (see Figure 5.14). Either adjust this lever to converge the eyes, or decrease the interpupillary distance by at least 5 mm to account for the convergence that naturally accompanies any accommodation. Hold the near vision test card about 50 cm in front of the patient's eye, ask the patient to fixate on the small print (5-point type), and move the test card toward the eye until the patient states that the print is blurred. This position, measured in meters, is the NPA and can be converted into diopters using the formula D = 1/f. For example, a patient who reports blur at 25 cm (0.25 m) has an NPA of 1/0.25, or 4 diopters.

Most refractors are equipped with an accommodation rule, such as the Prince rule. This combination of a near vision card with a ruler calibrated in centimeters and diopters provides a convenient method of measuring the NPA. The ruler can be attached to the front of the refractor or used separately.

To select the appropriate reading add, follow these steps:

1. Determine the accommodation requirements for the near vision task. For example, reading at 40 cm would require 2.50 diopters of accommodation (1/0.4 m = +2.50 D).
2. Measure the accommodative amplitude independently for each eye. A simple way to do this is to have the patient fixate on a reading target (eg, a 20/25 line of print held at 40 cm) with each eye. Stimulate accommodation by placing successively stronger minus spheres until the print blurs. Then relax accommodation by using successively stronger plus lenses. The print will clear, but as successively stronger plus lenses are added, the onset of blurring will again be noted. The sum of the 2 lenses used to reach the blur points is a measure of accommodative amplitude. For example, if the patient accepted –3.00 D to blur (stimulate accommodation) and +2.50 D to blur (relax accommodation), the amplitude would be 5.50 D.
3. From the measured accommodative amplitude, allow one-half to be held in reserve and consider one-half to be the available accommodation. Other techniques for more precise measurement of accommodative amplitudes and for measurements of binocular amplitude of accommodation are beyond the scope of this text, but in general a consideration of both the NPA and the patient's age will give a good prediction of the add that will be needed. Average accommodative amplitudes for different ages are summarized in Table 5.4.
4. Subtract the patient's available accommodation (step 3) from the total amount of accommodation required for the task at hand (step 1) for the tentative power of the add that will be needed.

Table 5.4 Average Accommodative Amplitudes for Different Ages

Age	Average Accommodative Amplitude[a]
8	1.40 (± 2 D)
12	13.0 (± 2 D)
16	12.0 (± 2 D)
20	11.0 (± 2 D)
24	10.0 (± 2 D)
28	9.0 (± 2 D)
32	8.0 (± 2 D)
36	7.0 (± 2 D)
40	6.0 (± 2 D)
44	4.5 (± 2 D)
48	3.0 (± 2 D)
52	2.5 (± 2 D)
56	2.0 (± 2 D)
60	1.5 (± 2 D)
64	1.0 (± 2 D)
68	0.5 (± 2 D)

[a] Continuing back from age 40, accommodation increased by 1 D for each 4 years. Beyond age 40, the decrease in accommodation is somewhat more rapid. From age 48 on, 0.5 D is lost every 4 years. Thus, one can recall the entire table by remembering the amplitudes at age 40 and age 48.

5. Add this extra plus power (the reading add) to the sphere of the distance refractive correction already in the refractor and again determine the patient's near visual acuity. If you are using a trial frame, make sure you have placed the distance sphere lens in the appropriate slot on the back of the frame, and the cylindrical lens in the front, as you would normally do for determining the distance correction. Put the appropriate plus lens as an *additional lens in front* of the lens combination already in place.

6. By moving the reading material closer to and then farther away from the patient, determine that the add allows the patient an adequate range for seeing near work clearly.

Guidelines for Prescribing Glasses

To help you avoid many common problems and get started with proper prescribing habits, this section presents general guidelines and tips on prescribing for myopia, hyperopia, and astigmatism as well as for presbyopia. Consult the detailed textbooks on this topic listed at the end of this chapter for more complete discussions than can be supplied here.

General Prescribing Guidelines

- If the patient has good vision and is asymptomatic, do not prescribe new glasses or change old ones (it is hard to improve the asymptomatic, happy patient).

- Don't prescribe minor changes (less than 0.50 D) unless the patient can definitely tell an improvement over his or her old spectacle correction.
- Specify vertex distance for lenses with power of greater than or equal to 5.00 D.
- Try to avoid changing cylinder axis more than 10°. If a greater change must be made, have the patient walk around wearing the prescription in a trial frame for 20 to 30 minutes, and warn the patient that an adjustment period probably will be necessary.
- Check the final eyeglass prescription using the duochrome test.
- Put the prescription in a trial frame and let the patient walk around in the waiting room if you think the prescription might be questionable, if this is a first prescription, or if there is a change from the previous prescription of more than 0.50 D.
- Check and recheck your prescription for accuracy. Errors are often made when copying the prescription from the refractor or trial frame into the medical record and onto a prescription pad.

Prescriptions for Myopia

The typical presentation of uncorrected myopia is blurred distance vision with good near vision. Patients often state that they need to squint to see objects far away.

- In general, give the manifest refraction for best acuity and do not overcorrect. Young myopic patients will often prefer more minus power in the manifest refraction than they need for best acuity, because the additional minus enhances the contrast of the dark test letters on the light chart background. During the subjective refraction, to help prevent overcorrection, ask the patient if the letters are actually clearer and if detail is more easily seen, or if the letters are just darker and smaller. Overcorrection causes the patient to accommodate, often leading to asthenopia (eyestrain).
- Use the results of cycloplegic retinoscopy and cycloplegic refraction to avoid overcorrecting.
- For adult myopic patients over the age of 40, make sure that increasing the minus power does not induce presbyopic symptoms. Check that all patients can read comfortably with their new distance prescriptions.

Prescriptions for Hyperopia

Most young children are hyperopic, but they can easily compensate for this ametropia by accommodating. Indications for correcting hyperopia in children include:

- Hyperopia greater than 5.00 D, or lesser degrees of hyperopia if symptomatic (asthenopia, or vague eye discomfort such as intermittent blurring or trouble reading)
- Decreased uncorrected acuity with improvement in acuity with hyperopic spectacles
- Anisometropia (prescribe glasses if a hyperopic error in 1 eye of 1.50 D or greater compared with the fellow eye is noted during the amblyogenic period—before the child is 6 or 7 years old—especially if there is any difference in measurable acuity)
- Esotropia

Hyperopic adults can partially compensate for their hyperopia by accommodating. The manifest hyperopia is the amount of plus power needed for sharp distance vision. After cycloplegia, an additional latent component of the hyperopia can be detected by both retinoscopy and refinement. This is the portion of the hyperopia that the patient overcomes by accommodating. Symptoms can occur because of inability to maintain the accommodation necessary to overcome hyperopia. Symptoms include decreased distance vision or intermittent blurring of distance vision as latent hyperopia becomes manifest; difficulty with near work as part of the loss of accommodation that accompanies the normal aging process; early presbyopia in young, uncorrected hyperopic adults; asthenopia or visual discomfort, including burning and tearing, and even bifrontal headaches exacerbated by near work; and fatigue after reading for short periods.

Children less than 4 years old who require hyperopic spectacles can usually accept the full cycloplegic measurement. Once a child reaches school age, consider reducing the plus for the refractive prescription by about one-third, but do not require the child to accommodate more than 2.50 D continually for the distance. If the child is cooperative, a manifest refraction can be useful, because the full hyperopic prescription can cause blur at distance. For adults, give the manifest refraction. Correct for infinity rather than the 20-foot examination room length by reducing the manifest refraction by –0.25 D.

Prescriptions for Astigmatism

Symptoms of uncorrected astigmatism include blur at both distance and near. Uncorrected astigmatic patients often report the need to squint for both distance and near to improve vision. The patient with uncorrected astigmatism might also complain of a bifrontal headache with prolonged near work. Observe the following prescribing guidelines in cases of astigmatism:

- For children under the age of about 4, prescribe the full astigmatic correction and advise full-time wear. In general, if more than 1.50 D of cylinder is detected, glasses are indicated.
- Be cautious about changing the axis of the astigmatic correction, especially in adults, because such changes are often poorly tolerated. Asking the patient to walk around for a few minutes wearing the prescription in a trial frame is helpful in this situation.
- Ascertain that any new astigmatic correction produces significant improvement in both distance and near acuity.
- Be wary of introducing new astigmatic correction in adults, as it can produce intolerable distortions for the patient even if measurable acuity is improved.
- Advise patients that a period of adjustment to the new correction could be needed.

Prescriptions for Presbyopia

The predominant symptom of uncorrected presbyopia is difficulty reading at near. Patients with early presbyopia also sometimes report that they need more light to read and that they can read well in the morning, but not at night after a long day of accommodative effort (close work). Patients experience difficulty reading fine print, such as a telephone directory, and threading a needle. Very early in presbyopia, patients note that their eyes are slow to focus on near print, and then slow to change focus as they look at more remote objects. The usual onset of presbyopia is approximately between 40 and 45 years old, but presentation can be younger in those with undercorrected hyperopia and older in those with undercorrected myopia. The following guidelines can be useful in determining presbyopic correction.

- Myopic patients with refractive errors under –3.00 D might not complain of difficulty with near tasks because they routinely remove their glasses for reading. Remember to ask about this habit, because these patients might have symptoms with accommodative effort if they wear their corrections full time.
- Various medications can exacerbate presbyopic symptoms. Some of these are barbiturates, tricyclic antidepressants, and antihistamines and decongestants (including nonprescription medications).
- Bifocals with adds of +0.75 D or less are rarely necessary, although they might be required for specific tasks, such as seeing a music stand.
- Alternatives for the presbyopic emmetropic patient are single-vision readers, bifocals with plano tops, and half glasses.
- Alternatives for presbyopic myopic and presbyopic hyperopic patients are separate glasses for reading and distance, and bifocals. Myopic patients also can remove their glasses or use half glasses when reading.

Several bifocal and trifocal styles are illustrated in Figure 5.20. In general, the type and the placement of the bifocal or trifocal segment is best left up to the optician, who will discuss the various options with the patient. The patient should be encouraged to tell the optician about specific near vision requirements, such as the need to view a computer screen at a particular distance. Most patients have heard about "bifocals without a line," by which they usually mean one of a number of the progressive addition lenses (see Figure 5.20H). These lens styles have no visible demarcation line and not only are more cosmetically acceptable for many patients, but also eliminate much of the image jump and displacement that can occur as gaze is shifted from the distance to the near segment. Although the patient might ask for a prescription by brand name (eg, Varilux), the available progressive bifocals are comparable, and the decision for the one used is often left to the optician. Because the correct fitting of these lenses is crucial to successful use, the fitter's personal expertise can be as important as the choice of the add power itself. Blended bifocals also lack a sharp demarcation line and are less expensive than progressive addition lenses, but they have an area of blur where the near and distance segments join. This is at approximately the same position that the patient might experience an image jump as fixation shifts from 1 segment of the bifocal to the other.

Trifocals can be useful for patients who have intermediate distance needs, such as computer use. Other special-need adds are sometimes used for particular purposes, such as reading music, reading blueprints, and viewing museum exhibits. Try to duplicate the special-needs situation when testing. It is useful to ask the patient to measure the distances for the tasks for which the glasses will be worn. This will allow you to determine a more appropriate add.

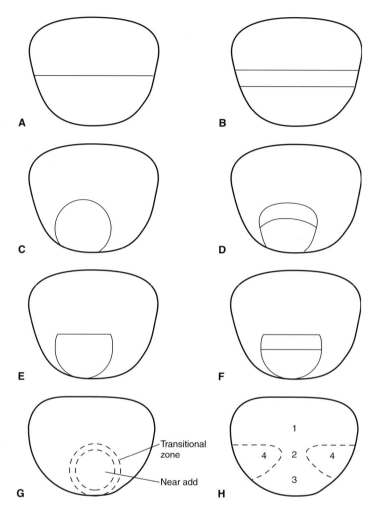

Figure 5.20 Common multifocal lens styles. **(A, B)** Executive bifocal and trifocal. **(C, D)** Round-top bifocal and trifocal. **(E, F)** Flat-top ("D" segment) bifocal and trifocal. **(G)** Invisible, or blended, bifocal. **(H)** Progressive addition multifocal lens. (1) Distance correction. (2) Corridor of increasing plus power. (3) Maximum plus power of near segment. (4) Zone of significant distortion.

Optical Fitting Considerations

Pantoscopic Tilt

Spectacle lenses in frames are tilted slightly to conform with the rotation of the eye on the optical axis of the spectacle lens. This minimizes the effect of oblique astigmatism, an aberration that would be induced with down gaze if the lens were fit perpendicular to the distance visual axis. Vertex distance changes are also minimized with this adjustment. The tops of the spectacle lenses are intentionally tilted forward, which helps achieve a plane that allows a more constant distance between the back surface of the spectacle lens and the front surface of the cornea. Pantoscopic tilt is not an exact measurement, but because most opticians incorporate this tilt when fitting spectacle lenses, it should be taken into account when using either a refractor or a trial frame. In general, most spectacles are fitted with a downward tilt of between 5° and 10° to the visual axis. This means the top of the spectacle lens is tilted slightly forward compared with the bottom of the spectacle lens.

Interpupillary Distance

It is important to know the distance between the 2 pupils so as to align and center spectacle lenses properly. Adjustments should be made for the interpupillary distance (IPD) measurement when using either a trial frame or a refractor. An effective and rapid method for measuring the IPD is to stand directly in front of the patient, hold a millimeter ruler at arm's length, and steady it on the base of the patient's nose, with the numbers facing you. Instruct the patient to look directly into your left eye and to maintain that gaze as you align the zero mark of the ruler with the nasal border of the patient's right pupil. Then, without moving the ruler, instruct the patient to look into your right eye. Note the position of the temporal border of the patient's left pupil. The distance between the nasal border of 1 pupil and the temporal border of the other is a usable estimate of the IPD. Remember to align your left eye with the patient's right eye and your right eye with the patient's left eye. Do not stand close enough to the patient to induce excessive convergence or you will underestimate the IPD by several millimeters. The IPD should be adjusted on the refractor or the trial lens frame before retinoscopy is performed. Most trial frames require each eyepiece to be adjusted separately, while most refractors have a single knob that adjusts the 2 eyepieces simultaneously.

More than 90% of adults will have interpupillary distances between 60 and 68 mm. This measurement is not exactly the same as the geometric IPD, which is of importance only when high-power lenses are being fit. If lenses over 4.00 D are decentered, prism will be induced, which can be sufficient to affect binocular viewing. Usually the nose is midway between the 2 pupils, but occasionally there is significant facial asymmetry. If this is the case, special fitting adjustments must be made. Clinical Protocol 9.2 presents instructions for measuring binocular IPD. More detailed discussion on IPD determination and optical centration measurements can be found in the reference books listed at the end of this chapter.

Pitfalls and Pointers

- The examiner's eyes and the patient's eyes must be properly aligned with each other for retinoscopy. If they are not, the examiner might develop back or neck strain after repeated examinations. In addition, if the eyes are misaligned, aberrations from the patient's lens, glare, and extraneous reflections will interfere with the accuracy of retinoscopic measurements.
- Retinoscopy is easier to perform if cycloplegia is used and the patient's pupils are dilated.
- Remember that retinoscopic "with" motion indicates the need for plus lenses to be added, whereas "against" motion indicates the need for minus power to be added.

- If an irregular reflex or a very dull reflex is noted in retinoscopy, suspect high myopia or hyperopia, keratoconus, corneal warpage syndrome, other surface irregularities, or a cataract.
- Manifest means without cycloplegia. This term is often incorrectly used as synonymous with subjective refraction. If the refraction is done under cycloplegia, this should be noted. Subjective refinement of all refractions is generally assumed unless the refraction is identified specifically as retinoscopy.
- Although retinoscopy and subjective refraction seem to be difficult techniques to perform, with practice they become manageable. Don't be discouraged if they seem bewildering at first.

Suggested Resources

Clinical Optics. Basic and Clinical Science Course, Section 3. San Francisco: American Academy of Ophthalmology; published annually.

Corboy JM. *The Retinoscopy Book: An Introductory Manual for Eye Care Professionals.* 5th ed. Thorofare, NJ: Slack; 2003.

Guyton DL. *Retinoscopy and Subjective Refraction* [DVD]. San Francisco: American Academy of Ophthalmology; 2007.

Guyton DL, West CE, Miller JM, Wisnicki HJ. *Ophthalmic Optics and Clinical Refraction.* 2nd ed. Baltimore, MD: Prism Press; 1999.

Milder B, Rubin ML. *The Fine Art of Prescribing Glasses Without Making a Spectacle of Yourself.* 3rd ed. Gainesville, FL: Triad; 2004.

Refractive Errors and Refractive Surgery [Preferred Practice Pattern]. San Francisco: American Academy of Ophthalmology; 2007.

Rubin ML. *Optics for Clinicians.* 25th Anniv. ed. Gainesville, FL: Triad; 1993.

Clinical Protocol 5.1  **Using the Manual Lensmeter**

Focusing the Eyepiece

The focus of the lensmeter eyepiece must be verified each time the instrument is used.

1. With no lens in place in the lensmeter, look through the eyepiece of the instrument. Turn the power drum until the mires (perpendicular crossed lines) viewed through the eyepiece are grossly out of focus.

2. Turn the eyepiece in a plus direction, normally counterclockwise. This will fog (blur) the target seen through the eyepiece.

Clinical Protocol 5.1 *(continued)*

3. Slowly turn the eyepiece in the opposite direction until the target is clear, then stop turning. This procedure focuses the eyepiece.

4. Turn the power drum to focus the mires. The mires should focus at a power drum reading of zero (plano). If not, repeat the procedure.

Positioning the Eyeglasses

1. Place the lower rim of the eyeglasses on the movable spectacle table with temple pieces facing away from you. You are now prepared to read the back surface of the lens, normally the appropriate surface from which to measure.

2. Looking through the eyepiece, align the eyeglass lens so that the mires cross in the center of the target by moving the eyeglass lens on the spectacle table.

Measuring Sphere and Cylinder Power

The following steps describe the plus cylinder technique:

1. Turn the power drum to read high minus (about −10.00 D).

2. Bring the closely spaced mires (often called *single lines*) into sharp focus by rotating the power drum counter-clockwise while at the same time rotating the cylinder wheel to straighten the single lines where they cross the widely spaced perpendicular set of mires (often called *triple lines*).

3. If the single lines and the triple lines come into focus at the same time, the lens is a sphere (Figure 1). If only the single lines focus, you have identified the sphere portion of a spherocylinder. Record the power drum reading at this point as the power of the sphere.

4. If cylinder power is present, after noting the power drum reading for the sphere, measure cylinder power by moving the power drum farther counterclockwise (less minus, or more plus), bringing the triple lines into sharp focus (Figure 2).

5. Calculate the difference between the first power drum reading for the focused single lines and the second power drum reading for the focused triple lines. Record this figure as the plus-cylinder power of the lens.

6. Read the axis of the cylinder from the cylinder axis wheel.

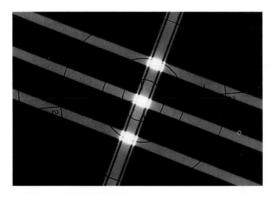

Figure 1   Measuring sphere.

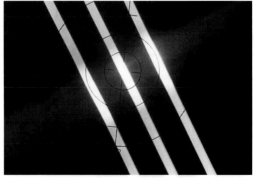

Figure 2   Measuring cylinder power.

Clinical Protocol 5.2 — Measuring Bifocal Power

1. After measuring the sphere and cylinder distance portion of a bifocal eyeglass lens, center the bifocal add at the bottom of the lens in the lensmeter gimbal (the ring-like frame) and refocus on the triple lines.

2. The difference between the distance reading of the triple-line focus and the new triple-line focus is the add, or bifocal power.

3. If the distance portion of the eyeglass lens is a sphere, just refocus the bifocal segment and calculate the algebraic difference between the power in the top segment and the power in the bifocal.

4. For a trifocal lens, follow the same procedure as for the bifocal segment to measure the trifocal segment directly. Customarily a trifocal is one-half the power of the bifocal.

Note: This method is applicable to standard bifocals. Progressive addition lenses (also known as *variable focus lenses* or *"lineless bifocals"*) are read according to the manufacturer's directions. Many have the power of the add imprinted on the lens itself.

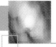

Clinical Protocol 5.3 — Measuring Prism Power and Orientation

The existence of prescribed prism power in a spectacle lens generally is revealed when the lensmeter mires cannot be centered in the central portion of the lensmeter target. Once you have determined the presence of a prism, measure prism power and determine orientation as follows:

1. With a nonpermanent marker, mark the position on the lens through which the patient is viewing while he is looking straight ahead. Center this mark in the lensmeter target.

2. Count the number of black concentric circles from the central cross of the lensmeter target to the center of the vertical and/or horizontal crossed mires (Figure 1). Each circle represents 1 prism diopter.

3. Record the direction of the thick portion (base) of the prism by determining the direction of the displacement of the mires. For example, if the mires are displaced upward, the prism base is base up; downward displacement indicates base-down prism; displacement toward the nose, base-in prism; and displacement toward the temples, base-out prism.

   Prism-compensating devices are incorporated into some lensmeters. Such devices permit the measurement of prism without using the concentric circles. To avoid recording prism power that is not actually present when using these devices, be sure the prism-compensating device is set to zero. Auxiliary prisms are available for use with some lensmeters to assist in measuring lenses with prism power greater than the number of concentric circles.

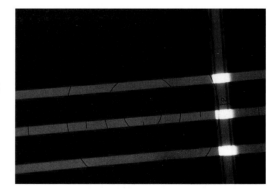

Figure 1 Measuring prism power.

Clinical Protocol 5.4

Measuring Optical Centration of Spectacle Lenses

At times, it is important to be able to note the proper position of the optical center of a spectacle lens, to see if it lines up appropriately with a patient's pupils. Most lensmeters have a marking or dotting device that can be used to mark temporarily the optical center of a spectacle lens. The technique for checking optical centers is as follows:

1. Place the spectacle lens against the lens stop of the lensmeter.

2. Make certain the eyeglasses frame sits squarely on the spectacle table, rim down, temple pieces away from you.

3. Focus the mires and center them with the focused eyepiece target (Figure 1). Use the dotting device to mark the lens while it is held in this position. The center mark (usually of 3 marks) is the optical center of the lens. If the lensmeter does not have a dotting device, use a nonpermanent marker to record the approximate center of the lens by noting where the lensmeter light source shines through the eyeglass lens and marking this point.

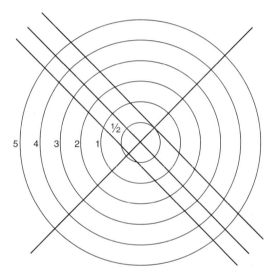

Figure 1   Measuring optical centration of the spectacle lens.

Clinical Protocol 5.5

Measuring Vertex Distance

1. Ask the seated patient to close both eyes.

2. Gently rest the fixed caliper arm of the distometer on the closed eyelid and carefully place the moveable caliper arm against the back surface of the trial lens, refractor lens, or the patient's eyeglass lens (see Figure 5.16).

3. Record the separation distance between these 2 surfaces from the millimeter scale on the distometer. (The scale allows for an average eyelid thickness.)

6

Ocular Motility Examination

In an ocular alignment and motility examination, the patient is tested for 3 principal properties of the visual system: binocularity (fusion), ocular alignment, and eye movement (motility). Because the subject is complex, this chapter begins with a discussion of commonly used terminology and basic extraocular muscle function before addressing specific examination techniques for assessing binocularity, alignment, and motility.

Strabismus Terminology

Strabismus is a general term used to describe a misalignment of the eyes in which both eyes are not directed at the object of regard. The Greek word *strabismus* means to squint, to look obliquely or askance, and in some countries other than the United States the terms *strabismus* and *squint* are used interchangeably. Strabismus can either cause or be caused by the absence of binocular vision. Strabismus can also lead to amblyopia.

Amblyopia is a term used to describe loss of vision due to abnormal visual input in childhood. In physiologic terms, amblyopia represents a failure of visual connections from disuse or inability to form a clearly focused retinal image during the first few years of life, a critical period in the development of the visual pathways. Neither amblyopia nor strabismus causes learning disabilities, although both can co-exist with learning disabilities.

Strabismus is measured with prisms and quantified in prism diopters. An ophthalmic prism is a wedge of clear plastic or glass with a triangular cross-section having an apex and a base (see Chapter 5). Prism power is measured by the number of centimeters of deflection of a light ray measured 1 meter from the prism and abbreviated as PD (for prism diopters) or by the superior delta symbol ($^\Delta$). The notation PD or $^\Delta$ is appended to the numeric measurement of the deviation. Plastic prisms and prism bars are calibrated according to the angle of minimum deviation, whereas glass prisms are calibrated according to Prentice's rule. The calibration of the prism dictates the orientation in which it must be held when measuring strabismus. Plastic prisms should be held with the rear surface perpendicular to the direction of the fixation object along the line of sight. This is the frontal plane position, and it closely approximates the angle of minimum deviation. Glass prisms should be held with the rear surface perpendicular to the eye's visual axis or parallel to the iris plane (Prentice position). Prisms are available singly or as bars of small horizontally or vertically oriented prisms attached to each other in increasing strength. Rotary prisms (Risley's prisms) produce a continuum of prismatic power.

A rotary prism may be handheld but is also mounted on the front of most refractors. Rotary prisms consist of 2 prisms of equal power that are counter rotated with respect to each other. The prismatic power produced varies from zero to the sum of the 2 powers.

A number of terms are used to classify and describe strabismus. Strabismus is called *comitant* when the angle of misalignment is approximately equal in all directions of gaze. Strabismus is called *incomitant* when the angle of misalignment varies with the direction of gaze.

Strabismus is further classified as either a heterophoria or a heterotropia. A *phoria* (or *heterophoria*) is a latent tendency toward misalignment that occurs only when binocularity is interrupted. During binocular viewing, the 2 eyes of a patient with a heterophoria are perfectly aligned. The term *strabismus* usually refers to a *tropia* (or *heterotropia*), a manifest deviation that is present when both eyes are open (Figure 6.1). A heterotropia that is present only part of the time is called *intermittent*, whereas one that is always present is called *constant*. Heterotropias and heterophorias are subdivided according to the direction of the deviation. *Esotropia*, a manifest strabismus in which the eye is deviated toward the nose, is the most common type of ocular misalignment of childhood. *Exotropia*, in which the eye deviates outward toward the temple, is more likely to be intermittent than esotropia. An upward deviation of an eye is called *hypertropia*. By convention, a vertical deviation is referred to as a *right* or *left* hypertropia according to the higher eye, whether or not that eye is the one used for fixation. In reality, if the patient uses the higher eye to fixate, the fellow eye will be hypotropic, but the term *hypotropia* is less commonly used. Table 6.1 summarizes the types of heterophorias and heterotropias. Table 6.2 lists clinical abbreviations commonly used in the evaluation of strabismus.

Figure 6.1 Types of heterotropia. **(A)** Esotropia. **(B)** Exotropia. **(C)** Left hypertropia. **(D)** Right hypertropia (left hypotropia).

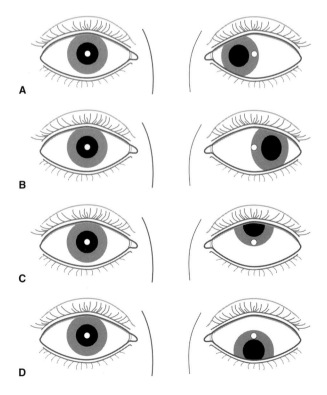

Table 6.1   Types of Heterophoria and Heterotropia

Prefix	Name of Disorder		Description
	-phoria (latent)	*-tropia (manifest)*	
eso-	esophoria	esotropia	inward deviation
exo-	exophoria	exotropia	outward deviation
hyper-	hyperphoria	hypertropia	upward deviation
hypo-	hypophoria	hypotropia	downward deviation

Table 6.2   Clinical Abbreviations Used in Evaluation of Strabismus

Alignment of the Eyes	Abbreviation	Usage
Esodeviations	E	Esophoria for distance
	ET	Esotropia for distance
	E(T)	Intermittent esotropia for distance
	E′ or ET′ or E(T)′	Esodeviations for near
Exodeviations	X	Exophoria for distance
	XT	Exotropia for distance
	X(T)	Intermittent exotropia for distance
	X′ or XT′ or X(T)′	Exodeviations for near
Hyperdeviations[a]	H	Hyperphoria for distance
	HT	Hypertropia for distance
	H(T)	Intermittent hypertropia for distance
	H′ or HT′ or H(T)′	Hyperdeviations for near
	Ortho	No deviation present
Extraocular muscles[a]	IO	Inferior oblique
	IR	Inferior rectus
	LR	Lateral rectus
	MR	Medial rectus
	SO	Superior oblique
	SR	Superior rectus
Other abbreviations	DHD, DVD	Dissociated horizontal deviation, dissociated vertical deviation
	IPD	Interpupillary distance
	NPA	Near point of accommodation
	NPC	Near point of convergence
	OA, UA	Overaction, underaction
	PD	Prism diopters or pupillary distance (meaning is clear from context)

[a] L (left) or R (right) generally precedes these abbreviations.

■ Motility Terminology

Eye movements can be monocular (1 eye only) or binocular (both eyes together). Monocular eye movements are called *ductions*, and 6 terms are used to describe them:

- *Adduction* (movement of the eye nasally)
- *Abduction* (movement of the eye temporally)
- *Elevation* (sursumduction; movement of the eye upward)
- *Depression* (deorsumduction; movement of the eye downward)

- *Intorsion* (incyclotorsion; nasal rotation of the superior vertical corneal meridian)
- *Extorsion* (excyclotorsion; temporal rotation of the superior vertical corneal meridian)

Binocular eye movements are described as versions and vergences. *Versions* are binocular eye movements in the same direction (eg, to the right, to the left, etc). One muscle of each eye is primarily responsible for the movement of that eye into a particular field of gaze. Two simultaneously acting muscles (1 from each eye) are called *yoke muscles*, and their movement is said to be *conjugate*; that is, they work at the same time to move the 2 eyes in the same direction. For example, the right medial rectus and the left lateral rectus work together to move the eyes to the left. The 6 positions of gaze in which yoke muscles act together, known as the *cardinal fields of gaze*, are right and up, right, right and down, left and up, left, and left and down.

Vergences are normal, disconjugate binocular eye movements in which the eyes move in opposite directions. The 2 primary types of vergences routinely evaluated are *convergence*, the movement of both eyes nasally, and *divergence*, the movement of both eyes temporally.

■ Function of the Extraocular Muscles

There are 7 extraocular muscles: 4 rectus muscles, 2 oblique muscles, and the levator palpebrae superioris muscle. The rectus and oblique muscles move the globe, whereas the levator muscle primarily moves the eyelid and only indirectly affects ocular motility. The relative positions of the extraocular muscles are shown in Figure 6.2.

The medial rectus and the lateral rectus muscles have only horizontal actions. Contraction of the medial rectus muscle results in adduction and contraction of the lateral rectus results in abduction. The superior rectus and the inferior rectus muscles originate nasally relative to their insertions and hence provide more complex motility action. The primary action of the superior rectus is elevation; its

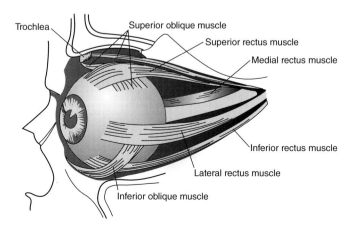

Figure 6.2 The extraocular muscles and the trochlea of the left eye.

Trochlea · Superior oblique muscle · Superior rectus muscle · Medial rectus muscle · Inferior rectus muscle · Lateral rectus muscle · Inferior oblique muscle

Table 6.3 Actions of Extraocular Muscles from Primary Position

Muscle	Action	Muscle	Action
Superior rectus	Elevation	Inferior rectus	Depression
	Adduction		Adduction
	Intorsion		Extorsion
Superior oblique	Intorsion	Inferior oblique	Extorsion
	Depression		Elevation
	Abduction		Abduction
Medial rectus	Adduction	Lateral rectus	Abduction

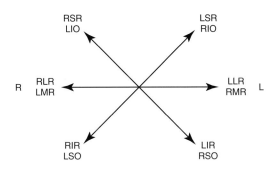

Figure 6.3 The cardinal positions of gaze and the yoke muscles acting in those positions.

secondary actions are adduction and intorsion. The primary action of the inferior rectus is depression; its secondary actions are adduction and extorsion.

The oblique muscles, as their names indicate, insert into the sclera at oblique angles. The superior oblique muscle passes through the trochlea, a cartilaginous pulley located on the superonasal orbital rim, before inserting in the posterosuperior quadrant of the globe. The primary action of the superior oblique muscle is intorsion; secondarily it provides depression (especially in adduction) and abduction. The inferior oblique inserts posterolaterally on the globe near the macula. Its primary action is extorsion; secondarily it provides elevation (especially in adduction) and abduction.

Table 6.3 summarizes the basic actions of the extraocular muscles; Figure 6.3 diagrams the paired yoke muscles in each eye that are primarily responsible for movement into the cardinal fields of gaze.

Ocular Motility Examination

A thorough history is an essential part of the examination of a patient suspected of having strabismus. As the history is obtained, the examiner has the opportunity to observe the patient in a relaxed, casual manner. Particular attention should be paid to the presence of any unusual head position or movement, noting its direction and whether it manifests as a head tilt or a face turn. It is also important to note any tendency of the patient to close 1 or both eyes partially or completely.

The examiner should obtain information about the birth history and subsequent development of the patient, especially if the patient is a child. Areas of particular interest regarding a child include a history of prematurity, rubella, or seizures. Also obtain information regarding any medications currently being used, or medications used by the mother during pregnancy. It is important to document the age of onset of the strabismus (old photographs can be invaluable in this regard), as well as whether it is constant or intermittent, present at distance or near or both, alternating or unilateral, or worse when the child is tired or ill. Previous treatment by patching, glasses, or surgery should be documented. In the case of an older patient, information should be obtained about double vision, the patient's general health, and any history of trauma or medical problems such as diabetes or thyroid disease. In all cases, the examiner should ask about any family history of strabismus or amblyopia.

Overview of Examination

If the patient is being seen for a routine examination, tests of visual acuity are usually done before motility is evaluated. If, however, the patient is being seen specifically for motility evaluation and strabismus is suspected, tests of binocularity are best performed before any test that involves covering 1 eye, since dissociation of the eyes by monocular occlusion can influence the results of tests of binocularity.

After the history and general inspection, the examiner should first perform tests of binocularity and fusion (see the next section). Next, the ocular alignment is assessed at distance and near fixation (later in this chapter). If a deviation is present, it is measured, preferably using the alternate prism and cover test. Finally, ocular movements into the cardinal and midline positions of gaze are evaluated.

■ Tests of Binocularity and Fusion

Subjective testing of the patient's fusional ability is an important part of the ocular examination. Such tests evaluate both stereopsis, or relative ordering of visual objects in depth (commonly called *3-dimensional viewing*), and gross binocular status. As noted earlier in this chapter, these tests are best performed prior to dissociative tests that require occlusion.

Stereopsis

The term *stereopsis* refers to the simultaneous use of the eyes to perceive details of depth, distinct from the monocular cues such as overlay of contours and sizes of known objects that allow appreciation of gross depth perception. In this way, we order things in space and judge relative nearness of objects. *Sensory fusion* describes the ability of the brain to blend (fuse) separate images from the 2 eyes into a single image. *Suppression* is active central inhibition of the images originating from 1 eye, which prevents diplopia in the presence of strabismus. Sensory fusion is necessary to achieve high-grade stereopsis, defined as at least 40 seconds of arc (stereoacuity is always quantified in seconds of arc). Patients without demonstrable fusion use monocular cues for depth perception, such as differences in sizes of familiar objects. The ability to identify correctly stereoscopic targets does not automatically indicate the presence of sensory fusion, but it implies that some degree of binocular viewing is occurring. It is possible to fuse without having high-grade stereopsis but not possible to have high-grade stereopsis without sensory fusion.

Some tests for stereopsis, such as the polarized Titmus stereotest and the random-dot stereograms, are designed for use at near; other less frequently used tests are designed for use at distance. For additional information on the Titmus stereotest, and instructions for performing it, see Chapter 4.

Other Tests of Binocular Status

Several other tests are performed for the evaluation of binocular status. Those most commonly used are the Worth 4-dot test, the Maddox rod test, and the 4^{Δ} base-out test. Because of the subjective nature of the responses to these tests, more than 1 type of test is often performed to confirm or refute the findings. The least dissociative test, or the one that allows the patient to see the same or very similar image with each eye, will give a response most closely approximating everyday seeing conditions.

Worth 4-dot test

The Worth 4-dot test, performed at both distance and near, provides information about the patient's gross binocular status. The patient wears a pair of eyeglasses with a red filter over 1 eye and a green filter over the other eye (Figure 6.4). Red light is visible to the eye behind the red lens, but green light is not visible because the red lens absorbs these wavelengths. Green light is visible to the eye behind the green lens, but red light is not visible because the green lens absorbs these wavelengths. The patient looks at a target composed of 4 lighted circles: 1 red, 2 green, and 1 white. Looking at the target in the distance tests central (foveal) fusion. When the patient views the test at 16 inches (40 cm), peripheral fusion is tested. Different responses can be obtained. Patients with normal ocular alignment and normal sensory status will report seeing a total of 4 lights, indicating fusion. If the eye behind the green lens is suppressed, a total of 2 red lights is reported. If the eye behind the red lens is suppressed, 3 green lights are seen. If the patient reports a

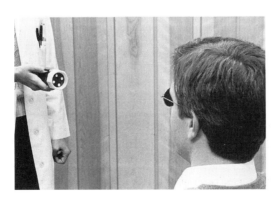

Figure 6.4 The Worth 4-dot test for near. The flashlight target, which illuminates the 4 dots, is held by the examiner. The same flashlight, or a wall-mounted illuminated target with a similar distribution of the 4 lights (not shown), can be used for the distance test. The patient wears the same red-and-green glasses for both tests.

total of 5 lights, 2 red and 3 green, the examiner should determine if all lights are seen simultaneously. If 2 red and 3 green are seen simultaneously, diplopia is present. If the red and green are seen in rapid succession, alternating suppression is present. If there is diplopia, it is classified as crossed or uncrossed. With crossed diplopia (noted in esotropia), images are seen to the left with the right eye and to the right with the left eye. In uncrossed diplopia (noted in exotropia), images are seen to the left with the left eye and to the right with the right eye. The single white light might be noted as red or green if 1 eye is strongly dominant. It might also be reported as pink or as a mixture of the 2 colors if there is no strong preference for either eye. Results are recorded (for both distance and near) either as fusion, suppression of 1 eye (right or left), or diplopia.

Maddox rod test

The Maddox rod test is a binocular test that can be used only with patients who are able to give reliable, subjective responses. It is performed at distance (20 feet) and at near (16 inches) using a muscle light for fixation. Patients wear their habitual corrective lenses for the test. A striated Maddox rod, usually a different color than the white fixation light, is placed before the patient's preferred eye, and the patient is instructed to fixate on the light. Placing the striations horizontally allows the patient to see the line vertically; placing them vertically allows the patient to see the line horizontally. The patient is asked if a line is seen while looking at the fixation light. There are 4 possible responses:

- The line is not seen (indicates suppression of the eye that is looking through the Maddox rod).
- The line goes through the light (indicates fusion and suggests that orthophoria is present).
- The line is above or below the light (indicates vertical diplopia and usually the presence of a vertical deviation).
- The line is to the left or to the right of the light (indicates horizontal diplopia and usually the presence of a horizontal deviation).

The examiner records the patient's responses for both distance and near as for the Worth 4-dot test.

The 4$^\Delta$ base-out test

The 4$^\Delta$ base-out test is useful to diagnose a foveal suppression scotoma in patients without strabismus, such as those with monofixation syndrome. A 4$^\Delta$ prism is placed base-out in front of 1 eye while the patient fixes on a target. The typical response in a normal patient is a version movement (both eyes) followed by convergence to reestablish fusion. A patient with a foveal suppression scotoma of the contralateral eye will demonstrate a version without convergence, whereas a patient with a suppression scotoma of the ipsilateral eye will show no movement. Several atypical responses to this test have been described, and it is not valid when acuity is poor in either eye. This test is discussed in greater detail in the resources listed at the end of this chapter.

■ Tests of Alignment

The most commonly used methods of assessing and quantifying ocular alignment are the red reflex (Bruckner) test, corneal light reflection test, and cover tests. Corneal light reflection tests are typically used with patients who have poor fixation or who are unable to cooperate sufficiently for cover testing. Cover tests require that the patient be able to cooperate and to fixate with each eye on a target so that accommodation can be controlled. For measuring a deviation, the examiner should choose the best test that the patient can perform, in descending order of (1) alternate prism and cover test, (2) Krimsky test, and (3) Hirschberg test.

Red Reflex Test

The red reflex test, also referred to as the *Bruckner test*, is the most rapid but the least sensitive test for detecting strabismus. It is particularly useful to screen for strabismus. It is performed by using the direct ophthalmoscope, with the bright white light and the lenses set to zero, to obtain a red reflex simultaneously in both eyes. If strabismus is present, the deviated eye will have a different reflex (lighter, darker, brighter, or dimmer) than that of the fixating eye, depending on the underlying problem (Figure 6.5). This test will also identify opacities in the visual axis and moderate to severe anisometropia.

Corneal Light Reflection Test

The corneal light reflection test compares the position of the corneal light reflection in both eyes. In normally aligned eyes, the reflections should be symmetric on the 2 corneas and in the same position relative to the pupil. Observation of the corneal light reflection constitutes an objective assessment of ocular alignment. For newborns and uncooperative children, this might be the only feasible way of testing for and measuring strabismus. The 2 most commonly used tests to measure corneal light reflection are the Hirschberg and Krimsky tests.

Hirschberg test

The Hirschberg test gives an estimation of ocular alignment by directly analyzing the angle of decentration of the corneal light reflection. Figure 6.6 illustrates

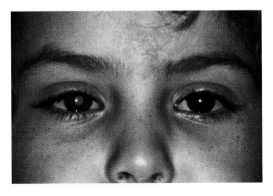

Figure 6.5   The red reflex test. This child has an esodeviation, as evidenced by the lighter, brighter reflex in the nonfixating eye.

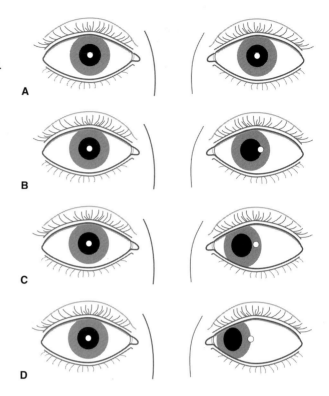

Figure 6.6 Hirschberg test of performing the corneal light reflection test to estimate deviation. **(A)** Normal alignment. **(B)** Pupillary margin, 30$^\Delta$ (15°) esotropia. **(C)** Mid-iris, 60$^\Delta$ (30°) esotropia. **(D)** Limbus, 90$^\Delta$ (45°) esotropia.

estimated deviations, and Clinical Protocol 6.1 describes how to measure ocular alignment using the Hirschberg test. This technique is based on the fact that every millimeter of decentration is equal to roughly 7°, or 15$^\Delta$, of deviation off the visual axis. A light reflection at the pupillary margin (2 mm from the pupillary center) is equal to approximately 15° (30$^\Delta$) deviation; a reflection in the middle of the iris indicates a deviation of about 30° (60$^\Delta$); and a reflection at the limbus is equivalent to a deviation of 45° (90$^\Delta$).

Krimsky test

The Krimsky test utilizes reflections from both corneas and is the preferred approach for assessing ocular deviation in a patient with poor vision in the deviating eye. Reflections from both eyes are produced by an appropriately placed penlight that is fixated by the patient's better eye. Prisms of increasing or decreasing power are placed in front of the fixating eye until the corneal reflection is centered in the deviating eye (Figure 6.7). Clinical Protocol 6.2 summarizes the modified Krimsky test for measuring corneal light reflection.

Cover Tests

For cover tests to be meaningful, the examiner must closely scrutinize the patient's eye movements when 1 eye is occluded. The validity of a cover test depends on the patient's ability to maintain constant fixation on an accommodative target. For a young child, the fixation target can be a toy or a small picture, and several different

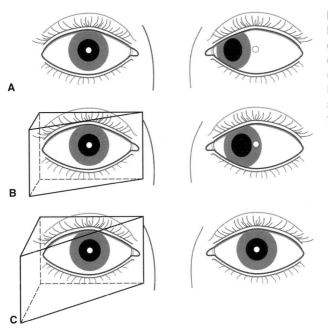

Figure 6.7 Modified Krimsky test of estimating deviation. A decentered corneal reflection in the left eye **(A)** is gradually centered by placing progressively stronger prisms in front of the fixating right eye **(B, C).**

targets presented in sequence might be needed to ensure good fixation. Each eye must be able to move adequately when fixating. These tests are performed at both distance and near, typically 20 feet (6 m) and 13 inches (33 cm). A standard occluder should be used, but at times the examiner might need to use his or her hand or fingers as the occluder.

Cover testing should be performed both with and without the patient's habitual refractive correction if the patient is hyperopic and only with correction if the patient is myopic. The results are recorded in universally accepted terms to assist other caregivers in understanding the patient's records and to allow valid comparisons with their findings.

The cover-uncover test is performed first to establish the presence of either a manifest deviation (heterotropia) or a latent deviation (heterophoria). The alternate cover test is then performed to measure the deviation.

Cover-uncover test

Clinical Protocol 6.3 describes how to perform the cover-uncover test. This test is usually done with the patient in an upright, seated position, but it can even be done with a bedridden patient. The only necessary condition is that the patient be able to maintain fixation with each eye individually on a target. As 1 eye is covered, observe the opposite, uncovered eye carefully for any movement. If there is movement of the uncovered eye to pick up fixation, a heterotropia is present. Concentrate on the uncovered eye and ignore any movement of the covered eye after the cover is removed. It is not necessary with this test to detect a heterophoria, as that will be found later with the alternate cover test. Some patients start with straight eyes prior to the cover-uncover test but develop an overt deviation with or after testing, which indicates that their fusion is easily disrupted. Such a patient has an intermittent heterotropia. The corresponding deviation should be denoted with parentheses, for example: X(T) or E(T), as appropriate.

Alternate cover test

The alternate cover test is performed by alternately covering each eye. A deviation that is detected by the alternate cover test that is not detectable by the cover-uncover test is by definition a phoria. When a tropia is present, the alternate cover test measures the total deviation, both latent (phoria) and manifest (tropia). The alternate cover test is a dissociative test; therefore, it often results in a deviation considerably larger than the amount initially noted with the cover-uncover test. Results of the alternate cover test are recorded as in the examples in Table 6.4. Clinical Protocol 6.4 describes the technique for performing the alternate cover test.

Simultaneous prism-cover test

In some patients, the amount of deviation measured by the alternate prism and cover test is considerably larger than the deviation that is usually manifest (ie, the deviation "builds" with the alternate cover test). In these cases, the simultaneous prism-cover test is helpful in determining the actual heterotropia present when both eyes are uncovered. It is performed by covering the fixating eye at the same time that the prism is placed in front of the deviating eye. The test is repeated using successively larger (or smaller) prism powers until the deviated eye no longer shifts when the fixating eye is covered.

Other Considerations With Alignment Tests

Parents of small children sometimes voice concern about an infant's ocular alignment when no true deviation is present. Often these parents have observed *pseudostrabismus*, which is an artificial appearance of misaligned eyes. Pseudoesotropia usually results from prominent epicanthal folds or a wide nasal bridge or both. In these cases, the corneal light reflection will be centered when measured by the Hirschberg test and there will be no deviation detectable by the cover-uncover test.

Pseudoexotropia usually results from *positive angle kappa*, which is a disparity between the visual axis and the anatomic axis of the eye (Figure 6.8). The corneal

Table 6.4 Sample Recording Results of Alternate Cover Testing

Example 1		Example 2	
c̄c̄	XT 30$^\Delta$	s̄c̄	RET′ 10$^\Delta$ builds to 30$^\Delta$
	X(T)′ 20$^\Delta$	c̄c̄	RE(T)′ 5$^\Delta$

This example describes a patient wearing corrective lenses (c̄c̄) who has a constant exotropia of 30 prism diopters at distance and intermittent exotropia of 20 prism diopters at near (near = ′).

This example describes a patient who, when not wearing glasses (s̄c̄), shows a constant right esotropia at near of 10 prism diopters that increases to 30 prism diopters with alternate cover. When this patient wears glasses, the right esotropia becomes intermittent and is reduced to 5 prism diopters.

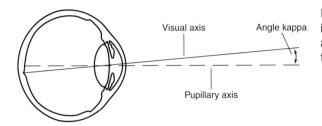

Figure 6.8 Positive angle kappa is a disparity between the visual and anatomic (pupillary) axes of the eye.

light reflection will appear to be decentered if angle kappa is present, but true strabismus is absent by cover testing. Nasal decentration simulates an exotropia (positive angle kappa) and temporal decentration simulates an esotropia (negative angle kappa). A mild degree of positive angle kappa is a common finding in many normal individuals.

Frequently a patient will present with an anomalous head position that is caused by strabismus. Head tilts and face turns should be noted in the patient's record. Many schemes have been devised for recording the findings of alignment testing. Two examples are illustrated in Figure 6.9. Notation can be made on such a schematic drawing, but the patient's head should be properly aligned before cover test measurements are taken. When measurements are taken with the patient assuming another head position, even if it is their habitual position, it should be noted.

At times the examiner will intentionally tilt the patient's head to obtain measurements, most often as part of the evaluation of cyclovertical muscles. This technique is particularly useful to diagnose superior oblique palsies as part of the 3-step test, which involves an assessment of the alignment of the eyes in primary position, in far right and far left gaze, and with the head tilted to the right and to the left.

The presence of any *nystagmus* (involuntary rhythmic eye movements) should be noted. Latent (occlusion) nystagmus is a conjugate, horizontal jerk nystagmus that occurs under monocular viewing conditions. In this condition, when 1 eye is occluded (as is done for cover testing) nystagmus develops in both eyes, with the fast phase directed toward the uncovered eye.

Accommodative convergence of the visual axes occurs as part of the near reflex. A fairly consistent increment of accommodative convergence (AC) occurs for each diopter of accommodation (A), and the relationship can be expressed as the accommodative convergence/accommodation (AC/A) ratio. The normal AC/A ratio is 3^Δ

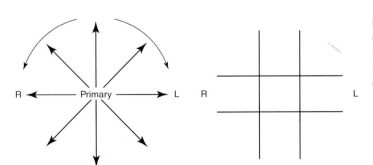

Figure 6.9 Two different schemes used to record the results of ocular alignment and motility examinations.

to 5$^\Delta$ of accommodative convergence for each diopter of accommodation. Abnormalities of this ratio are common and are an important cause of strabismus. If the AC/A ratio is abnormally high, the excess convergence tends to produce esotropia during accommodation or focusing on near targets. If the AC/A ratio is abnormally low, the eyes will tend to have an exodeviation when the individual looks at near targets. Clinical Protocol 6.5 describes 2 techniques of measuring the AC/A ratio. For other methods and detailed discussion of the clinical implications of this interrelationship, refer to comprehensive resources such as those referenced at the end of this chapter.

Evaluation of Eye Movements (Motility)

Clinical Protocol 6.6 describes the assessment of ocular motility. The phrase *diagnostic positions of gaze* is applied to the composite of these gaze positions or movements. The positions of gaze are referred to as follows:

- *Primary position* (straight ahead)
- *Secondary positions* (straight up, straight down, right gaze, and left gaze)
- *Tertiary positions* (the 4 oblique positions of gaze: up and right, up and left, down and right, and down and left)
- *Cardinal positions* (up and right, up and left, right, left, down and right, down and left)
- *Midline positions* (straight up and down from the primary position)

Pitfalls and Pointers

- Visual acuity testing for detection of amblyopia is critical in all cases of suspected strabismus.
- A very small angle deviation might not be possible to detect with the corneal light reflection test and might even be difficult to detect with cover tests in very young children.
- The examiner must use ingenuity to keep a very young patient interested and fixating on a target. Such ploys as brightly colored toys, pictures, and storytelling about the objects are useful. A good general rule is "1 toy, 1 look." A well-prepared examiner will have several interesting toys or pictures always at hand.
- When performing cover tests, the examiner must ensure that the patient is actually fixing on the object of regard with each eye. Inaccurate results are obtained if the patient is unable to fix reliably on an object due to poor visual acuity or inattention.
- When testing binocularity with the Titmus test, the examiner should ensure that the stereophotograph is clean (no scratches or fingerprints) and that the polarization of the viewing eyeglasses is effective.

Suggested Resources

Adult Strabismus Surgery [Clinical Statement]. San Francisco: American Academy of Ophthalmology; 2003.

Amblyopia [Preferred Practice Pattern]. San Francisco: American Academy of Ophthalmology; 2008.

Esotropia and Exotropia [Preferred Practice Pattern]. San Francisco: American Academy of Ophthalmology; 2008.

Pediatric Ophthalmology and Strabismus. Basic and Clinical Science Course, Section 6. San Francisco: American Academy of Ophthalmology; published annually.

Veronneau-Troutman S. *Prisms in the Medical and Surgical Management of Strabismus.* St Louis: CV Mosby Co; 1994.

von Noorden GK, Campos EC. *Binocular Vision and Ocular Motility: Theory and Management of Strabismus.* 6th ed. St Louis: CV Mosby Co; 2001.

Wright WW, Spiegel PH, eds. *Pediatric Ophthalmology and Strabismus.* 2nd ed. New York: Springer; 2002.

Clinical Protocol 6.1  **Performing the Corneal Light Reflection (Hirschberg) Test**

1. Have the patient seated facing you with head straight and eyes directed in primary gaze.

2. Hold a penlight in front of the patient's eyes at a distance of approximately 2 feet, directing the light at the midpoint between the 2 eyes of the patient. Align yourself with the light source. Instruct the patient to look directly at the light.

3. Compare the position of the 2 corneal light reflections and record the estimated result as prism diopters or degrees of deviation. Make a notation in parentheses beside the measurement: (by Hirschberg).

Clinical Protocol 6.2 **Performing the Krimsky Test**

1. Position the patient, the penlight, and yourself as for the Hirschberg test above.

2. Choose a prism of a power estimated by the Hirschberg test of estimating deviation.

3. Place the trial prism in front of the fixating (not the deviated) eye, with the apex of the prism (narrower end) pointing in the direction of the deviation. If a prism bar is available, use it with the flat (back) surface toward the patient, and the apices of the prisms pointed in the direction of the deviation, as with single prisms.

(continued)

Clinical Protocol 6.2 *(continued)*

4. Increase or decrease the strength of the trial prism until the light is reflected from each cornea symmetrically.

5. Record the strength of the prism used, noting (by Krimsky) in parentheses beside the measurement. For example, if it was necessary to use a 30$^\Delta$ prism to center the corneal reflections for a patient with an exotropia, record the results as follows:

   XT 30$^\Delta$ (by Krimsky)

Clinical Protocol 6.3 **Performing the Cover-Uncover Test**

1. Make sure that the patient's usual refractive correction is in place.

2. Have the patient look at a distance fixation target, and position yourself directly opposite the patient, within arm's reach, without obstructing the patient's view.

3. Swiftly cover the fixating eye with an occluder or your hand, and observe the other eye for any movement. Carefully note its direction.

4. Uncover the eye and allow about 3 seconds for both eyes to be uncovered.

5. Swiftly cover the other eye and observe its fellow eye for any movement.

6. Ensure that the patient is maintaining fixation on the same point as established for step 1.

7. Note results but do not record them until other cover testing is completed.

8. Repeat the test for near, using a near fixation point.

Clinical Protocol 6.4 **Performing the Alternate Prism and Cover Test**

1. With the patient seated upright and looking at a distance fixation point, rapidly shift the occluder from 1 eye to the other several times, not allowing any interval of binocularity. Make sure that each eye fixes on the target after each movement of the cover. The examiner should be seated slightly to the side of midline, facing the patient and at arm's length from the patient.

2. Place a trial prism over 1 eye (usually the patient's dominant eye), while continuing to shift the cover from 1 eye to the other. Remember to orient the prism with the apex toward the direction of deviation. Choose the strength of the initial trial prism to approximate the deviation estimated by the position of the corneal light reflections.

3. Continue to place prisms of progressively higher power in front of the eye until no movement is noted in either eye (neutralization). Additional prisms may be introduced until a reversal of movement is noted. The use of both horizontally and vertically placed prisms is often necessary to neutralize the shift completely. For large deviations, 2 horizontal or 2 vertical prisms should not be stacked on each other because it causes measurement errors. Instead, prisms should be placed in front of both eyes.

4. Record the results as noted in the examples in Table 6.4; in addition you may diagram the results in the various diagnostic positions of gaze (see examples in Figure 6.9).

5. Repeat the test for near.

Clinical Protocol 6.5 — Determining Accommodative Convergence/Accommodation Ratio

Gradient Method

1. Measure deviation in proper refractive correction using an accommodative target at one-third meter.
2. Remeasure deviation with +3.00 D lenses over the glasses.
3. Remeasure deviation with −3.00 D lenses over the glasses.
4. Calculate AC/A = $(\Delta_{-3.00} - \Delta_{+3.00})/6D$

Heterophoria Method

1. Measure deviation at distance fixation, with refractive correction in place.
2. Remeasure deviation at 1/3 m (33 cm).
3. Calculate AC/A = $1/3 (n^\Delta - d^\Delta)$ + interpupillary distance (cm).

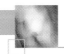

Clinical Protocol 6.6 — Assessing Versions

1. Sit facing the patient. Hold a small fixation target at eye level about 10 to 14 inches in front of the patient, with the patient looking in primary position (straight ahead).
2. Ask the patient to follow the target as you move it into the 6 cardinal fields and then up and down along the midline. Elevate the upper eyelid with a finger on your free hand to observe movements in down gaze.
3. Note whether the amplitude of eye movements is normal or abnormal in both eyes. To record the relative underaction or overaction in each gaze position, designate normal as 0 (no overaction or underaction) and use the numeral 4 to designate maximum underaction or overaction. Underactions thus are rated using a scale from −1 to −4, while overactions are rated from +1 to +4.

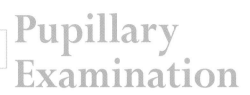

Pupillary Examination

7

The pupil is the window to the inner eye, through which light passes to reach retinal photoreceptors. Because of its potential to reveal serious neurologic or other disease, examination of the pupil is an important element of a thorough ophthalmic evaluation, requiring meticulous attention to detail. Pathologic disorders can alter the size, shape, and location of the pupil, as well as the way the pupil reacts to light and near-focus stimulation. The patient who has a pupillary abnormality generally comes to the attention of the ophthalmologist because of anisocoria (difference in size between the 2 pupils) or reduced pupillary light reaction.

This chapter provides a brief, basic background about pupillary pathway anatomy as well as instructions for the principal tests to evaluate pupillary responses. It also gives a brief overview of the pupillary abnormalities that are most commonly encountered through pupillary evaluation and testing.

Anatomy of Pupillary Pathways

Disorders of the pupil generally arise from dysfunction of the afferent or efferent pupillary pathways. The afferent pathway is composed of optic nerve axons emanating from the retina and optic disc, passing through the chiasm, and exiting the optic tract before the lateral geniculate body to synapse in the dorsal midbrain. The efferent pathway includes the parasympathetic and the sympathetic input to the iris muscles.

The size of the pupil is controlled by the opposed actions of the sympathetic and parasympathetic nervous systems that control the tone of 2 smooth muscles, the pupillary sphincter muscle and the pupillary dilator muscle. The pupillary sphincter muscle is supplied by cholinergic fibers of the parasympathetic system through the third cranial (oculomotor) nerve; the pupillary dilator muscle is supplied by adrenergic fibers of the sympathetic system. Additionally, the pupils tend to be smaller in infants and larger in children and young adults, becoming smaller again with advancing age.

Parasympathetic Pathway (Light-Reflex Pathway)

The pupillary parasympathetic pathway subserves the pupillary light reflex (Figure 7.1). The afferent arc begins in the retina and ends in the midbrain tectum. When light stimulates the retinal photoreceptors (rods and cones), electrical impulses are transmitted through the retina by way of retinal ganglion cell axons, which include pupillomotor fibers. The pupillary and visual fibers pass through the optic nerve to the chiasm, where hemidecussation occurs, and then to the optic

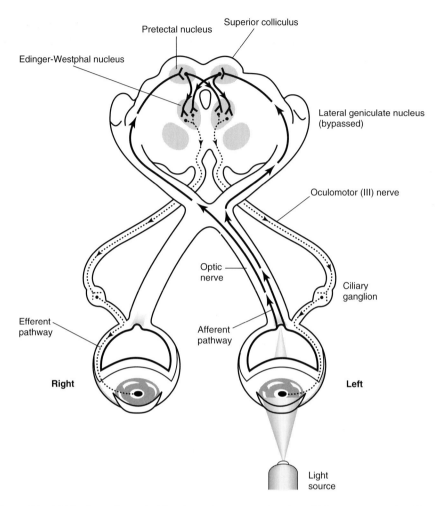

Figure 7.1 Light reflex pathway. In this schematic cross-section, the solid line represents the afferent pathway and the dotted line represents the efferent pathway. A light stimulating the left retina will generate impulses that travel up the left optic nerve and divide at the chiasm. Some impulses continue up the left tract; some cross and travel up the right tract. The impulses arrive at each pretectal nucleus and stimulate cells, which in turn send impulses to the Edinger-Westphal nuclei and down the third cranial nerve to each iris sphincter, causing each pupil to constrict. Because of the double decussation, the first in the chiasm and the second between the pretectal nuclei and the Edinger-Westphal nuclei, the direct pupil response in the left eye equals the consensual response in the right eye. (Reprinted from *Immediate Eye Care: An Illustrated Manual*, Ragge NK, Easty DL, p. 185, © 1990, with permission from Elsevier.)

tract. They bypass the lateral geniculate body, where the visual fibers synapse, to enter the midbrain. The first synapse occurs at the pretectal nuclei, near the superior colliculus. The fibers then decussate a second time in the posterior commissure and synapse at both the ipsilateral and contralateral Edinger-Westphal nuclei, the parasympathetic motor center of the oculomotor nerve.

The efferent fibers from the Edinger-Westphal nuclei then travel superficially in the oculomotor nerve as it leaves the brain stem and enter the orbit within the inferior division of the oculomotor nerve to synapse at the ciliary ganglion. Postganglionic fibers then travel within the short posterior ciliary nerves, passing through the suprachoroidal space to innervate the pupillary sphincter muscle and the ciliary muscle. This complex anatomic pattern, with partial crossings at the chiasm and in the posterior commissure, results in the symmetry of the direct and consensual pupillary responses.

Near-Reflex Pathway

The near-reflex pathway subserves pupillary constriction when fixating a target at near. It is less well defined than the light-reflex pathway. The final common pathway is mediated through the oculomotor nerve with a synapse in the ciliary ganglion. Its central fibers are located more ventrally in the midbrain than those of the light-reflex pathway; that is, ventral to the Edinger-Westphal nuclei. Unlike the light-reflex pathway, which is entirely subcortical, the near-reflex pathway sends fibers to the cerebral cortex bilaterally.

Sympathetic Pathway

Pain, fear, and certain other psychic stimuli lead to pupillary dilation through the sympathetic innervation of the pupillary dilator muscle. The oculosympathetic pathway consists of a 3-neuron arc (Figure 7.2). The first-order neurons of the sympathetic pathway originate in the posterior hypothalamus, descend to the intermediolateral gray column of the spinal cord, and synapse at the ciliospinal center of Budge at spinal levels C8 to T2. Preganglionic second-order neurons arise from the intermediolateral column, leave the spinal cord by the ventral spinal roots, and enter the rami communicans. They pass though the area of the apex of the lung and join the paravertebral cervical sympathetic chain and ascend through this chain to synapse at the superior cervical ganglion. Postganglionic third-order neurons originate in the superior cervical ganglion, entering the cranium with the internal

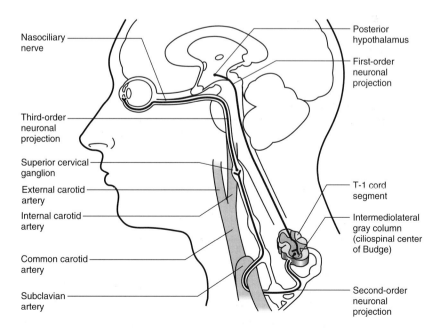

Figure 7.2 Oculosympathetic pathway.

carotid artery. The fibers join the ophthalmic division of the fifth cranial (trigeminal) nerve within the cavernous sinus, reaching the ciliary muscle and pupillary dilator muscle by means of the nasociliary nerve and the long posterior ciliary nerves. Some sympathetic fibers might transiently join the sixth cranial (abducens) nerve within the cavernous sinus.

■ Examination of the Pupils

A pupillary examination begins with a general observation of the pupils. The pupillary reflexes are tested by way of the light-reflex test and the swinging flashlight test (to evaluate the direct and consensual pupillary reflexes) and the near-reflex test (to evaluate the near vision response).

General Pupillary Observation

In a room with standardized ambient light, begin a general observation of the pupils by noting the shape of each pupil and the color of the irides. Have the patient fixate a distance target across the room to minimize accommodation and the accompanying miosis. Sit on 1 side of the seated patient and diffusely illuminate both pupils from below the nose with a handheld light (eg, muscle light), using the least amount of light necessary to discern pupil size (Figure 7.3). Carefully measure the pupil diameter in both eyes with a millimeter ruler, the pupil gauge usually printed on the near vision chart, or an Iowa pupil gauge. Record the size in millimeters in the patient's chart. Refer to "Size (mm)" in Figure 7.4 for an example.

If the patient has anisocoria, the pupillary diameters should be measured under both dim and bright illumination. A subtle degree of anisocoria (usually less than

Figure 7.3 Pupils can be seen in dim light by shining a handheld light on the patient's face from below while the patient looks into the darkness. (Reprinted with permission from Thompson HS, Kardon RH. Clinical importance of pupillary inequality. *Focal Points: Clinical Modules for Ophthalmologists*, Vol. 10, Module 10. San Francisco: American Academy of Ophthalmology; 1992.)

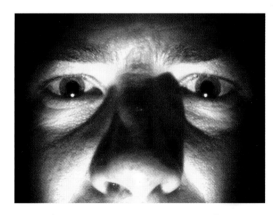

Figure 7.4 Example for recording principal pupillary testing measurements.

	Size (mm)	Briskness of Light Reaction	RAPD	Near Reaction
Pupil OD	4.5	3+		3+
Pupil OS	4.5	2+	2+	3+

1 mm) can be a normal finding and then is called *essential*, or *physiologic*, anisocoria. In physiologic anisocoria, the inequality in pupillary size remains the same under all lighting conditions, and the pupillary light reflexes are equally brisk.

If anisocoria is present, the examiner must document the size in millimeters of the palpebral fissure and note the presence and *degree* of any ptosis. Ptosis found on the side of a larger, sluggish pupil suggests the possibility of oculomotor nerve paresis. Ptosis found on the side of a smaller pupil requires pharmacologic testing to rule out Horner syndrome, which results from a lesion affecting the sympathetic pathway.

Light-Reflex Test

Shining a light in 1 eye normally causes both pupils to constrict equally, a result of the hemidecussation of pupillomotor fibers in both the chiasm and the midbrain tectum. The pupillary reaction in the illuminated eye is called the *direct reflex*, and the reaction in the nonilluminated eye is called the *consensual reflex*. Clinical Protocol 7.1 describes the basic test used to evaluate these light reflexes as they occur in both eyes simultaneously.

Swinging Flashlight Test

The swinging flashlight test is done after the light-reflex test to compare the direct and consensual responses in each eye individually (Clinical Protocol 7.2). This test is used to detect the presence of a relative afferent pupillary defect (also called the *Marcus Gunn pupil*), a critical neuro-ophthalmic sign. During the swinging flashlight test, the examiner briskly alternates illumination from 1 eye to the other several times, noting pupillary response. A normal response is for the pupils to become initially constricted and to remain so as the light is swung from eye to eye. However, if 1 pupil consistently dilates and the other constricts as the light is alternated, a relative afferent pupillary defect is present ipsilateral to the pupil that dilates (Clinical Protocol 7.2).

A relative afferent pupillary defect can be detected even when 1 pupil is bound down by adhesions, paralyzed, or pharmacologically dilated, as long as the contralateral pupil is not. Swinging the light to the eye with optic nerve disease might show no pupillary change in that eye if the pupil is immobile. In such a situation, the degree of consensual response in the normal eye reflects optic nerve activity in the affected eye, and swinging the light to the intact eye should result in further pupillary constriction.

Near-Reflex Test

When a person looks at a near target, 3 reactions normally occur:

- Accommodation (contraction of the ciliary muscle, resulting in increased lens thickness and curvature)
- Convergence (contraction of the medial rectus muscles)
- Miosis (by contraction of the pupillary sphincter)

This combination of actions is called the *near synkinesis*. The term *synkinesis* indicates concurrent or simultaneous movements or contractions. The pupillary near reflex should be normal if the light reflex is normal, but the opposite is not true (see light-near dissociation below). Clinical Protocol 7.3 describes the near-reflex test.

Abnormal Pupils

Pupillary evaluation can reveal a variety of ophthalmic and neurologic abnormalities, including iris muscle damage, lesions of the sympathetic or parasympathetic pathways, optic nerve or retinal pathology, and dorsal midbrain lesions. This section discusses the primary findings commonly encountered when examining the pupils and the implications of those findings. Table 7.1 summarizes the characteristics of pupils in a variety of clinical situations.

Iris Abnormalities

Trauma, surgery, inflammation, or ischemia can damage the iris and alter its appearance. The pupil can be somewhat dilated, sluggishly reactive, and irregular because of traumatic sphincter rupture. There might be notches in the pupillary margin. Additional sequelae of trauma include iritis and reactive miosis. Inflammation can result in anterior and posterior synechiae, affecting the appearance and reactivity of the pupil. Various disorders can cause iris neovascularization with closure of the chamber angle. Developmental anomalies and genetic disorders can be associated with such iris abnormalities as coloboma (congenital absence of part of an ocular tissue), aniridia (absence of the iris), polycoria (more than 1 pupillary opening in the iris), Brushfield spots (white spots on the peripheral iris, usually in Down syndrome), Lisch nodules (melanocytic nodules of the iris in neurofibromatosis), or iris transillumination. Iris abnormalities are best observed at the slit lamp.

Relative Afferent Pupillary Defect

A relative afferent pupillary defect (RAPD), or Marcus Gunn pupil, is detected with the swinging flashlight test, described earlier. An RAPD indicates unilateral or asymmetric damage to the anterior visual pathways (eg, optic nerve disease or extensive retinal damage). Thus, the absence of a RAPD means there is either symmetric damage to the afferent visual system or no damage. It is not seen with symmetric damage to the anterior visual pathways and it is not present in patients with cataract or other media opacities, refractive errors, functional visual loss, or cortical lesions. The RAPD is often proportional to the amount of visual loss. It is graded from +1 to +4, with +4 designating an amaurotic pupil, an extreme example in which the eye shows no direct light reaction as a result of profound optic nerve damage.

Light-Near Dissociation

Light-near dissociation refers to a case in which the patient has significantly better pupillary near reflex than light reflex. Light-near dissociation can result from damage to bilateral structures that constitute the afferent limb of the pupillary light reaction (eg, bilateral optic atrophy) or from damage to the fibers that mediate the pupillary light reflex in the dorsal aspect of the midbrain. Mesencephalic fibers for the near reflex are located more ventrally than fibers for the light reflex. Thus, the

Table 7.1 Pupillary Findings in Common Clinical Situations

Clinical Entity	General Features	Neuroanatomic Site of Lesion	Response to Light and Near Stimulation	Anisocoria?	Response to Mydriatics	Response to Miotics	Response to Other Pharmacologic Agents
Essential (physiologic) anisocoria	Round, regular	Benign, normal finding	Both brisk	No change	Dilates	Constricts	Normal
Traumatized iris	Irregular, notched pupil border on slit-lamp examination	Pupillary iris sphincter muscle	Both variable; depend on extent of damage	Greater in light	Dilates	Variable constriction; depends on extent of damage	NA
Relative afferent pupillary defect (Marcus Gunn pupil)	Round, regular; positive swinging flashlight test	Optic nerve or extensive retinal damage	Affected pupil shows better consensual than direct light reaction	No change	Dilates	Constricts	Normal
Midbrain pupils	Mid-dilated bilaterally	Dorsal midbrain	Poor to light, better to near	No change	Dilates	Constricts	NA
Tonic pupil (Adie's syndrome)	Acutely dilated, eventually can become miotic; sector pupil palsy, vermiform movement	Ciliary ganglion	Absent to light, tonic redilation	Greater in light	Dilates	Constricts	Pilocarpine 0.1% constricts; Mecholyl 2.5% constricts
Pharmacologically dilated pupil	Very large, round, unilateral	Iris sphincter	Fixed at 8–9 mm	Greater in light	Already maximally dilated	No constriction	Pilocarpine 0.5%–2% will not constrict
Oculomotor palsy (nonvascular)	Mid-dilated (5–7 mm), mild to severe ptosis, unilateral	Third cranial nerve; suspect aneurysm	+/– fixed	Greater in light	Dilates	Constricts	Pilocarpine 0.5%–2% will constrict
Horner syndrome	Small, round, mild ptosis, unilateral	Sympathetic pathway	Both brisk	Greater in darkness	Dilates	Constricts	Cocaine 4%–10%: poor or no dilation; Paredrine 1%: poor or no dilation if third-order neuron damage, dilates otherwise
Argyll Robertson pupil	Small, irregular, bilateral	Midbrain	Poor to light, better to near	No change	Poor	Constricts	NA

near-reflex fibers are sometimes spared from the effect of compressive or superficial inflammatory lesions involving the dorsal midbrain.

Light-near dissociation is evident in dorsal midbrain (Parinaud) syndrome, which arises most commonly from a pineal-region tumor compressing the dorsal midbrain but can be caused by multiple sclerosis, stroke, or hydrocephalus. The patient has mid-dilated pupils with light-near dissociation, up-gaze palsy, eyelid retraction, and convergence-retraction nystagmus. The light-near dissociation arises from compression of the superficially located fibers needed for the light reflex; the more ventral near fibers are spared.

Another syndrome that shows light-near dissociation is Argyll Robertson pupil, a rare but classic sign of neurosyphilis (particularly tabes dorsalis). Unlike dorsal midbrain compression, both pupils are miotic. Other causes of light-near dissociation include Adie's tonic pupil (see later in this chapter), severe afferent damage, and Wernicke encephalopathy. Certain disorders such as diabetes mellitus (probably the most common cause of light-near dissociation) and amyloidosis cause light-near dissociation because of their associated peripheral autonomic neuropathies.

Horner Syndrome

Horner syndrome results from damage to ocular sympathetic fibers at any level along the sympathetic pathway (central, preganglionic, or postganglionic neurons). Features of this syndrome include

- Mild ptosis (due to paresis of Müller's muscle)
- Miosis (due to paralysis of the pupillary dilator muscle)
- Ipsilateral decrease in facial sweating (anhidrosis or hypohidrosis)
- Apparent enophthalmos
- Heterochromia iridis (usually in congenital cases)

Other signs include lower eyelid reverse ptosis (the margin of the eyelid is higher than normal) and transient decrease in intraocular pressure. The associated anisocoria is more apparent in dim illumination. A dilation lag is noted when shifting from bright to dim illumination.

Testing

Pharmacologic testing to confirm the diagnosis of Horner syndrome consists of the instillation of a drop of 4% to 10% cocaine solution in each eye, which dilates the normal eye only. It works by blocking the reuptake of norepinephrine from sympathetic nerve endings, allowing the norepinephrine to remain in contact with its effector muscle longer. If the sympathetic pathway on 1 side is interrupted at any level, norepinephrine is not released from the nerve endings; the cocaine will have no effect; and the pupil on that side will remain relatively miotic.

Once the diagnosis of Horner syndrome is confirmed with the cocaine test, hydroxyamphetamine can be used to differentiate central and preganglionic lesions from postganglionic lesions. The hydroxyamphetamine test cannot be performed on the same day as the cocaine test because cocaine interferes with the action of hydroxyamphetamine. One drop of hydroxyamphetamine (Paredrine 1%) is instilled in each eye. Because hydroxyamphetamine stimulates the release of norepinephrine from sympathetic postganglionic nerve terminals, it will fail to dilate the pupil in patients who have postganglionic lesions but will dilate the pupils in those with central or preganglionic lesions.

Differentiation of lesions is clinically useful because central and preganglionic lesions are more likely to be harbingers of serious disease than are postganglionic lesions. For example, central lesions arise from central nervous system vascular events and tumors. Preganglionic lesions are caused by apical lung tumors (Pancoast tumors), chest surgery, and thoracic artery aneurysm. The causes of postganglionic lesions include cluster headaches, dissection of the internal carotid artery, and neck trauma.

Do not perform applanation tonometry, test corneal sensation, or otherwise irritate or touch the corneas before pharmacologic testing; any resulting epithelial defect can lead to unequal absorption of the diagnostic drops and perhaps a false-negative or a false-positive test result.

The Fixed and Dilated Pupil

The differential diagnosis of a fixed, dilated pupil is important to master. This sign can be seen in the following conditions:

- Adie's tonic pupil
- Oculomotor nerve palsy
- Pharmacologic blockade
- Traumatic iris sphincter rupture
- Angle-closure glaucoma

Adie's tonic pupil

Adie's tonic pupil is typically seen as unilateral mydriasis in an otherwise healthy young woman. Acutely the pupil is large, but it diminishes in size over months to years and can become miotic eventually. The pupil shows sluggish, sectoral or no reaction to light and a better response to an accommodative target. Redilation after the near response is tonic (slow). When present, slow, wormlike (vermiform) contractions of the iris help in making the diagnosis. The precise cause of the disorder is unknown. Postganglionic parasympathetic denervation is present, and the lesion is thought to localize to the ciliary ganglion or short posterior ciliary nerves. Many patients with Adie's tonic pupil show impaired knee or ankle jerks and corneal hypesthesia. The condition can be diagnosed by its hypersensitivity to weak miotic drops (*denervation supersensitivity*); an Adie's tonic pupil constricts to 0.05% to 0.1% pilocarpine drops, which affect a normal pupil only minimally.

Oculomotor nerve palsy

Compression of the third cranial (oculomotor) nerve results in the typical features of oculomotor nerve palsy, which include severe ptosis; deficits in elevation, depression and adduction; and a dilated, fixed pupil on the affected side. Because the parasympathetic fibers are located in the peripheral (superficial) portion of the oculomotor nerve as it exits the brain stem, they are typically affected by a compressive lesion (eg, tumor, aneurysm) and spared by a vasculopathic lesion (eg, diabetes mellitus). When acute third cranial nerve palsy is accompanied by pupillary mydriasis, an aneurysm at the junction of the internal carotid and posterior communicating arteries must be vigorously and urgently investigated with appropriate neuroimaging. Other causes of oculomotor palsy include brain tumor, basal meningitis, or uncal herniation. Vasculopathic (diabetic, hypertensive) oculomotor nerve palsy usually spares the pupil.

Pharmacologic blockade

Pharmacologic blockade is one of the most frequent causes of a dilated and fixed pupil in an otherwise healthy patient. It results from purposeful or inadvertent instillation of atropine-like drugs into the eyes. It can be differentiated from a dilated pupil accompanying third cranial nerve palsy or Adie syndrome by the absence of ptosis and motility abnormalities and by failure of the pupil to constrict upon instillation of pilocarpine 1% drops into the eye. These drops would cause constriction of a mydriatic pupil accompanying an oculomotor palsy.

Other causes

Another cause of pupillary mydriasis is traumatic iris sphincter rupture. Careful slit-lamp examination will reveal irregular pupillary borders at the sites of sphincter rupture. Acute angle-closure glaucoma classically presents with a mid-dilated and poorly reactive pupil; look for a red eye with corneal edema and increased intraocular pressure.

Pitfalls and Pointers

- Unilateral blindness, or a unilateral relative afferent pupillary defect, does not cause anisocoria. Whereas the pupil on the defective side might react only sluggishly or not at all to direct light stimulation, it will constrict consensually when the normal contralateral eye is stimulated (due to the double decussation of pupillomotor fibers).
- A relative afferent pupillary defect indicates that the afferent visual pathway is defective on 1 side in comparison with the contralateral pathway (the adjective relative emphasizes this). There is no such thing as a bilateral relative afferent pupillary defect.
- When performing the swinging flashlight test, be careful to spend equal time with the light illuminating each pupil to avoid differential bleaching of photoreceptors and possible artifactitious relative afferent pupillary defect. Marked anisocoria or prolonged occlusion can also cause differential photoreceptor bleaching that can confound pupillary testing.
- Recognize that pupil-involving oculomotor nerve palsy is often a harbinger of cerebral aneurysm. Perform the workup expeditiously, and obtain a neurosurgical consultation immediately; delay in diagnosis can have life-threatening consequences.
- When performing pharmacologic pupillary testing, instill drops in both eyes for comparison.
- Media opacities such as cataract or even dense vitreous hemorrhage almost never cause a relative afferent pupillary defect.
- Do not administer hydroxyamphetamine on the same day as cocaine (for diagnosis of Horner syndrome), because cocaine interferes with the action of hydroxyamphetamine.

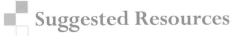

Suggested Resources

Burde RM, Savino PJ, Trobe JD. *Clinical Decisions in Neuro-Ophthalmology.* 3rd ed. St Louis: Mosby-Year Book; 2002.

Neuro-Ophthalmology. Basic and Clinical Science Course, Section 5. San Francisco: American Academy of Ophthalmology; published annually.

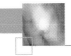

Clinical Protocol 7.1 **Performing the Light-Reflex Test**

1. Under dim room illumination, ask the patient to maintain fixation on a distance target, such as a large letter on the Snellen acuity chart.

2. Shine a bright handheld light directly into the right eye by approaching it from the side or from below. Do not stand in front of the patient or allow the patient to look directly at the light, which would stimulate the near reflex and preclude accurate light-reflex testing.

3. Record the direct pupillary response to light in the right eye in terms of the briskness of the response, graded from 0, indicating no response, to 4+, indicating a brisk response (see "Briskness of Light Reaction" in Figure 7.4).

4. Repeat steps 1 to 3 for the left eye.

5. Repeat steps 1 and 2 in the right eye, observing the consensual reflex by noting the response to the light of the nonilluminated (left) pupil. The rapidity of the response and change in pupil size should normally be equivalent to that seen in the direct light reaction and is graded on the same numeric scale.

6. Repeat steps 1, 2, and 5 in the left eye.

Clinical Protocol 7.2 **Performing the Swinging Flashlight Test**

1. Under dim room illumination with the patient fixating a distance target, illuminate the patient's right eye directly with a bright handheld light, in a manner identical to that used when testing the light reflex (Figure 1A). Note the pupillary constriction in both eyes.

2. Move the light beam immediately and swiftly over the bridge of the patient's nose to the left eye, noting the pupillary response in that eye. Take care to illuminate each pupil from the same angle. Normally, the pupil will either constrict slightly or remain at its previous size (Figure 1B). If, instead, the pupil dilates when the light illuminates it (ie, the direct light reflex is weaker than the consensual reflex), a relative afferent pupillary defect is present, which usually indicates a disorder of the optic nerve or severe retinal pathology (Figure 1C).

3. Quickly swing the light back to the right eye and evaluate the response. A normal response is again a mild constriction or no change in size at all. Net pupillary constriction or dilation is an abnormal response.

4. Repeat steps 1 to 3 rhythmically, spending equal intervals illuminating each pupil, until it is clear whether pupillary responses are normal or whether 1 pupil consistently dilates.

5. Record a relative afferent pupillary defect (RAPD) as 1+ to 4+, with 1+ indicating a mild afferent defect and 4+ indicating an amaurotic pupil, a severe defect in which the affected eye shows no direct light response (see "RAPD" in Figure 7.4).

(continued)

Clinical Protocol 7.2 *(continued)*

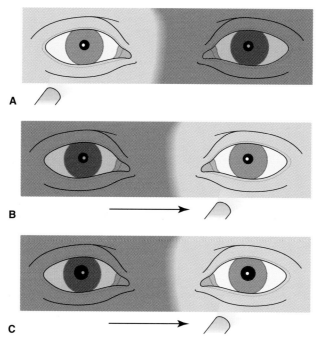

Figure 1   Swinging flashlight test. **(A)** Illuminating the patient's right eye. **(B)** Illuminating the patient's left eye. **(C)** Dilation indicating a relative afferent pupillary defect.

Clinical Protocol 7.3  **Performing the Near-Reflex Test**

1. Under normal room illumination, ask the patient to fixate a distance target.

2. While seated next to the patient, move a detailed target toward the patient's line of vision at near. (The patient's thumb is sometimes an excellent near target, providing proprioceptive as well as visual near clues to ensure adequate near efforts.) A flashlight should not be used for this purpose.

3. Instruct the patient to shift fixation to the near target. If using the patient's thumb as a target, the examiner holds the patient's thumb and moves it, asking the patient to view it intently.

4. Observe the pupillary reflex when the patient shifts fixation to the near target. Normal pupils constrict upon viewing the near target.

5. Repeat steps 1 to 4 several times.

6. Record the near reaction in terms of the briskness of the response, graded from 0, for no response, to 4+, for brisk response (see "Near Reaction" in Figure 7.4).

Visual Field Examination

8

The field of vision is that portion of a subject's surroundings that is visible at any one time. The visual field properly includes central fixation or foveal vision, conventionally measured by visual acuity tests, and extrafoveal (or peripheral) vision. Visual acuity, or foveal vision, and the peripheral visual field are tested in different ways and provide information on different aspects of visual function. Visual acuity testing measures the eye's greatest resolution, the ability to identify forms. Visual field testing measures peripheral sensitivity, the ability to detect light or motion at different locations.

The visual field of each eye can be tested separately by 1 or more tests. The visual fields are routinely screened with the confrontation fields test. If macular disease is suspected to be causing a central visual field defect, a device called an *Amsler grid* is used to test the central area of each eye's visual field. If a visual field defect is detected by screening, or symptoms suggest a high likelihood of peripheral field loss, further evaluation is conducted by manual or automated procedures known as *perimetry*. Perimetry is used to document the presence and severity of a visual field defect and to monitor progression of previously known visual field loss.

■ The Visual Field

The visual field is an inverted and reversed map of corresponding retinal points. The normal visual field extends about 50° superiorly, 60° nasally, 70° inferiorly, and 90° temporally from fixation. The visual field can be divided into central, intermediate, and peripheral zones. The central zone includes an area from the fixation point to a circle 30° away (a 5 mm radius from the fovea). The central zone contains the temporal physiologic blind spot, which corresponds to the optic nerve head centered about 15° nasally from the fovea. The intermediate zone extends from 30° to 50° and the peripheral zone is the area beyond 50°.

A *scotoma*, one type of *visual field defect*, is a place in the visual field where an object cannot be seen, surrounded by normal visual field. A *relative scotoma* is an area in the visual field where test objects of low luminance cannot be seen, but larger or brighter ones can. An *absolute scotoma* is an area where no test object can be seen (eg, the physiologic blind spot). Other types of visual field defects include arcuate defects and hemianopias.

Perimetry is the measurement of the visual field using either moving objects (kinetic perimetry) or stationary test stimuli (static perimetry). In kinetic perimetry, points along the edge of the visual field are determined by finding the weakest light stimulus (visual threshold) that evokes a visual sensation. The line that joins points having the same threshold is called an *isopter*. In static perimetry, the use of static targets that change in brightness gives a threshold map of different points.

The normal field of vision varies with the size, color, brightness, and movement of the test stimulus, or target; with the background illumination; and with a patient's alertness and familiarity with the test. Unlike all other portions of the ophthalmic examination, visual fields are conventionally recorded on charts that represent the field as the *patient sees it* (ie, the temporal field of the right eye is to the right), and the field for the right eye is always placed to the right when comparing the visual field maps of both eyes.

The visual field is a 3-dimensional concept that is presented in 2 dimensions (Figure 8.1A). Different types of perimetry give maps with different appearances. A visual field performed by kinetic perimetry (eg, with the Goldmann perimeter) is plotted on polar graph paper (Figure 8.1B) with radial meridians (measured counterclockwise from 0° at the right-hand horizontal) and circles of eccentricity (concentric rings every 10° out from fixation). With such a map obtained by kinetic perimetry, the examiner looks down onto the "hill of vision," with its contours represented by isopters. Most maps produced by automated static perimetry present an array of sensitivity values; these values can also be pictured by the program in gray tones—the gray scale. (Figure 8.1C). Darker shading indicates less visual sensitivity.

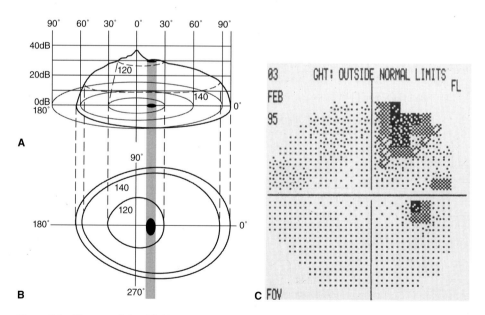

Figure 8.1 The normal visual field and the maps produced by different types of perimetry. **(A)** Three-dimensional model of the right eye's "island of vision surrounded by a sea of blindness." The horizontal plane indicates degrees (circles) of eccentricity and meridians. The vertical axis is plotted in decibels of visual sensitivity. **(B)** Topography of the visual field represented by plotting isopters on polar coordinates using kinetic perimetry. **(C)** Grayscale rendering computed by automated perimetry.

■ Screening Tests

Visual field screening is routinely done at a patient's initial eye examination. The confrontation fields test can screen for moderate to severe visual field defects, but confrontation testing is often unreliable for detecting mild visual field loss, as in early glaucoma. The Amsler grid, used when the patient has symptoms of central distortion or loss, helps evaluate macular function. Both screening tests are discussed in the following sections.

Confrontation Fields Testing

Confrontation testing of a patient's visual fields is done in a face-to-face position at a distance of about 1 meter (3 feet). By convention, the right eye is tested first, although if there is a marked difference in visual acuity it is advisable to begin with the better eye. The eye not being tested must be completely occluded, by using a handheld or press-on occluder, by putting a folded facial tissue under an elastic eye occluder, or by asking the patient to cover the eye with the palm of the hand. When the patient's left eye is covered, the examiner's right eye should be closed, and vice versa, to permit comparison. The examiner presents fingers midway between himself or herself and the patient, testing all 4 quadrants (Figure 8.2).

To assess the patient's visual field, patient's responses are compared to the examiner's normal visual field. To outline the visual field determined by the confrontation screening method, the examiner's hand is slowly brought inward from different directions, testing each of the patient's meridians. Clinical Protocol 8.1 provides instructions for performing the confrontation fields test.

Amsler Grid Test

The Amsler grid is used to test the central 10° to 20° of each eye's visual field. It helps test for suspected macular disease that produces a central scotoma, or metamorphopsia (distortion). The Amsler grid is a white or red pattern of lines with a central spot printed on a black background (Figure 8.3A). When viewed at a

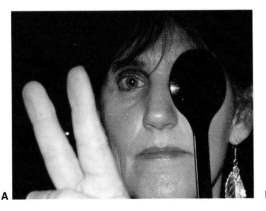
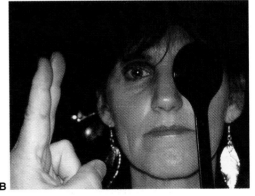

A   **B**

Figure 8.2   The confrontation fields test. **(A)** Correct presentation of fingers, side by side frontally. **(B)** Incorrect presentation, so that 1 finger hides the other. (Reprinted by permission from Walsh TJ, ed. *Visual Fields: Examination and Interpretation.* 2nd ed. Ophthalmology Monograph 3. San Francisco: American Academy of Ophthalmology; 1996.)

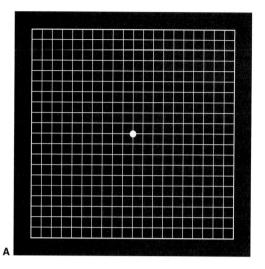
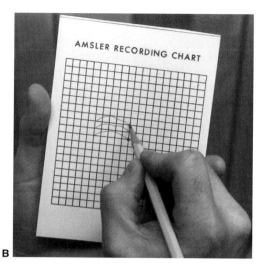

A   B

Figure 8.3   The Amsler grid. **(A)** The test pattern has white or red lines on a black background. **(B)** The patient draws the central field defect on the preprinted pad that has black lines on a white background.

distance of 30 cm (about 12 inches) using near correction, the lines are 1° apart. A patient with no abnormalities perceives the lines as straight and complete. Patients with abnormalities report distorted or missing lines, which they can record themselves on a preprinted black-on-white version of the grid (Figure 8.3B). Clinical Protocol 8.2 gives instructions for Amsler grid testing.

Special Situations

Confrontation testing to screen for visual field defects might not be possible in infants, obtunded patients, and patients with optic nerve disease. Alternative screening methods for such patients are described in the following sections.

Reflex eye movement test for infants

Test the visual field of infants and toddlers by making use of their involuntary fixational reflexes. First get the child's attention in a frontal gaze. While the child is watching your face, silently bring an interesting toy or other object from the periphery to elicit fixational head and eye movements.

Blink reflex test for obtunded patients

Quickly flicking your hand toward a sighted patient's open eye normally elicits a blink reflex. This test can help find a dense hemianopia or quadrantanopia.

■ Manual Perimetry

A perimeter is an instrument that measures the visual field by the patient's subjective responses. A perimeter is used to quantify or confirm a visual field defect discovered or suspected through screening, to detect subtle field defects not detected

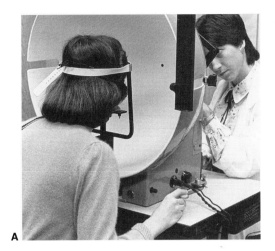
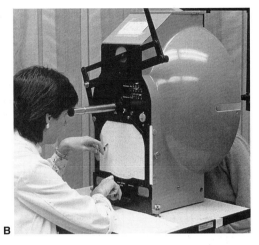

A   B

Figure 8.4   Goldmann perimetry. **(A)** From the patient's side. **(B)** From the examiner's side.

by confrontation testing, such as those associated with early glaucomatous damage, and to monitor changes in a previously known condition. The Goldmann perimeter is used to perform kinetic perimetry.

The Goldmann perimeter tests the entire visual field, using different target sizes and intensities. The Goldmann perimeter plots the visual field in degrees of arc.

The Goldmann perimeter is a hemispheric dome with a white background that is illuminated near the lower limit of photopic vision. A movable pantographic device permits a light target to be projected within the dome, continuously or intermittently, at various sizes and brightness levels (Figure 8.4). The examiner directly observes the patient's visual fixation from behind the dome through a telescope, and the patient responds to stimuli with a buzzer.

Six different target sizes are available, each 4 times the size of the previous target: 0 (0.0625 mm²), I (0.25 mm²), II (1 mm²), III (4 mm²), IV (16 mm²), and V (64 mm²). Target brightness (intensity) is measured in decibels (dB). Gray filters allow the brightness of the target to be reduced in 0.5 dB steps from 4 to 1 and in 0.1 dB steps from e to a. Perimetry almost always begins with target size I and intensity 4e (this isopter line would be labeled I4e on the diagram). Larger targets (II to V) are chosen if this isopter is revealed to be constricted. The choice of targets is usually limited to 2 or 3 of the following: I2, I4, II4, IV4, and V4.

■ Automated Perimetry

Automated static perimetry can often detect smaller or shallower defects than kinetic perimetry. Because the testing is tedious and time consuming, most modern static perimeters are computerized, and new automated instrumentation continues to be developed. Humphrey visual field analysis is the most commonly used computerized system, with an elaborate software package to perform various statistical evaluations. Automation has the ability to compare results statistically with normal individuals of the same age group and with previous tests for the same patient. Also, automated perimetry does not require as highly skilled operators as are needed for manual perimetry, and it eliminates certain operator errors. Some patients, such as young children and individuals who need vigorous encouragement to maintain fixation, might not be good candidates for automated perimetry.

Test Targets and Strategies

The standard target size for automated perimetry is equivalent to a Goldmann size III (4 mm²) white target. The number of points tested determines test time. Since automated static perimetry is fatiguing for the patient, the number of test points should be limited as much as possible. The most commonly used tests explore 50 to 120 test points. Different software programs test different areas of the visual field, depending on the specific disorder known or suspected. Program selection depends on whether the visual field examination is done for diagnostic testing of a suspected defect or for followup of a progressive condition. For example, a glaucoma test includes extra points to detect such common glaucomatous visual field defects as a nasal step or an arcuate defect, whereas neurologic visual field testing emphasizes points along the vertical meridian and within the central field, where many neurologic visual field defects may be found.

For most patients with glaucoma or a neuro-ophthalmologic condition, a 30° or a 24° field is appropriate. The Central 30-2 test is an example of a program that evaluates the central 30° with 76 points. It is commonly used for monitoring glaucoma patients and for detecting neurologic visual field defects. The 24-2 test (54 points) provides a 24° field from fixation with an extension of the nasal field to 30°, using a 6° grid. The 2 in the designation 24-2 test indicates a grid that straddles the horizontal and vertical meridians. The 24-2 test is generally preferred for testing most patients (instead of a 30-1 or 24-1 test, which align the grid onto the vertical and horizontal meridians).

Deficits less than 6° in diameter or located in the far periphery may be missed by the 30-2 and 24-2 tests. For patients with central visual field loss, the Central 10-2 test may be appropriate for sequential testing, because it tests the central 10° field with a 2° grid. For patients with peripheral visual field defects, Goldmann perimetry may be useful.

Interpretation of a Computerized Printout

Printed test results show basic patient information such as age and pupillary diameter. The raw data from automated static perimetry are shown as reliability measures and as the numeric plot, the actual sensitivity values at each tested point (Figure 8.5). The printout also presents statistical calculations showing how the patient varies from the expected normal. The examiner must look at the reliability measures, the numeric plot, the probability maps, and the global indices.

The reliability measures are the proportion of fixation losses, false-positive errors, and false-negative errors. Fixation loss is the proportion of times that the patient responded inappropriately, because of wandering fixation, to a stimulus at the presumed blind spot. The false-positive error rate is the proportion of times that the patient responded when no stimulus was presented. The false-negative error rate is the proportion of times that the patient did not respond when a suprathreshold

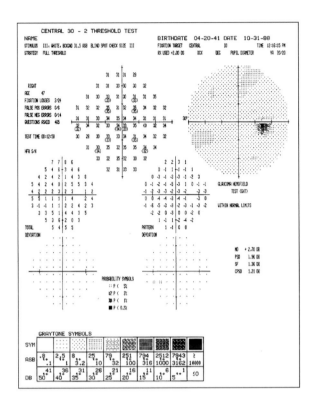

Figure 8.5 Computerized printout record of automated static perimetry. (Courtesy California Pacific Medical Center.)

stimulus (ie, a luminance that had been seen earlier in the test) was presented. The printout flags these parameters with *xx* when low reliability is suspected. The examination is unreliable if 3 or more of the following parameters occur:

- Total questions ≥ 400
- Fixation loss ≥ 20%
- False-positive responses ≥ 33%
- False-negative responses ≥ 33%
- Short-term fluctuation ≥ 4.0 dB (described in the following paragraphs)

The numeric plot gives the measured threshold values at each test point. Recall that a higher number means a dimmer light, and thus a more sensitive visual area. Repeated determinations are given in parentheses under the retested value. The darker the area, the greater the loss of sensitivity for a given target size. Because data between test points are extrapolated, the grayscale might not be accurate.

The global indices are MD (mean deviation from age-corrected normal), PSD (pattern standard deviation), SF (short-term fluctuation), and CPSD (corrected pattern standard deviation). MD is the average decibel value of the entire total deviation plot and is flagged if there is substantially depressed sensitivity, whether generalized or localized. PSD is a measure of the variability across the total deviation plot. SF is a measure of the variability of repeated determinations at 10 standard locations. SF of greater than 4.0 dB is considered to be an unreliable examination. CPSD is derived from PSD and SF to indicate the variability between adjacent points that could be due to disease rather than test-retest error. For each global index, the statistical significance is given, which is the probability of finding the obtained value in a healthy person.

Automated visual field results are not self-explanatory. The examiner must distinguish artifact from disease to account for an abnormal test.

■ Common Visual Field Defects

An abnormal visual field test result should be described in the medical record according to which eye is involved, the shape of the field abnormality, its location, and its symmetry. These attributes, and certain typical perimetric patterns, help to localize a lesion along the visual pathway. Table 8.1 lists some common descriptions of visual field defects, some of which are discussed in the next paragraphs.

Figure 8.6 shows a variety of commonly seen shapes of visual field defects together with a diagram of their anatomic origins. One of the most common shapes is a scotoma, a localized defect surrounded by detectable visual field. Some examples of common scotomas associated with glaucoma are shown in Figure 8.7. These scotomas often extend from the blind spot or appear to make the visual field smaller (peripheral constriction).

A Bjerrum scotoma, a monocular isolated paracentral defect, is an example of an arcuate scotoma, so called because it yields an arc-like shape when plotted. This crescentic form is caused by the normal course of the retinal ganglion cell nerve fibers. Defects in the arcuate zone can connect with the blind spot (Seidel scotoma), appear as 1 or more scattered paracentral scotomas, or end at the horizontal raphe (Rønne's nasal step). A nasal step is a scotoma that, when plotted, abuts onto the horizontal meridian and appears as a step-like loss of vision at the outer limit of the nasal field. An altitudinal defect is one that causes loss of the upper or lower visual field. There also can be generalized depression in which visual sensitivity is diffusely reduced.

A binocular visual field defect in each eye's hemifield is called a *hemianopia*. Incomplete hemianopias are referred to as *quadrantanopias* and *sectoral defects*. A chiasmal or retrochiasmal lesion produces visual field defects that respect the vertical meridian and that remain in 1 hemifield of each eye (see Figure 8.6). Retinal

Table 8.1 Terms Used to Describe Visual Field Defects

Type of Defect	Terms
Monocular field defects	Localized defects: wedge-shaped temporal field defect, arcuate nasal field defect, central scotoma, enlarged blind spot, cecocentral scotoma, annular scotoma Generalized defects: generalized depression, peripheral constriction
Binocular field defects	Homonymous hemianopias: with macular splitting, with macular sparing, with unilateral sparing of temporal crescent Bitemporal hemianopias Binasal hemianopias Quadrantanopias

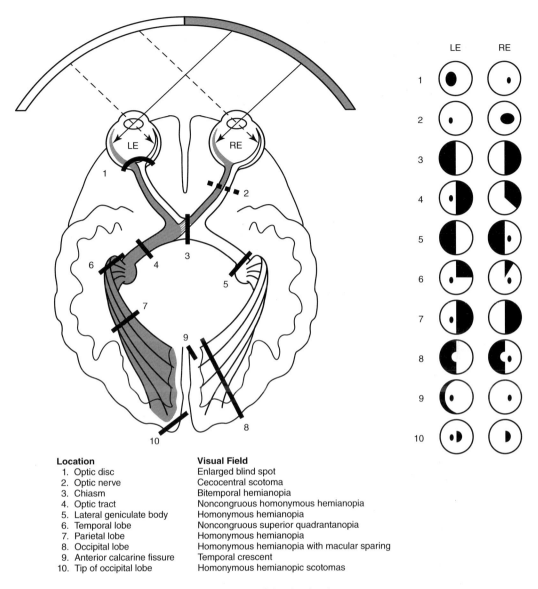

Location
1. Optic disc
2. Optic nerve
3. Chiasm
4. Optic tract
5. Lateral geniculate body
6. Temporal lobe
7. Parietal lobe
8. Occipital lobe
9. Anterior calcarine fissure
10. Tip of occipital lobe

Visual Field
Enlarged blind spot
Cecocentral scotoma
Bitemporal hemianopia
Noncongruous homonymous hemianopia
Homonymous hemianopia
Noncongruous superior quadrantanopia
Homonymous hemianopia
Homonymous hemianopia with macular sparing
Temporal crescent
Homonymous hemianopic scotomas

Figure 8.6 Abnormal visual fields produced by lesions of the visual pathways.

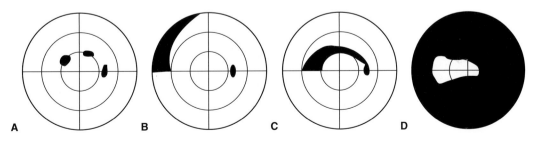

Figure 8.7 Visual field defects produced by glaucomatous optic neuropathy (right eye). **(A)** Paracentral scotomata. **(B)** Superior nasal step. **(C)** Arcuate scotoma. **(D)** Advanced peripheral constriction.

and optic nerve lesions produce visual field defects that can cross the vertical meridian (see Figure 8.7).

A hemianopia can be homonymous (ie, impairing visual function on the same side of each eye), bitemporal, or binasal. Quadrantanopias and altitudinal defects are described as being superior or inferior.

Retrochiasmal field defects that are similar between the 2 eyes are called *congruous*, and defects that are asymmetric or differently sized for each eye are *incongruous*. Because corresponding fibers from the 2 retinas lie close together as they near the visual cortex, lesions of the posterior radiations tend to be congruous, while anterior retrochiasmal lesions are more frequently incongruous.

Localizing Visual Field Defects

The physician needs to know the typical patterns obtained in perimetry to determine the probable location of a lesion. A decision-making approach based on knowledge of neuroanatomy helps the examiner make an accurate medical interpretation. Figure 8.8 depicts a variety of common perimetric defects and their likely anatomic origins.

Progression

Visual fields often must be tested on several occasions to get a reliable picture of the patient's status. Chronic diseases such as glaucoma can produce progressive visual field loss that might be detected before optic nerve or other changes are visible (Figure 8.9).

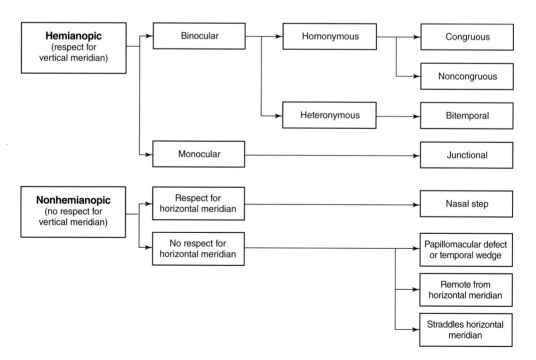

Figure 8.8 Interpretation tree for visual field defects. (From Trobe JD, Glaser JS. *The Visual Fields Manual: A Practical Guide to Testing and Interpretation.* Gainesville, FL: Triad; 1983.)

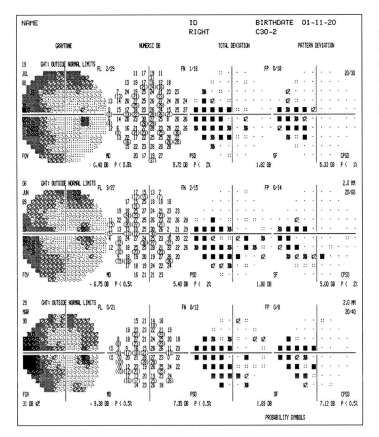

Figure 8.9 Progressive visual field loss as detected by repeat automated perimetry in a patient with chronic glaucoma.

Pitfalls and Pointers

Remember the "rules of the road" when interpreting visual field defects:

- Unilateral optic nerve disease causes unilateral visual field defects.
- Nasal retinal nerve fibers cross in the chiasm to go to the contralateral optic tract while temporal retinal nerve fibers remain uncrossed.
- Lesions involving the chiasm and retrochiasmal pathways cause visual field defects that respect the vertical meridian.
- Retrochiasmal lesions produce a contralateral homonymous hemianopia.
- The more posterior the lesion occurs in the post-chiasmal pathway, the more likely the defects to be congruous.

Suggested Resources

Anderson DR, Patella VM. *Automated Static Perimetry*. 2nd ed. St Louis: CV Mosby; 1999.

Choplin NT, Edwards RP. *Visual Field Testing With the Humphrey Field Analyzer*. Thorofare, NJ: Slack; 1999.

Glaucoma. Basic and Clinical Science Course, Section 10. San Francisco: American Academy of Ophthalmology; published annually.

Henson DB. *Visual Fields.* New York: Oxford University Press; 1993.

OTAC Glaucoma Panel. *Automated Perimetry* [Ophthalmic Technology Assessment]. San Francisco: American Academy of Ophthalmology; 2002.

Walsh TJ, ed. *Visual Fields: Examination and Interpretation.* Ophthalmology Monograph 3. 2nd ed. San Francisco: American Academy of Ophthalmology; 1996.

Clinical Protocol 8.1 — Performing the Confrontation Fields Test

Test Setup

1. Seat the patient and occlude the eye not being tested.

2. Facing the patient at a distance of about 1 m, close your eye that is directly opposite the patient's occluded eye.

3. Ask the patient to fixate on your nose or on your open eye.

Check for Scotoma

1. *Finger counting.* Hold your hands stationary midway between yourself and the patient in opposite quadrants about 30° from central fixation (60 cm [24 inches] from your mutual axis). Quickly present then retract a finger or fingers on 1 hand in 1 quadrant of the monocular field, asking the patient to state the number. To avoid confusion, limit the number of fingers shown to 1, 2, and 5, and hold the fingers side by side in the frontal plane. Repeat in all 4 quadrants, testing at least 2 times per quadrant.

   a. Test patients who cannot count fingers by waving your hand and asking if the patient perceives the motion. With patients who can perceive only light, test for the ability to determine the direction of light projection by pointing a muscle light or penlight toward the pupil while keeping the patient's other eye completely shielded. Repeat in all 4 quadrants.

   b. Test young children with a finger-mimicking procedure. First teach the child to hold up the same number of fingers as you do, then conduct the test as usual. Test rapidly, because a child will soon glance directly at your hand (although this involuntary movement can also indicate a normal response).

2. *Simultaneous finger counting.* Present fingers simultaneously in opposite quadrants, asking the patient to state the total number, using the following combinations: 1 and 1, 1 and 2, and 2 and 2. This test can reveal a more subtle field defect than finger counting in each quadrant separately. Sometimes a patient with a relative scotoma can detect fingers presented to the defective hemifield but has problems with simultaneous targets.

3. *Simultaneous comparison.* Hold both palms toward the patient, close to the line of sight, in opposite superior, then inferior, quadrants. Ask the patient to state whether 1 hand appears darker or less distinct. This test is very subjective and relies on equal illumination but can reveal a subtle defect in a hemifield.

   a. A similar test can be done by asking the patient to compare the relative hue or intensity of 2 identically colored objects, such as the red caps of 2 eyedropper bottles. Hold the targets in separate quadrants. If there is a hemianopia, the patient might describe 1 cap as red and the other as faded or colorless. This test can also be done with 1 colored item by bringing it across from a defective to a normal area, to determine whether there is a sudden change in intensity.

   b. Check a central scotoma by comparing central and eccentric locations, using hands or other identical objects.

Clinical Protocol 8.1 *(continued)*

Diagram the Confrontation Field

1. If an abnormality is detected, sketch a 360° visual field chart, labeled for right and left eye and temporal and nasal field, and plot the visual field as the patient sees it (Figure 1). If the patient can count fingers in all 4 quadrants, one may record the results as *counts fingers × 4*.

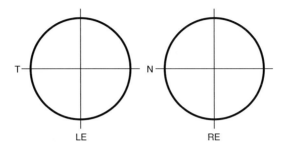

Figure 1 Sample chart for plotting the visual field as the patient sees it.

Clinical Protocol 8.2 **Performing the Amsler Grid Test**

Test Setup

1. With the patient wearing appropriate reading spectacles or trial lenses for near correction, ask the patient to hold the testing grid perpendicular to the line of sight, approximately 30 cm (about 12 inches) from the eye. Occlude the eye not being tested.

Check for Scotoma

1. Ask the patient to fixate steadily at the central spot of the grid.
2. Ask the patient whether any of the straight lines appear distorted or missing.

Diagram the Test Result

1. Have the patient draw the area of visual distortion or loss on the preprinted Amsler grid notepad (see Figure 8.3B). Be sure to note the date, patient's name, and tested eye. Test both eyes and record all results, whether abnormal or not.

External Examination

The external ocular examination consists of a 3-part stepwise sequence that focuses the examiner's senses on the patient: inspection (looking), palpation (feeling), and auscultation (listening). These methods are accompanied by specific clinical measurements as necessary. A fixed sequence of examination steps helps ensure that the examiner has covered all anatomic details and physiologic functions of the external eye. With experience, screening a patient's external features will occur almost automatically. The patient's history and appearance should lead the examiner to the appropriate testing techniques, so the many available examination tasks described in this chapter need not be applied in their entirety to every patient.

A thoughtful and thorough external examination can yield considerable information that directs the course of the rest of the examination. This chapter details the application of the 3 principal steps in the external ophthalmic examination and provides instruction in a variety of measurement and evaluation techniques that are commonly used in this part of a comprehensive ophthalmic examination.

■ Situating the Patient

The patient usually sits in the examining chair for the examination. Young children often do well sitting on their parent's lap. An uncooperative infant or toddler can be laid flat on a bed or padded table and immobilized by having the parent hold the child's upstretched arms firmly against the sides of the child's head while leaning against the child's legs and body. Very young infants can be swaddled (Figure 9.1).

■ General Observation

Before the detailed external ocular examination begins, the examiner usually conducts a brief visual survey of the entire patient, being attentive for signs of medical, dermatologic, and neurologic disease. This general physical observation may occur during casual pre-examination conversation or history taking. By observing the patient's specific actions and appearance, especially the facial features around the eyes, the examiner can often find clues to the patient's attitude, overall well-being, and general physical or ocular problem. Sometimes an examiner can recognize a disease pattern by an initial intuition. Other times, the history will direct the examiner's attention to a specific abnormality.

Observing the patient in a lighted room before the stepwise ocular inspection gives many clues to anatomic deformities and illness. During this observation,

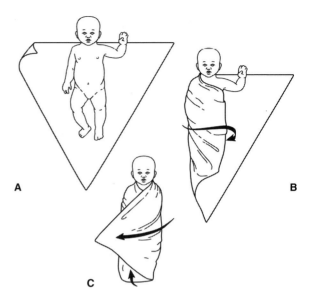

Figure 9.1 How to bundle a baby for an eye examination. **(A)** Fold a sheet into an equilateral triangle and lay the supine infant on it, with the infant's head just above the top edge. **(B)** Fold 1 side over the infant to pin 1 arm against the body, tucking the edge of the sheet under the child's body and tucking the bottom flap of the sheet up over the baby's feet. **(C)** Hold the other arm against the baby's side while pulling the other edge over the baby's body and tuck the edge underneath the child.

note the patient's demeanor, mental status, complexion, and apparent nutritional health, along with any abnormal movements, disabilities, or stigmata. Some conditions with obvious features are quickly recognizable, such as albinism and Down syndrome. The extremities, especially the hands, can give clues to systemic diseases, such as rheumatoid arthritis. Focusing on the face and ocular adnexa can reveal skin conditions, such as rosacea, and other disorders that can affect the eyes.

During the external examination, the examiner looks for any disturbance in the following sequence:

- Head and face: bones, muscles, nerves and blood vessels; skin; lymph nodes; mouth, nose, and paranasal sinuses
- Orbit
- Eyelids
- Lacrimal system
- Globe

■ Inspection

The inspection is a visual survey of the external eye and, like the general observation, often begins while talking to the patient. The basic equipment for the external examination should be readily available (Table 9.1). Clinical measurements that are taken during the external examination are assessed for symmetry and compared with expected values. Each visible or palpable mass is measured in the longest dimension and its perpendicular.

Head and Face

Obtain different perspectives of the person's head and face, beginning at a talking distance and then proceeding to closer inspection and magnified views. A sketch

Table 9.1   Equipment for Examining the External Eye

Equipment	Use
Illuminators:	
Room light or natural sunlight	Gross observation of skin abnormalities and other diseases; globe evaluation
Finnoff transilluminator ("muscle light")	Evaluation of masses or lesions of eyelid and globe; transscleral illumination; estimation of anterior chamber depth
Penlight or pocket flashlight	Diffuse illumination at bedside; evaluation of masses or lesions of eyelid and globe; near PD measurement
Handheld illuminator with slit aperture	Assessment of axial and peripheral anterior chamber
Blue or UV light source	Tear outflow testing with fluorescein
Direct ophthalmoscope	Transpupillary retroillumination; magnified examination of skin or eye lesions
Retinoscope	Detection of refractive changes caused by abnormal corneal topography and lens opacities
Magnifiers:	
Condensing lens	Assessment of eyelid lesions
Loupes (2×–3×)	Assessment of eyelid and eye lesions
Slit-lamp biomicroscope	Assessment of skin and external ocular lesions
Measuring devices:	
Millimeter ruler	Measurement of lesion dimensions, lid positions, intercanthal and interpupillary distances, globe displacement, and corneal diameter
Exophthalmometer	Measurement of exophthalmos and intercanthal distance
Calipers or gauge	Measurement of corneal diameter
Ophthalmodynamometer	Measurement of ophthalmic arterial pressure
Listening devices:	
Stethoscope	Auscultation of orbit, neck, and chest
Blood pressure cuff	Measurement of brachial arterial pressure
Retractors:	
Cotton-tipped applicators	Raising and lowering eyelids; lid eversion
Metallic retractors	Eyelid double eversion; opening eyelid in young child
Pharmaceuticals and supplies:	
Fluorescein solution or strips	Tear film testing and ocular surface status
Schirmer strips	Tear film testing
pH indicator paper	Tear pH testing
Anesthetic eyedrops	Tear film testing and easing pain
Anesthetic gel	Lacrimal probing
Wire swab	Nasal examination
Tongue depressor	Mouth and throat examination
Lacrimal set:	
Punctal dilator	Punctal dilation
Lacrimal probes	Lacrimal probing
Lacrimal cannula with 3mL syringe	Lacrimal irrigation
Nasal speculum	Nasal examination
Protective devices:	
Examination gloves	Examiner and patient protection
Safety spectacles	Examiner protection

or photograph of the patient's face can be made to document any abnormalities. Measuring the occipitofrontal circumference of the head with a tape measure, along with other growth measurements such as height and weight, helps to assess children with developmental delay.

Inspect the face for symmetry and craniofacial bone development, looking for evidence of old trauma, clefting syndromes, and hemifacial atrophy. Following this, evaluate the mobility of the facial muscles. Any suspected motor or sensory abnormality is tested by special techniques (Clinical Protocol 9.1). Corneal sensation may be tested at this time, if indicated.

Inspect the facial skin for dermal and vascular changes. Observe the skin's color, texture, tone, and moisture. A magnifying lens such as the +20 D condensing lens used in indirect ophthalmoscopy, the direct ophthalmoscope, 2× to 3× binocular loupes, and low magnification with the slit-lamp biomicroscope can help in assessing individual skin lesions. Common skin abnormalities are classified by the most distinctive characteristic (Table 9.2). The distinguishing attributes of skin abnormalities that should be noted are size, elevation, color, margination, depth of involvement, distribution, surface changes, and degree of tissue destruction.

Lymph nodes are normally not visible or palpable. Gross enlargement of any node should be noted. The examiner may palpate for preauricular and cervical lymph nodes before inspecting other external features, particularly when considering infection, granulomatous disease, or malignancy.

Examine the inside of the mouth and nose with a penlight to look for changes in the oral and nasal mucous membranes. Note whether the parotid or other salivary glands are enlarged or tender.

Table 9.2 Common Abnormalities and Characteristics of the Skin

Abnormality	Characteristics
Erythema	Dilated blood vessels
Macule	Focal area of dilated blood vessels, without palpable elevation
Papule	Focal area of dilated blood vessels, with elevated accumulation of inflammatory and other cells
Nodule	Solid inflammatory lesion extending into deep dermis
Vesicle	Small blister filled with clear fluid
Bulla	Large blister filled with clear fluid
Pustule	Blister or abscess filled with pus
Cyst	Encapsulated lesion filled with liquid or viscous fluid
Papilloma	Hypertrophied epidermis and vessels with normal surface
Verruca	Papillomatous growth covered by keratotic epidermis
Hyperkeratosis	Accumulation of keratinizing epidermal cells
Scaling	Dried squamous cells
Crusting	Dried blood, pus, or sebum
Eczema	Crusts on an erythematous base
Erosion	Ruptured vesicle or bulla
Ulcer	Loss of epidermis and papillary layer of dermis
Fissure	Linear ulcer
Eschar	Hemorrhagic ulceration

Sinus examination is feasible if the light source is very bright and the room is completely dark. To examine each frontal sinus, point the transilluminator upward through the supraorbital ridge while covering the orbit with your hand. To examine each maxillary sinus, point the transilluminator downward behind the infraorbital rim and look into the patient's open mouth and through the palate to see the glow of light from clear, air-filled sinuses.

Orbit

The anatomic relationship between the 2 orbits should be noted. Common measurements to be taken for this purpose are the intercanthal distances and the interpupillary distance.

A millimeter ruler is used to measure the intercanthal distances (ie, the distance between the 2 medial canthi and the distance between the 2 lateral canthi). The normal distance between the medial canthi (about 30 mm) is nearly one-half the interpupillary distance. The distance between the lateral canthi is routinely measured during exophthalmometry (discussed later).

The interpupillary distance (IPD, or PD) is the distance between the centers of both pupils. The PD is routinely obtained during spectacle lens fitting using the corneal reflection pupillometer, an optical instrument that measures the distance between the 2 corneal reflections (assuming orthophoria). In the clinic, it is convenient to use a millimeter ruler to measure the distance between either the temporal pupillary border or limbus of 1 eye and the nasal pupillary border or limbus of the other eye as the patient stares at a distance target (Figure 9.2). Clinical Protocol 9.2 describes the binocular technique. The average distance PD is about 61 mm, with sex and ethnic differences; the corresponding near PD is about 4 mm less.

Check the position of both globes, first by looking directly at the patient. Look for apparent exophthalmos or enophthalmos by the following technique:

1. Ask the patient to tilt the head forward.
2. Look over the patient's forehead and eyebrows from above, sighting along the plane of the face. The examiner might need to stand up.
3. Elevate both upper eyelids as the patient maintains primary position.
4. Note the position of the front of each globe in relationship to the other. Record any disparity between the 2 eyeballs of more than 2 mm.

Measurement of the axial (anteroposterior) position of the globes by exophthalmometry is important to document and follow orbital disease. An

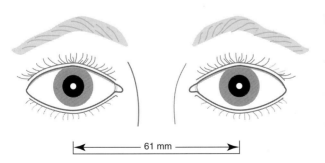

Figure 9.2 Measuring the interpupillary distance by recording the distance between the 2 corneal light reflections. IPD can also be measured between the nasal limbus of 1 eye and the temporal limbus of the other eye.

61 mm

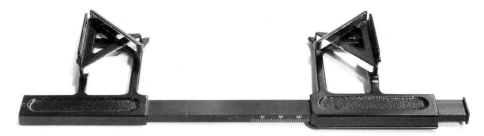

Figure 9.3 Exophthalmometer. (Reprinted by permission from Vaughan DG, Asbury T. *General Ophthalmology.* 10th ed. Stamford, CT: McGraw-Hill/Appleton & Lange, 1983. Reproduced with permission of the McGraw-Hill Companies.)

exophthalmometer measures the distance from the lateral orbital margin to the corneal apex (Figure 9.3). An average value is 17 mm. Measurements are greater in tall people, in those with a large skull or small orbits, and in some patients with axial myopia. While absolute values help in following an individual patient, the most important initial measurement is the difference between the 2 eyes. *A difference of more than 2 mm is considered abnormal.* The examiner must make sure that the orbital rims are stable and symmetric, because trauma and facial deformities can affect the measurements. Clinical Protocol 9.3 includes instructions for performing exophthalmometry.

Orbital masses might not only produce proptosis but also displace the globe vertically or horizontally. The examiner should measure displacement of the globe in any direction. Instructions for doing so are in Clinical Protocol 9.4. Pulsation of the globe should also be noted. Frequently, the patient has to be examined in various seated and supine positions to make ocular pulsations apparent.

Eyelids

Evaluate the symmetry and relative position of the eyebrows. Check to see whether there is any compensatory lifting or wrinkling on 1 side compared with the other. Note the position of the eyelashes relative to the globe, the number or density of the lashes, and their color. Note the position, movement, and symmetry of the eyelids, including the presence of any scars from previous surgery or injury.

Specific abnormalities of the lids and lashes are described, drawn, or photographed for the medical record. Shining a transilluminator through the eyelid can help differentiate a solid from a cystic lid mass. Table 9.3 lists common eyelid abnormalities.

With the eyelids open, the upper eyelid usually hides the top 1.5 mm of the cornea. The lid creases of the upper and lower eyelids divide the lid skin into adherent tarsal portions and loosely attached preseptal portions. The lower lid crease is more evident in the young. The nasojugal and malar folds of the lower lid become more prominent with aging. Table 9.4 lists many normal adult values relative to eyelid structure and function.

To assess eyelid closure, ask the patient to blink and then gently to close both eyes. Normal lid movements are necessary for the lacrimal pump to draw tears into the puncta, canaliculi, and lacrimal sac. Any gap that allows exposure of the ocular surface (ie, lagophthalmos) is noted and measured.

Table 9.3   Common Abnormalities of the Eyelids, Eyelashes, and Eyebrows

Abnormality	Description
Abnormal eyelid position or function:	
Lagophthalmos	Insufficiency or weakness of eyelid closure
Blepharospasm	Involuntary contraction of the orbicularis oculi muscle
Blepharoptosis	Abnormal drooping of the eyelid (owing to congenital, mechanical, myogenic, aponeurotic, or neurogenic causes)
Protective ptosis	Drooping of the upper eyelid (owing to ocular surface discomfort or inflammation)
Pseudoptosis	An eyelid that appears to sag (owing to contralateral lid retraction, a small or displaced globe, or an overhanging brow)
Brow ptosis	Drooping of the eyebrow
Ectropion	Outward turning of the eyelid margin (owing to involutional, cicatricial, or paralytic causes)
Entropion	Inward turning of the eyelid margin (owing to involutional, cicatricial, or spastic causes)
Lid lag	Delayed movement of the upper lid during downward pursuit of the eye
Abnormal eyelashes or eyebrows:	
Trichiasis	Misdirection of 1 or more eyelashes
Madarosis	Patchy or diffuse loss of eyelashes
Poliosis	Whitening of lashes
Distichiasis	Extra row of eyelashes
Synophrys	Confluent eyebrows that meet in the midline
Abnormal eyelid fold:	
Dermatochalasis	Redundant eyelid skin
Blepharochalasis	Chronic lymphedema with wrinkled eyelid skin
Epicanthus	Vertical fold at the medial canthus
Epiblepharon	Horizontal fold near the lower eyelid margin

Table 9.4   Normal Adult Values of Eyelid Structure and Function

Blinking rate	15–16 blinks per minute
Palpebral tissue length	25–30 mm
Palpebral fissure height	8–12 mm
Distance from upper lid margin to corneal light reflex	35 mm
Distance from upper lid margin to upper lid crease	8–11 mm
Levator excursion	8–15 mm

Eyelid position relative to the cornea is estimated by observing the position of the upper and lower eyelid margins relative to the superior and inferior corneal limbus, respectively. Judging the margin–limbus distances is useful for screening. For any patient with blepharoptosis, the examiner must measure interpalpebral fissure height, upper lid margin–corneal reflex distance, upper lid crease position, and levator function. Clinical Protocol 9.5 outlines these steps. Figure 9.4 illustrates a method of noting the results of these measurements in the medical record. The degree of blepharoptosis is graded as listed in Table 9.5.

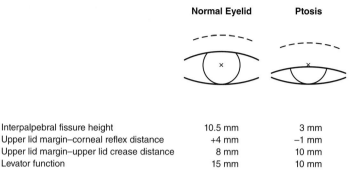

Figure 9.4 Method of recording ptosis measurements.

	Normal Eyelid	Ptosis
Interpalpebral fissure height	10.5 mm	3 mm
Upper lid margin–corneal reflex distance	+4 mm	−1 mm
Upper lid margin–upper lid crease distance	8 mm	10 mm
Levator function	15 mm	10 mm

Table 9.5   Method of Grading Degree of Upper Eyelid Blepharoptosis

Severity	Interpalpebral Fissure Height	Margin–Reflex Distance
Mild	7 mm	+1.5 mm
Moderate	6 mm	+0.5 mm
Severe	5 mm	−0.5 mm

Upper eyelid retraction is assessed with the patient's gaze in the primary position by noting where the upper lid margin crosses the globe in relation to the superior limbus. Lid retraction is classified as listed in Table 9.6. Patients with lid retraction might also exhibit lid lag (von Graefe sign), which is a delayed or fluttering lid movement on downward pursuit.

To detect lower lid retraction, first have the patient fixate on a target, such as your finger. While you look at the eye you suspect to be affected, have the patient follow your finger as you move it downward until the lower lid margin of the patient's other eye rests at the lower limbus. Observe whether any sclera shows between the lid margin and limbus of the involved eye, an indication of lid retraction.

Lacrimal System

Observe the lacrimal gland by raising the patient's upper lid and instructing the patient to look downward and medially, thereby prolapsing the palpebral lobe. The orbital lobe is sometimes palpable at the superotemporal orbital rim. Observe and note any lacrimal gland masses (see also "Lacrimal System" under "Palpation" later in this chapter).

Observe the lacrimal puncta for apposition to the globe and patency. Look for punctal eversion, stenosis, occlusion, and functional obstruction by redundant

Table 9.6   Method of Grading Degree of Upper Eyelid Retraction

Severity	Upper Lid Margin Position
Mild	Lid margin intersects the upper limbus
Moderate	Up to 4 mm of sclera of the superior globe is visible
Severe	More than 4 mm of sclera shows

conjunctiva. Inspect the area of the lacrimal sac for swelling and erythema. Note whether there is an overflow of tears.

Globe

To examine the entire ocular surface and sclera, hold the eyelids open and ask the patient to look up, down, right, and left. Twirling a cotton applicator at the upper and lower lid creases helps to raise and lower the lids and avoids direct touching of the lids or globe with the fingers. This technique is illustrated in Figure 9.5.

The volume of the tear meniscus should be assessed by inspection. Indicator paper can be used after a chemical injury to check the tear pH.

Inspect the bulbar conjunctiva. Note the type and extent of any conjunctival discharge and classify it as watery, serous, mucoid, mucopurulent, or purulent.

The palpebral conjunctiva is first examined inferiorly. Ask the patient to look up while you gently pull the lower lid downward. Evaluate the tarsal conjunctiva, normally about 3 to 4 mm wide at its central portion, and as much of the remaining lower palpebral conjunctiva as possible. To expose the upper tarsal conjunctiva, evert the upper lid as the patient looks down. Clinical Protocol 9.6 presents several techniques for lid eversion. The central upper tarsus is normally 9 to 10 mm wide, and the overlying tarsal conjunctiva generally is the best place to evaluate conjunctival papillae and follicles. Exposure of the retrotarsal conjunctiva and upper fornix might require the use of an eyelid retractor (double eversion of the eyelid).

Examine the anterior globe in sufficient ambient lighting. Subtle color changes of the conjunctiva and sclera (eg, icterus, age-related hyaline plaques at the insertion of horizontal rectus muscles) are better seen with the naked eye in natural sunlight than with slit-lamp illumination. One or more intrascleral nerve loops are often present, usually 4 mm from the superior limbus.

Measurements of the corneal diameter, when needed, are usually obtained with a millimeter ruler, although calipers and gauges give a more accurate reading. The observer must sight exactly perpendicular to the ruler to avoid parallax error.

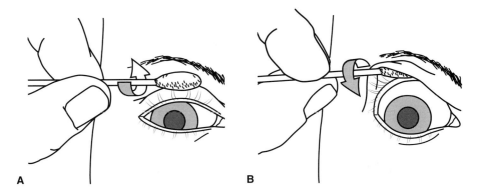

A **B**

Figure 9.5 No-touch technique for raising upper eyelid. **(A)** Apply a cotton-tipped applicator to skin of upper eyelid at the lid crease as the patient looks down. **(B)** Twirl the applicator stick between the thumb and forefinger to bunch up the excess lid skin and elevate the upper lid margin, then elevate the lid skin by raising the applicator stick toward the superior orbital rim.

Table 9.7   Method of Grading the Anterior Chamber Angle

Angle Grade	Diffuse Light Yields	Slit Light Shows	Gonioscopy Shows
IV	Full illumination of nasal iris	AC depth = corneal thickness	Ciliary body
III	2/3 illumination of nasal iris	AC depth = 1/2 corneal thickness	Scleral spur only
II	1/3 illumination of nasal iris	AC depth = 1/4 corneal thickness	Trabecular meshwork only
I	< 1/3 illumination of nasal iris	AC depth < 1/4 corneal thickness	No trabecular meshwork

The horizontal corneal diameter is about 10 mm in the newborn and reaches the adult length of 11 to 12 mm by 2 to 3 years of age. The vertical diameter is more difficult to assess because the exact location of the superior and inferior limbus is harder to define. The corneal diameter is measured in patients suspected to have a developmental disorder of the globe.

Better ways than gross inspection are available to evaluate corneal topography, but a quick look from the patient's side, aligning your view along the iris plane, helps to discern severe ectasia, as in keratoconus. Another way to detect a corneal deformity is to look at the contour of the lower eyelid border as the patient looks down. For example, Munson's sign is the angular curvature of the lower lid produced by keratoconus. The retinoscope and direct ophthalmoscope can also be used to detect refractive changes caused by abnormal corneal topography.

The depth of the anterior chamber can be checked during the external examination. Diffuse and narrow-beam penlight techniques for doing so are described in Clinical Protocol 9.7. In the penlight technique, the angle of the anterior chamber is classified by the relative positions of the anterior iris and the posterior cornea (Table 9.7). Gonioscopy is performed whenever an anterior chamber angle abnormality is suspected (see Chapter 11).

Suspected lesions inside the eye can be assessed by using a transilluminator or bright penlight. Clinical Protocol 9.8 describes specific techniques of transscleral illumination and transpupillary retroillumination.

■ Palpation

Feeling for abnormalities involves tactile, proprioceptive, and temperature senses. The considerate examiner avoids sudden, unexpected touches on or around the eyes, particularly in patients with poor vision and in sighted people who have their eyes closed. Explaining the examination's goals helps to reassure patients during palpation.

A screening examination is done routinely as follows:

1. Use the middle fingers to check for preauricular lymph nodes.
2. Use the index fingers and thumbs to open the eyelids wide apart.
3. Ask the patient to gaze in different directions to expose most of the ocular surface as you inspect the globe.
4. Judge and record any mass according to its size, shape, composition, tenderness, and movability.

A more detailed examination is done when necessary, such as in suspected trauma or with a congenital anomaly. Cranial nerve function might also need to be assessed (see Clinical Protocol 9.1).

Head and Face

Note frontal bossing and other anomalous bony changes. Tenderness over the maxillary or frontal sinus can be a sign of paranasal sinusitis.

Palpation of the temporal artery in elderly patients might reveal tenderness with hardening and tortuosity during acute episodes of giant-cell arteritis. Palpation of the neck vessels is done to check for carotid arterial pulses and for a jugular venous hum (Figure 9.6).

Certain types of infections produce enlarged lymph nodes. Palpation for an enlarged preauricular (superficial parotid) lymph node is done by placing the fingers below the patient's temple, just in front of the tragus. This node is normally neither tender nor palpable. Palpate the submandibular lymph nodes located under the angle of the jaw. Superficial cervical lymph glands—the jugular, post-sternocleidomastoid, and supraclavicular nodes—are palpated in patients with suspected lymphadenopathy. The locations of these lymph nodes are shown in Figure 9.7.

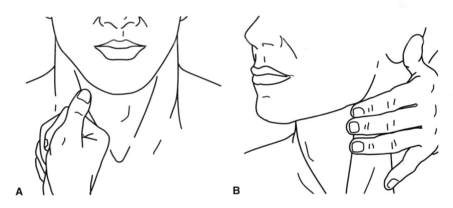

A **B**

Figure 9.6 Palpation of the carotid pulse. **(A)** Placement of the examiner's thumb from the front. **(B)** Placement of the examiner's fingers from behind.

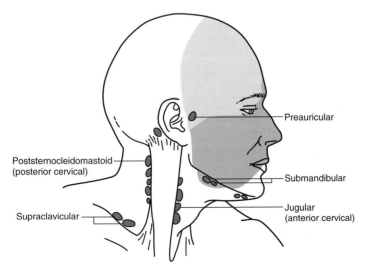

Poststernocleidomastoid (posterior cervical)

Supraclavicular

Preauricular

Submandibular

Jugular (anterior cervical)

Figure 9.7 Lymph nodes inspected or palpated during the external ophthalmic examination. Shaded areas show the lymphatic drainage of the ocular adnexa to the preauricular and submandibular nodes.

Orbit

Clinical Protocol 9.9 describes the methods of palpating the orbital margins and contents of patients with head trauma who might have fractures. A step-off can indicate a facial fracture. Simultaneous palpation of both sides makes it easier to identify abnormalities. In all cases of suspected orbital trauma, the examiner must first be certain of the integrity of the globe before any manipulations are done. If a ruptured globe is suspected, do not palpate directly. Instead, hold the eyelids of an injured eye open by directing the upper lid onto the brow and the lower lid onto the cheek without pressing on the globe. Note discrepancies from the normal anatomy in the medical record.

Eyelids

Gentle palpation of the closed lids is done by sliding the examining finger over the eyelid skin. This maneuver can be helped by stretching the skin and having the patient rotate the globe so the examiner does not press on the cornea. A mass can sometimes be felt even when it is difficult to see. The examiner should note the presence of an eyelid mass and whether the eyelid margin or conjunctiva is involved. The dimensions of an eyelid lesion should be measured with a millimeter ruler. Generally, the longest diameter and its perpendicular are recorded, along with the lesion's consistency and movability.

To test for the presence of a Bell's phenomenon (activated superior rectus function when efforts are made to close the eyelids against resistance), ask the patient to shut the eyelids and to keep them closed while you gently pry the eyelids open and peek at the position of the globes. Determining what part of the globe lies behind the interpalpebral fissure is important if there is incomplete eyelid closure (so as to know whether corneal exposure is occurring).

Lacrimal System

Any mass of the lacrimal gland or lacrimal sac is evaluated for size and tenderness. A patient with epiphora should undergo compression of the sac to learn if material can be expressed from the puncta. Clinical Protocol 9.10 describes lacrimal sac compression and the dye disappearance test, which are the principal diagnostic tests for a patient with excess tears.

Globe

Applying fingertip pressure onto the eyeball through the eyelid can help determine whether congested vessels can be blanched (suggesting conjunctival vascular dilation) or not (such as with ciliary flush or episcleritis) and whether a nodule is movable (suggesting a conjunctival phlyctenule or episcleral nodule) or not (such as with nodular scleritis). The location of any focal tenderness should be noted.

Schirmer testing, used for patients with dry eye, is described in Clinical Protocol 9.11. The examiner uses sterile filter paper strips (30 mm long, plus a 5 mm wick) to assess the amount of tear fluid. The Schirmer test *without* anesthetic measures both basal tears (from the accessory lacrimal glands) and reflex tears (from the main lacrimal gland). The test *with* anesthetic measures predominantly basal tear secretion. The examiner usually selects only 1 of these 2 tests. Each test measures the relative degree of aqueous tear production, because the amount of conjunctival mucus and meibomian gland lipids collected by the test strips is negligible. A measurement (with anesthetic) of >10 mm/5 min is regarded as indicating normal tear production. A measurement of 5 to 10 mm/5 min is equivocal and could be normal or abnormal, because tear production varies by age and other factors. A value of <5 mm/5 min suggests a dry eye state. Measurements without anesthetic tend to be about 5 mm/5 min greater because the strips cause some irritation.

■ Auscultation

Auscultation for an orbital bruit is performed by placing the bell of the stethoscope over the closed eyelids as the patient briefly holds his or her breath. A small pediatric bell works well. The noise of eyeball movement can be eliminated by instructing the patient to open the eyelids of the opposite eye and fixate on a straight-ahead target. The stethoscope bell can also be placed over the frontal sinus and on the temple to listen around the orbit.

Faint rumbling sounds heard over the globe can be normal. An orbital bruit can signify the presence of a carotid-cavernous fistula or an arteriovenous malformation. The bruit is usually accentuated during systole and decreases with compression of the ipsilateral carotid artery or both jugular veins.

The neck can be examined for a carotid bruit by listening over the carotid bifurcation just below the jaw angle. Chest auscultation is necessary to ensure that a cardiac murmur is not being transmitted to the neck. Some ophthalmologists include blood pressure measurement in their initial eye examination.

Pitfalls and Pointers

- Be professional and nonjudgmental during the external examination. The patient is also examining the examiner and is sensitive to offhand remarks and nonverbal signs that could be misinterpreted. Conversing with the patient helps to distract the patient from your observation and palpation tasks.
- Wash your hands between all patients. Washing your hands in the room just before starting the examination shows the patient you follow recommended precautions and often alleviates some anxiety. Warm, dry, clean, and manicured hands are appreciated by everyone.
- Don't rush to examine the obvious lesion and ignore the rest of the external examination. Sit back, get an overview, and proceed carefully and thoroughly through the stepwise procedure.
- Don't forget to compare the abnormal eye with the fellow one. Back-and-forth comparisons between the 2 sides of the face can reveal a subtle asymmetry.
- Compare your findings with previous records. Looking at old photographs, including driver's licenses, can reveal an unrecognized but long-standing ptosis or asymmetry. If necessary, have the patient bring in old photographs from home. The examiner should also have photographs taken whenever possible to document trauma, presurgical appearance, and any lesion that might be growing.

- Be careful when measuring the lid fissure height. The position of the eyelids will change depending upon eye position, facial muscle activity, alertness, and external stimuli such as phenylephrine eyedrops. Check the palpebral fissure in primary position with eyes gazing at a distance target. Don't forget to observe the brow for ptosis, compensatory elevation, and wrinkling.
- Be gentle. Pressure on the globe can elicit the oculocardiac reflex and produce bradycardia in susceptible individuals. Be sure to warn the patient about what to expect during procedures such as lid eversion.

Suggested Resource

Orbit, Eyelids, and Lacrimal System. Basic and Clinical Science Course, Section 7. San Francisco: American Academy of Ophthalmology; published annually.

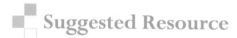

Clinical Protocol 9.1

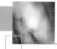

Performing a Neurosensory Examination of the Head and Face

Assessing Facial Nerve Function

1. Ask the patient to squeeze the eyes closed forcefully and note whether the orbicularis oculi muscles completely bring the eyelids together.

2. Compare the relative strength of both orbicularis oculi muscles by using your fingertips to pry the eyelids open. The needed force should be the same for both sides.

3. Ask the patient to smile and show his or her teeth. Note the symmetry of the facial expression.

4. When there is weakness of 1 side of the lower face, check for a supranuclear lesion by asking the patient to raise both eyebrows and to wrinkle the forehead. A central facial palsy spares the forehead and orbicularis oculi muscles; a peripheral lesion often does not.

Eliciting Blink Reflexes

1. Without mentioning it to the patient, note the frequency and completeness of normal blinks. Expect to see a complete blink every 4 seconds.

2. If voluntary blinks are not present, swat your hand toward the patient to elicit a blinking movement.

3. Tap on the patient's glabella if a central nervous system disorder is suspected. A normal response produces only a few blinking movements; repetitive blinks (as in parkinsonism) are abnormal.

Assessing Facial Sensation

1. Using your fingertip, tissue paper, or cotton wisp, lightly touch 1 side of the patient's face and then the contralateral, corresponding side. Ask the patient to compare the affected side with the normal side (eg, by asking how much the affected side is worth if the normal side equals $1). Repeat for all 3 trigeminal nerve dermatomes and for the distribution of each principal sensory nerve (Figure 1).

2. Map the area of reduced sensation (eg, the zone of hypesthesia resulting from an infraorbital nerve damaged by an orbital floor fracture).

3. Perform simultaneous testing of both sides of the face if abnormal cortical function is suspected.

Clinical Protocol 9.1 *(continued)*

Testing Corneal Sensation

1. Without touching the eyelashes or stimulating the visual startle reflex, touch the cornea with a clean cotton wisp, facial tissue wick, fragment of dental floss, or puff of air from a small syringe. A brief touch should produce a reflex blink with a faint subjective sensation. The response may be graded on a scale of 0 to 4+.

2. Use an esthesiometer, an instrument that has a nylon filament of adjustable length, to quantify the degree of sensation for patients in whom recovery or further loss is anticipated.

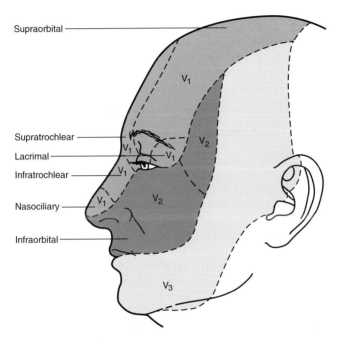

Figure 1   Assessing facial sensation.

Clinical Protocol 9.2

Measuring Binocular Interpupillary Distance

1. Ask the patient to fixate a distance target.

2. Facing the patient at an arm's length distance, position yourself just below the patient's gaze. Align your eyes with the patient's eyes as the patient maintains distance fixation over your head.

3. Rest the millimeter ruler lightly across the bridge of the patient's nose.

4. Close your right eye and use your left eye to line up the zero point of the ruler with the temporal limbus of the patient's right eye (Figure 1).

(continued)

Clinical Protocol 9.2 *(continued)*

5. Keep the ruler steady. Close your left eye and open your right eye.

6. Read the measurement that aligns with the nasal limbus of the patient's left eye (Figure 2).

7. Repeat the above sequence to confirm a reproducible reading.

8. Near PD is measured in a similar way by having the patient stare at your nose instead of the distance target.

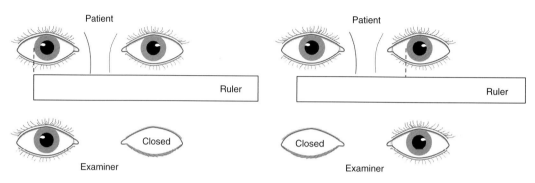

Figure 1   Aligning with the patient's right eye.   **Figure 2**   Aligning with the patient's left eye.

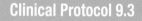

Clinical Protocol 9.3   **Performing Exophthalmometry**

1. Position yourself directly in front of the patient. Your left eye measures the patient's right eye, and your right eye measures the patient's left eye.

2. Hold the exophthalmometer so that the angled mirrors are oriented upwards, above the fixation foot plates.

3. If a patient's previous intercanthal reading is known, set the last recorded distance between the patient's lateral canthi on the scale. If this is the patient's first reading, place the instrument so that the foot plates rest on both lateral orbital rims at the level of the outer canthi (Figure 1).

4. With your left eye, sight along the right-hand mirror of the instrument at the reflection of the patient's right eye.

5. Instruct the patient to occlude his or her left eye with a hand or occluder and to look toward your eye to achieve straight-ahead alignment.

6. Using your open left eye, align the instrument's 2 vertical markers (usually a long vertical line in the center of the proptosis scale and a corresponding mark or line on the instrument's base).

7. Read the distance from the lateral orbital rim to the corneal apex by noting where the mirror image of the patient's anteriormost corneal curvature falls along the mirror's millimeter ruler (Figure 2). Note that you see the anterior corneal surface from the side, and the reading is the anterior extent of the corneal apex on the gauge.

8. Obtain a similar measurement for the patient's left eye by using your right eye to align the appropriate vertical markers on the opposite mirror of the instrument.

9. Record the readings for each eye and the distance between the lateral canthi as shown below.

Clinical Protocol 9.3 *(continued)*

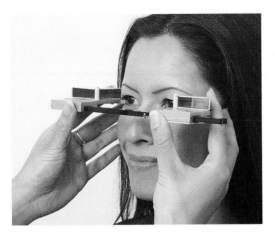

Figure 1 Position of the foot plates.

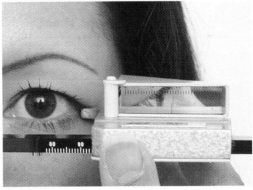

Figure 2 The mirror image of the corneal curvature is visible on the ruler.

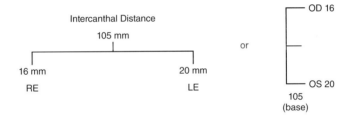

Figure 3 Recording exophthalmometry results.

Clinical Protocol 9.4 **Measuring Globe Displacement**

Horizontal Displacement

1. Imagine a vertical straight line down the middle of the patient's face that aligns the center of the glabella and the philtrum of the upper lip.

2. Hold a millimeter ruler horizontally across the bridge of the patient's nose, perpendicular to the imaginary vertical line (Figure 1).

3. Measure the distance from the center of the nasal bridge to the medial limbus of the right eye as the patient stares at a distance target. Occlude the contralateral eye if strabismus is present.

(continued)

Clinical Protocol 9.4 *(continued)*

4. Repeat the measurement for the left eye. The difference between the 2 measurements is the amount of horizontal displacement.

Vertical Displacement

1. Hold a straightedge horizontally along the patient's nasal bridge to align visually the lateral canthi.

2. Hold a millimeter ruler vertically, perpendicular to the horizontal straightedge, to pass through the center of the pupil of the patient's right eye.

3. Measure the distance from the edge of the horizontal straightedge to the pupillary center (or corneal light reflex).

4. Repeat the measurement for the left eye. The difference between the 2 measurements is the amount of vertical displacement.

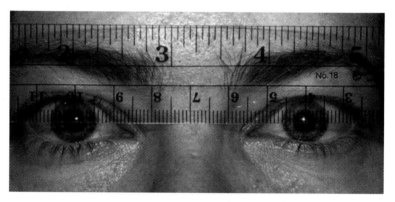

Figure 1 Horizontal displacement measurement. (Reprinted, with permission, from *Clinical Tests: Ophthalmology* by Huber and Reacher, 1989. Mosby-Wolfe Limited, London, UK.)

Clinical Protocol 9.5  **Measuring Eyelid Position**

Interpalpebral Fissure Height

1. Ask the patient to fixate a penlight in primary gaze position.

2. Hold a millimeter ruler vertically, close to the patient's open eye, to measure the distance between the center of the upper and lower eyelid margins (Figure 1).

3. Record the interpalpebral fissure height in millimeters for each eye.

4. To recheck the measurements, obtain and add together the following 2 measurements:

    a. The distance between the upper eyelid margin and the corneal light reflex (normally about 4 mm).

    b. The distance between the lower eyelid margin and the corneal light reflex (normally about 6 mm).

Clinical Protocol 9.5 *(continued)*

Upper Lid Margin–Corneal Reflex Distance

1. Hold a penlight directly in front of the patient, so that the patient observes it in primary gaze and a corneal light reflex is present.

2. Use a millimeter ruler to measure the distance between the center of the upper eyelid margin and the corneal light reflex (Figure 2).

3. Record the margin–reflex distance for each eye. Use a negative number if the light reflex is obstructed by the eyelid.

Upper Lid Crease Position

1. Use a penlight or other near target to bring the patient's gaze into the primary position.

2. Measure the distance between the upper eyelid margin and the upper eyelid crease (Figure 3).

3. Record the upper lid crease position for each eye. Note if the upper eyelid crease is absent and cannot be accurately measured.

Levator Function

1. Either hold a thumb on the brow or place the palm of your hand against the patient's forehead. This maneuver prevents the frontalis muscle from assisting with upper eyelid elevation, thereby isolating the action of the levator muscle.

2. Ask the patient to look down, and align the zero point of the millimeter ruler with the patient's upper eyelid margin, taking care not actually to touch the patient's lids or lashes (Figure 4A).

3. Do not move the ruler. Ask the patient to look up as far as possible. Keeping the ruler steady, measure the new location of the upper eyelid margin (Figure 4B). The difference between the 2 measurements (ie, the total amount of upper lid excursion) gives the levator function.

4. Record the levator function in millimeters for each eye.

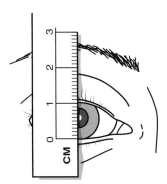

Figure 1   Measuring the interpalpebral fissure height.

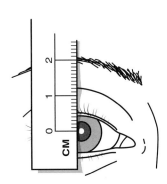

Figure 2   Measuring the upper lid margin–corneal reflex distance.

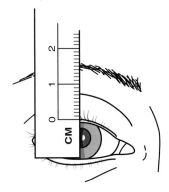

Figure 3   Measuring the upper lid crease position.

(continued)

Clinical Protocol 9.5 *(continued)*

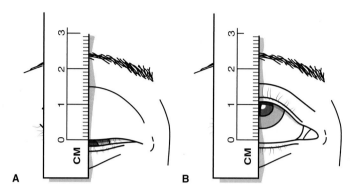

Figure 4   Measuring levator function. **(A)** Aligning with patient's upper eyelid margin. **(B)** Aligning the new location of the upper eyelid margin.

Clinical Protocol 9.6   **Everting the Eyelid**

Examining the Lower Conjunctiva and Fornix

1. With the patient looking down, press the skin below the lower lid with your thumb or forefinger against the maxillary bone and tug down (Figure 1A).

2. Ask the patient to look up, which allows the lower fornix to prolapse and exposes most of the lower palpebral conjunctiva (Figure 1B).

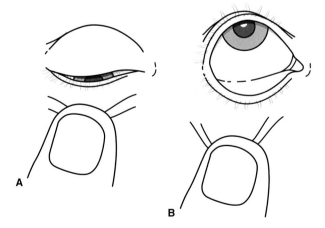

Figure 1   Examining the lower conjunctiva and fornix. **(A)** Lower lid position. **(B)** The patient is asked to look up.

Clinical Protocol 9.6 *(continued)*

Examining the Upper Conjunctiva

Steps for the 2-hand method:

1. Using your thumb and forefinger to grasp some eyelashes, pull the upper lid margin away from the globe (Figure 2A).

2. Place an applicator stick horizontally at the upper lid crease, along the upper border of the tarsus, to act as a fulcrum (Figure 2B). Hold the applicator stick in the hand that is temporal to the eye being examined.

3. Pull the upper lid margin outward and upward to fold the upper lid over the applicator stick (Figure 2C). Withdraw the applicator stick and hold the lid margin in place against the skin overlying the superior orbital rim with the thumb to view the upper tarsal conjunctiva (Figure 2D). Eversion of the upper eyelid is easier if the patient is looking down.

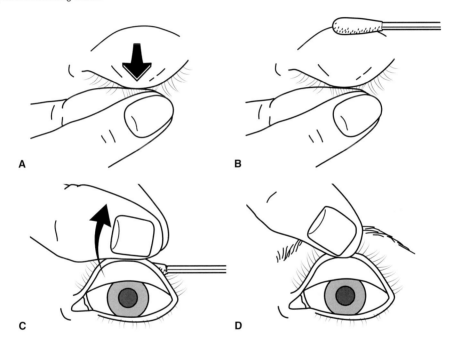

Figure 2 Examining the upper conjunctiva, 2-hand method. **(A)** Upper lid position. **(B)** Applicator stick acting as a fulcrum. **(C)** Upper lid folding over the applicator stick. **(D)** Lid held in place with the thumb.

Steps for the 1-hand method:

1. With the patient looking upward, use your hand that is temporal to the eye being examined and place your thumb against the lower lid to hold it in place (Figure 3A).

2. Place the tip of the index finger against the upper lid to hold the upper lid upward and instruct the patient to look down and to hold that gaze (Figure 3B).

3. Pinch the upper and lower lids together, an action that should permit the upper lid to hang over the lower lid margin (Figure 3C).

4. Lay the side of your index fingertip across the upper lid just above the upper border of the tarsus and push on the upper tarsal border.

5. Pinch the upper lid outward between your index finger and thumb (Figure 3D).

(continued)

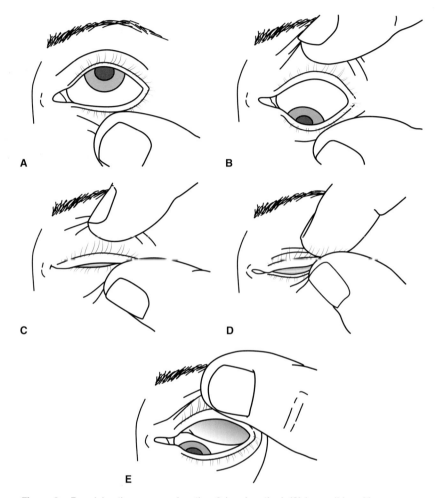

Figure 3 Examining the upper conjunctiva, 2-hand method. **(A)** Lower lid position. **(B)** Examiner's fingers holding the lids apart. **(C)** Bringing the lids back together. **(D)** Pinching the upper lid outward. **(E)** Everting the upper lid.

6. With finger and wrist rotation, flip the upper lid over to expose the upper palpebral conjunctiva. The index finger maintains a steady downward pressure on the upper lid crease as the finger is pulled away. The thumb provides the upward rotary action that turns the lid over. The thumb holds the upper lid margin in place against the superior orbital margin (Figure 3E).

Exposing the Upper Fornix

Steps for the 1-hand method:

1. Evert the upper lid by the 2-hand or 1-hand method.

2. Firmly hold the upper lid margin against the superior orbital margin with your thumb.

3. With your free hand, use your forefinger to press the lower lid upward over part of the cornea and backward against the globe. This action should compress the orbital contents sufficiently to cause most of the upper fornix to protrude.

Clinical Protocol 9.6 *(continued)*

Steps for the retractor method:

1. With the patient looking down, use your thumb and forefinger to grasp some eyelashes of the upper lid and pull the lid margin away from the globe.

2. With your free hand, place the edge of a lid retractor at the upper border of the tarsus of the upper eyelid, with the retractor handle facing down (Figure 4A).

3. Rotate the handle of the retractor upward and hold the retractor in place to view the upper tarsal conjunctiva (Figure 4B).

4. Continue to rotate the retractor and allow its curved end to press the cul-de-sac outward. This action everts the eyelid and exposes the upper fornix by suspending the upper lid on the retractor (Figure 4C). Pressing on the globe from below accentuates the protrusion of the upper fornix.

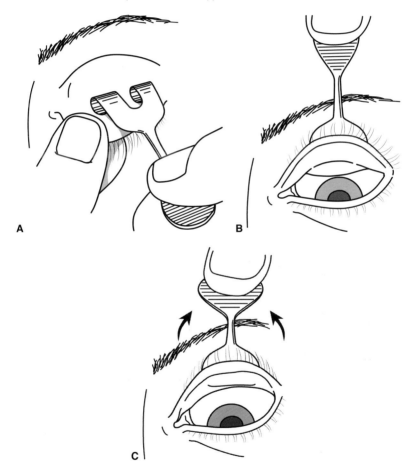

Figure 4   Exposing the upper fornix, retractor method. **(A)** Placing the lid retractor.
(B) Rotating the handle upward. **(C)** Continued rotation presses the cul-de-sac outward.

Clinical Protocol 9.7 — Estimating Anterior Chamber Depth

Flashlight With Diffuse Beam

1. While facing the patient, hold a penlight near the temporal limbus, and shine the light across the front of the right eye toward the nose. Keep the beam parallel to the plane of the normal iris.

2. Observe the medial aspect of the iris. Normally, the iris is completely illuminated (Figure 1A). An eye with a shallow anterior chamber will have two-thirds of the nasal portion of the iris in shadow (Figure 1B).

3. Grade the angle as open (grade IV or III), intermediate (grade II), or narrow (grade I).

4. Repeat the test for the left eye.

Flashlight With Slit Beam

1. Direct the slit beam perpendicular to the peripheral cornea.

2. View the anterior chamber angle at a 60° angle from the beam.

3. Grade the peripheral angle width by comparing the distance between the corneal endothelium and the iris with the corneal thickness. In an open angle, the peripheral chamber depth equals the corneal thickness. When the peripheral depth is one-fourth or less of the normal corneal thickness, gonioscopy should be done to evaluate the angle.

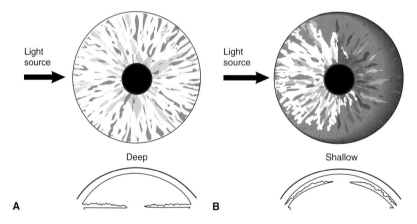

Figure 1 Estimating anterior chamber depth. **(A)** Normal iris with complete illumination. **(B)** Iris with shadow, indicating shallow anterior chamber.

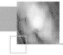

Clinical Protocol 9.8 — Illuminating the Inner Eye for External Viewing

Illumination Through the Sclera

1. In a darkened room, place the tip of the transilluminator against the eyelid. The light could also be held directly against the patient's anesthetized globe if the bulb is not hot.

2. Identify the red reflex, normally seen exiting through the dilated pupil and glowing through most of the sclera.

3. If a corneal opacity is present that obscures a clear view of the inner eye, note the shape of the pupil.

Clinical Protocol 9.8 *(continued)*

4. Look for a mass in the eye wall using transscleral illumination. Move the light source over the surface of the globe while examining the light reflected through the pupil and sclera. The pupil will be dark when the trans-illuminator is placed over a solid lesion. A solid lesion inside the eye wall will also obscure the faint scleral glow when the light is held against the adjacent or opposite sclera.

Illumination Through the Pupil

1. Shine a coaxial bright light, such as the direct ophthalmoscope, into the patient's eye from a distance of about 50 cm.

2. Look for any obscuration of the reflected light. Opacities near the pupillary axis appear as dark shadows at the pupillary plane against the normal red reflex.

3. Localize an opacity by asking the patient to look slowly up and down or by shifting the direction of the light; opacities visible against the red reflex will shift with eye movements according to their position relative to the pupillary plane (Figure 1). Determine which direction the opacity appears to move in relationship to the pupillary axis:

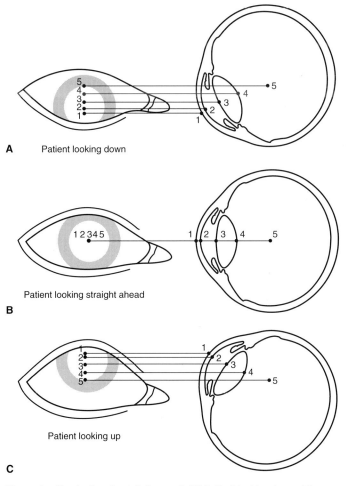

A   Patient looking down

     Patient looking straight ahead

B

     Patient looking up

C

Figure 1   Illumination through the pupil. **(A)** Patient looking down. **(B)** Patient looking straight ahead. **(C)** Patient looking up.

(continued)

Clinical Protocol 9.8 *(continued)*

   a. No movement. An opacity in the pupil, such as an anterior lens opacity, will remain stationary.

   b. Same direction. An opacity anterior to the pupil (eg, in the cornea) shifts in the same direction as the patient's direction of gaze.

   c. Opposite direction. An opacity posterior to the pupil (eg, in the posterior lens or vitreous) shifts in the opposite direction.

 Clinical Protocol 9.9   **Palpating the Orbit**

Orbital Rim

1. Palpate the anterior portion of the orbit by placing a finger between the orbital margin and the globe. Standing behind the patient can make it easier to roll the small finger around the orbital rim.

2. Begin laterally. The lateral orbital margin is generally about 5 mm from the lateral canthus.

3. Slowly move upward (clockwise on the patient's right orbit and counterclockwise on the left orbit). Locate the supraorbital notch or foramen by gently moving your fingertips along the orbital rim, at the junction of the medial one-third and lateral two-thirds of the superior orbital margin.

4. Move your fingertips medial to the supraorbital notch. Feel for the trochlea, normally palpable 4 mm posterior to the orbital margin. The upper border of the medial canthal ligament can be felt just below this point.

5. Move your fingertips along the inferior orbital margin, which should form a smooth, continuous contour. A vertical line extending from the supraorbital notch intersects the palpable infraorbital foramen, 4 mm below the inferior orbital margin.

6. Move your finger along the outer orbital rim and feel the marginal tubercle of the zygomatic bone. Approximately 6 mm above this point is the junction of the frontal and zygomatic bones, which is palpable at the supraorbital margin. The frontozygomatic suture is about 10 mm from the lateral canthus.

Orbital Contents

1. After completing the circumference of the orbital rim, gently touch the patient's closed eyelids.

   a. Any thrill or pulsation movement should be noted.

   b. If a sinus fracture is suspected, move the fingers around the globe to detect any crepitus within the confines of the orbital margin.

   c. Press gently into the periocular tissues to feel for the anterior extension of a retrobulbar or anterior orbital mass.

2. Judge the resiliency of the retrobulbar tissues by cautiously pushing the globe posteriorly through the patient's closed eyelids. Normally the eye can be displaced into the orbital fat about 5 mm. By comparing the 2 orbits, the degree and ease of globe retropulsion are assessed.

3. Ask the patient to perform a Valsalva maneuver. Judge whether any pressure is transmitted to the orbits by keeping your fingertips pressed onto both globes through the patient's closed eyelids during the maneuver.

Clinical Protocol 9.10 — Measuring Lacrimal Outflow in the Tearing Patient

Lacrimal Sac Compression

1. Apply pressure by gently pushing your index finger or a cotton-tipped applicator stick over the lacrimal fossa inside the inferomedial orbital rim (not on the side of the nasal bone).

2. Note any mucus or mucopurulent material that can be expressed back through the canaliculi and puncta. Reflux confirms a completely obstructed nasolacrimal duct (Figure 1). If no reflux is found, then proceed with the dye disappearance test.

Dye Disappearance Test

1. Instill fluorescein into both eyes using a moistened fluorescein strip or a drop of fluorescein solution.

2. Observe the tear film, preferably with a cobalt-blue light, to ensure that fluorescein is visible in the preocular tear film of both eyes.

3. Wait 5 minutes. The patient may blink normally but should avoid wiping the eyes.

4. Use a cobalt-blue light to examine the tear meniscus.

   a. The tear film should be clear, indicating complete disappearance of the fluorescein dye.

   b. If the tears are still tinged yellow, the lacrimal outflow system has a functional or anatomic blockage (Figure 2).

   c. Record any asymmetric clearance by indicating which side retains the dye longer.

5. For patients with delayed clearance of fluorescein, determine the level of occlusion by lacrimal probing and irrigation.

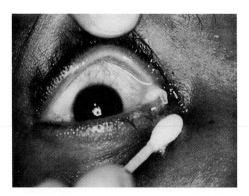

Figure 1 Lacrimal sac compression. (Photograph courtesy of Francis C. Sutula, MD. Reprinted from *Orbit, Eyelids, and Lacrimal System*, Basic and Clinical Science Course, 1996.)

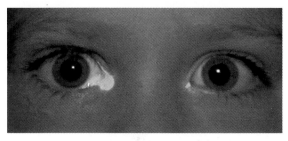

Figure 2 Dye disappearance test. (Reprinted from *Orbit, Eyelids, and Lacrimal System*, Basic and Clinical Science Course, 1996.)

Clinical Protocol 9.11

Conducting Tear Production Tests for the Dry Eye

Schirmer I Test ("Schirmer Without Anesthetic")

1. Seat the patient in a dimmed room with the back of the head stabilized against the headrest of the examining chair.

2. Remove any excess moisture from the patient's eyelid margin and cul-de-sac with a facial tissue or cotton-tipped applicator. Do not instill any eyedrops into the eye before the test.

3. Fold a packaged, sterile filter paper strip at the indentation mark. To avoid contaminating the sterile strips, bend the round wick end of the test strips at the notch 120° before opening the pouch.

4. Open the pouch and remove a strip. Use the strip with the angled end for the right eye. Grasp the strip by the non-wick end to avoid contaminating the wick end with your fingertips.

5. Ask the patient to look up. Draw the lower lid gently downward, checking to make sure that the lid margin has been adequately dried with a cotton-tipped applicator. By convention, the strip with 1 corner cut off is used for the right eye.

6. Hook the rounded, bent end of the test strip over the lower eyelid margin of each eye and release the lower lid to hold the strip in place. The strip is typically placed at the junction of the inner two-thirds and the outer one-third of the eyelid margin. It should not touch the cornea. The notch should point toward the lateral canthus. Check to make sure that the short end of the strip is inserted all the way to the notch.

7. Ask the patient to gaze slightly above the midline with the eyelids open in subdued light (Figure 1). The patient may continue normal blinking. Patients are permitted to keep their eyes closed during the test, but squeezing should be discouraged.

8. Note the time. After 5 minutes have elapsed, remove both strips.

9. Measure the distance between the indentation mark and the farthest extent of wetting. Standardized strips are packaged in an envelope with a millimeter scale. Do not include the bent wick end in the final measurement.

10. Record the result in the chart as follows: Schirmer I testing (without anesthetic): right eye: X mm/5 min; left eye: Y mm/5 min. If complete wetting occurs before 5 minutes, this time may be noted.

Basic Secretion Test ("Schirmer With Anesthetic")

1. Instill 1 drop of proparacaine 1% eyedrops into both eyes.

2. Wait 1 minute while the patient keeps both eyes closed.

3. Gently blot the cul-de-sac dry with a tissue or cotton swab.

4. Proceed with steps 1 to 10 of the Schirmer I test.

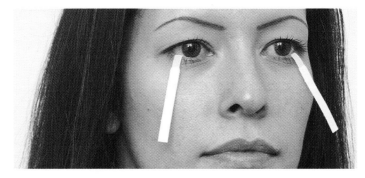

Figure 1 Schirmer test.

10 Slit-Lamp Biomicroscopy

The slit-lamp biomicroscope (commonly called the *slit lamp*) is an instrument that permits magnified examination of the eye using various kinds of illumination. A unique feature of the slit lamp is that its slit-shaped beam of light allows the examination in cross-section of living ocular tissues that are transparent or translucent. The slit lamp enhances the external examination by allowing a binocular, stereoscopic view; a wide range of magnification (10× to 500×); and illumination of variable shapes and intensities.

This chapter discusses the uses of the slit lamp in general and its parts and their functions in detail, including the principles of slit-lamp illumination. Various diagnostic and measurement techniques conducted with a slit lamp also are covered. Specific applications of slit-lamp techniques to the anterior segment examination are discussed in Chapter 11; detailed instructions for performing Goldmann applanation tonometry with the slit lamp appear in Chapter 12; instructions for indirect slit-lamp biomicroscopy of the posterior segment are included in Chapter 13.

Uses of the Slit Lamp

The slit lamp is indispensable for the detailed examination of virtually all tissues of the eye and some of its adnexa. It is routinely used for examination of the anterior segment, which includes the anterior vitreous and those structures anterior to it. Most of the anterior segment tissues (except the anterior chamber angle and the posterior surface of the iris) are directly visible with the slit lamp alone, without special variations in technique or nonstandard attachments or lenses. Optical constraints of the instrument and the eye to be examined prevent useful visualization of the angle of the anterior chamber and those structures that are posterior to the anterior vitreous unless various attachments or accessories are used (as discussed later in this chapter and in Chapters 11 and 13).

In addition to physical (visual) examination, the slit lamp is often used for tonometry, linear measurement of tissues or lesions, ophthalmic photography, and laser therapy. It can also be used in contact lens fitting, although this topic is beyond the scope of this manual.

Parts of the Slit Lamp

A typical slit lamp is illustrated in Figure 10.1. The Haag-Streit 900 model is shown because it is the most commonly encountered; several other fine slit lamps are available whose differences from the Haag-Streit instrument are usually relatively minor or are easily mastered.

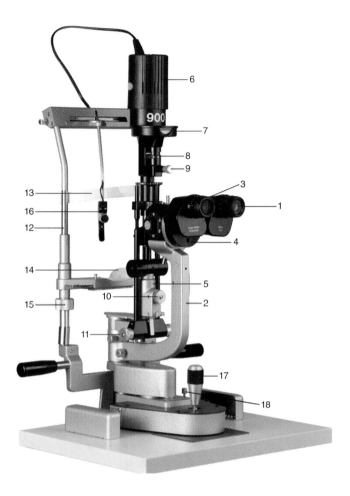

Figure 10.1 Parts of the slit lamp (Haag-Streit 900). The numbers correspond to descriptions given in the text. (Courtesy Haag-Streit USA Inc.)

The slit-lamp biomicroscope consists of 3 principal portions: the viewing arm, containing the eyepiece and magnifying elements; the illumination arm, containing the light source and many of its controls; and the patient-positioning frame. These portions are connected to a base, which has a joystick that the examiner uses to move the viewing and illumination arms about. The entire unit is wired to a transformer power source on a supporting platform. The specific parts of the instrument are detailed below; numbers in parentheses correspond to the numbers in Figure 10.1.

The Viewing Arm

The examiner looks through a pair of eyepieces (1), also known as oculars, mounted on top of the viewing arm (2); oculars are available that provide 10×, 16×, or 25× magnification, depending on the examiner's preference. A knurled focusing ring around each ocular can be twisted to suit the examiner's refractive error, and the 2 oculars can be pushed together or spread apart, much like the eyepieces of field binoculars, to accommodate the examiner's interpupillary distance. The oculars are attached to a housing containing the instrument's magnification elements (3). Below this housing is a lever (or sometimes a knob) for adjusting magnification (4).

The Illumination Arm

The illumination arm (5) and the viewing arm are parfocal; that is, the image of the source of illumination and the image being viewed by the examiner are both in focus at the same location at any given time when focus for viewing has been established. The illumination arm can also be swung 180° side to side on its pivoting base, allowing the examiner to direct the light beam anywhere between the nasal and the temporal aspect of the eye being examined. Atop the illumination arm is a lamp housing (6) containing the light bulb that is the instrument's light source. At the base of the housing, a window exposes a disk showing a calibrated scale (7) that indicates the length of beam being used; this scale is also used to measure lesions. In a separate housing below the scale is a lever for varying the brightness of the light beam (8); on some instruments, this lever also allows access to various filters, including the cobalt-blue and red-free filters. At the base of this housing is a projecting knurled knob (9). When twisted, this control varies the length (height) of the light beam; on some models, this knob activates the cobalt-blue filter as well. The rod to which this knob is connected can be pushed side to side to vary the light beam's orientation and rotation.

On the principal lower frame of the illumination arm, a knob facing the examiner (10) can be loosened to decenter the illuminating arm nasally or temporally (that is, made not parfocal with the illuminating arm); this feature is useful for retroillumination from the fundus and for the sclerotic scatter lighting technique. Accessible by either hand, knurled dual knobs for changing the width of the light beam (11) are located at the bottom of each side of the metal shafts supporting the lamp housing and are attached to the lower frame of the illumination arm. With this control, the beam can be varied from a narrow slit to 8 mm wide.

The Patient-Positioning Frame

The patient-positioning frame (12) consists of 2 upright metal rods to which are attached the forehead strap (13), for the patient to rest the forehead against during examination, and the patient chin rest (14). Often a pad of disposable papers is attached to the chin rest; the papers are torn off one by one to provide a hygienic surface for each new patient. Just below the chin rest is a knob for adjusting its height (15). A fixation light (16) is attached to a swing arm projecting from a crosspiece above both rods that form the patient positioning frame; the examiner positions this light in front of the eye not being examined to direct the patient's gaze during biomicroscopy. Alternatively, the patent may simply be asked to look at the examiner's ear.

The Base

The slit lamp's joystick control (17) is located on the base of the instrument within easy reach of the examiner who is looking through the oculars. The joystick is used to shift the viewing and illumination arms forward, backward, laterally, or diagonally. On some instruments, the joystick is twisted and rotated to lower and elevate the light beam. A locking knob (18) in the base near the common support of the viewing and illumination arms can be loosened to allow mobility of focus. The knob is tightened to prevent the slit lamp from shifting when it is not in use. Under the instrument supporting platform is a knob for turning the slit lamp's power transformer on and off (not shown); it usually also has 3 settings for degrees of brightness, although the lowest (5 V) is the most commonly used, and prolonged use of the highest can lead to early bulb failure.

Other Attachments

Various additional devices can be attached to the slit lamp, such as an applanation tonometer for measuring intraocular pressure and a Hruby lens for examining the fundus. These are not shown in Figure 10.1 but are discussed later in this chapter, and instructions for their use are provided in Chapters 12 and 13, respectively.

■ Preparing and Positioning the Patient

The patient's head is positioned and steadied for slit-lamp examination by means of the chin rest and forehead strap. The chin rest usually consists of a concave plastic cup to which is attached a stack of disposable tissue papers. The tissue on which the last patient's chin rested is torn away to expose a fresh tissue for the patient to be examined, preferably in view of the patient so that he or she knows that a clean chin rest is being provided. The chin rest occasionally consists only of the plastic cup, without the tissues; in this situation patients often appreciate seeing the physician clean the cup with a wipe of an alcohol swab or tissue. Rarely, patients want to see the forehead strap cleaned.

With the patient's forehead and chin firmly in place, the height of the chin rest can be raised or lowered by means of a nearby knob; in this way, the patient's eye is brought level with the black demarcation line on a supporting rod of the patient-positioning frame just below the level of the forehead strap.

The patient's chin should be well seated in the chin rest and the forehead pressed firmly against the forehead strap. Some patients tend to drift backward and might need to be helped, or encouraged, by the examiner or an assistant to keep the forehead forward. The slit lamp's viewing and illumination portions should be well back from the chin rest and forehead strap before attempting to position the patient; otherwise, the patient's nose, or even eye, can be bumped by the slit-lamp apparatus.

It can be difficult to position the slit lamp and its headrest close to obese patients, because their upper bodies tend to push everything away. Such patients can be accommodated by keeping the slit lamp farther away, requiring them to lean forward and to extend their necks to some degree.

Patients who have relatively short torsos often cannot be set well into the headrest because the table on which the instrument is mounted applies uncomfortable pressure to their thighs or knees. In such cases it can be useful either again to have the patient lean forward more or to fold up the footrest on the patient's chair so that the patient's legs can be dangled (providing more room above the thighs and knees). You might instead ask the patient to twist to one side (or rotate the patient's chair away from the angle of approach of the slit lamp) to enable you to bring the slit lamp in from an angle (instead of from straight ahead) and to have the patient's legs to the side of the slit-lamp table. Children often have difficulty reaching the chin rest and forehead strap and can do so more easily if they kneel on the seat of the examination chair.

Adjust the settings on the slit lamp so that the patient is not initially subjected to uncomfortably bright light when the instrument is turned on. This can be accomplished by setting the instrument to provide a very narrow beam of light, or by providing illumination that is filtered by the cobalt-blue or red-free (green) filter, or by dimming the light source if it is set to provide diffuse illumination.

It is always considerate to ask if the patient is comfortable before beginning the examination. Patients often want the chin rest raised or lowered slightly. The stool on which the examiner sits should be adjusted to a comfortable height, and the slit lamp's oculars should be adjusted for the examiner's interpupillary distance.

■ Principles of Slit-Lamp Illumination

The slit lamp is capable of illuminating the tissues of the eye in several different ways, any or all of which can be useful, depending on the clinical situation. The beginning ophthalmology resident should strive early to master all of these techniques of illumination, so as to be able to use the slit lamp to its full advantage.

The slit lamp offers 6 main illuminating options, each with its own special properties and particular uses:

- Diffuse illumination
- Direct focal illumination
- Specular reflection
- Transillumination, or retroillumination
- Indirect lateral illumination
- Sclerotic scatter

In addition, moving the slit beam by oscillating it allows the examiner to observe properties of certain ocular tissues that cannot be viewed with static lighting alone. All of these illumination techniques are described in detail below.

Diffuse Illumination

Diffuse illumination is used mainly for obtaining an overview of ocular surface tissues (eg, bulbar and palpebral conjunctiva), although it can also be useful for examining intraocular structures (iris, lens capsule). It may be used with white light or with the cobalt-blue or red-free filters. Diffuse illumination with white light calls for the use of a full-height, broad beam that is directed onto the surface of the eye or adnexa from either the temporal or nasal side (Figure 10.2). The brightness

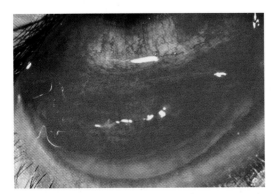

Figure 10.2   Diffuse illumination with white light. The beam has been widened to its fullest extent, here to evaluate membranous (adenoviral) conjunctivitis.

Figure 10.3 Diffuse illumination with the cobalt-blue filter (to enhance the fluorescence of fluorescein dye) is used here to demonstrate irregular breakup of the tear film with anterior-membrane corneal dystrophy. The stained tear film has pulled away to form dry spots (the areas of breakup; thus, no fluorescence).

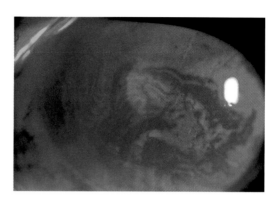

level needs to be lowered, or the broad beam will be uncomfortably bright for the patient.

The cobalt-blue filter produces blue light in which fluorescein dye fluoresces with a yellow-green color. Diffuse illumination with blue light is used for evaluating fluorescein staining of ocular surface tissues or the tear film (Figure 10.3) and to discern the fluorescein pattern during Goldmann applanation tonometry (see Chapter 12).

The red-free filter produces light-green light, facilitating the evaluation of rose-bengal staining (Figure 10.4).

Direct Focal Illumination

Direct focal illumination is achieved by directing a full-height, medium-width, medium-bright beam obliquely into the eye and focusing it on the cornea so that a quadrilateral block of light (parallelepiped, or corneal prism) illuminates the cornea (Figure 10.5).

The anterior surface of the parallelepiped represents the anterior surface of the cornea; the posterior surface represents the posterior surface of the cornea; and the other 2 faces of the parallelepiped (perpendicular to the surface faces) show the cornea in cross-section. The same kind of illumination may be used to

Figure 10.4 Diffuse illumination with red-free (green) filter is here used to enhance visibility of rose-bengal red dye, which has stained keratin in intraepithelial (squamous) neoplasia.

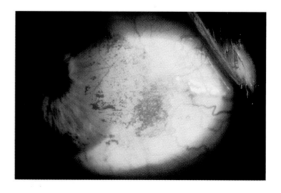

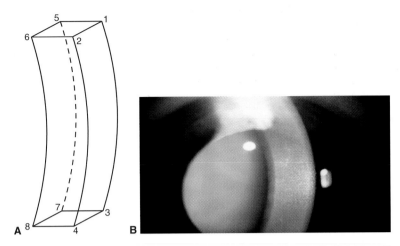

Figure 10.5 **(A)** The corneal parallelepiped (medium-width beam) achieved with direct focal illumination; face 1-2-3-4 represents the surface of the corneal epithelium; face 5-6-7-8 is the corneal endothelium; and faces 2-6-4-8 and 1-5-3-7 represent cross-sections of the cornea. **(B)** Clinical photograph of corneal parallelepiped originating from the nasal direction (right eye) and showing anterior-membrane (map-dot-fingerprint) corneal dystrophy.

examine the anterior chamber and the crystalline lens. When the beam is reduced to 1 × 1 mm, direct focal illumination is used for grading flare and cell in the anterior chamber (see Chapter 11).

Following direct focal examination with the medium beam, the parallelepiped is narrowed so that its anterior and posterior surface components become very thin, leaving only the cross-sectional illumination of the cornea. This thin beam, called an *optical section*, is especially useful for judging the depth of lesions (Figure 10.6) and examining the crystalline lens. The corneal epithelium appears as a thin, optically empty (black) line at the surface of the optical section. The rest of the cornea, the lens, and (to a lesser extent) the vitreous are relucent (reflective of light) and so have a silvery appearance. The anterior chamber normally is optically empty, or nearly so.

Direct focal illumination, with either a medium beam or an optical section (or both), is the most frequently used kind of slit-lamp illumination.

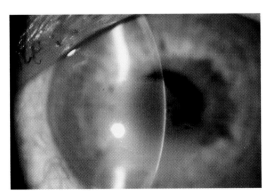

Figure 10.6 The optical section provides a purely cross-sectional view. Here it is used to visualize superficial (intraepithelial) keratin in corneal intraepithelial (squamous) neoplasia.

Specular Reflection

Specular reflection, or reflected illumination, is used mainly for examination of the corneal endothelium, although it can also be used for examining the anterior surface of the cornea or lens. It depends on creating a zone of specular reflection, which is an area of very bright illumination produced by the reflection of light directly to the examiner's eyes. Zones of specular reflection exist, for example, on the surface of a sunlit lake. Most of the surface of the lake appears relatively dark because the sunlight is reflected somewhere other than straight to the observer; but very bright patches are seen on the lake in locations from which sunlight is reflected directly to the observer—the zones of specular reflection. When such an area of reflection is established on the corneal endothelium, it is actually possible for the examiner to see individual endothelial cells and their cellular outlines. This is because minute irregularities in the tissue cause some of the light in the zone of reflection not to be reflected to the examiner, and the irregularities then stand out as dark areas in an otherwise bright zone.

To achieve specular reflection, the examiner directs a medium to narrow beam of light (it must be thicker than an optical section) toward the eye from the temporal side. The angle of illumination should be wide (50° to 60°) relative to the examiner's axis of observation (which should be slightly nasal to the patient's visual axis). A bright zone of specular reflection will be evident on the temporal, midperipheral corneal epithelium. Placing the surface of the parallelepiped on this zone of epithelial reflection will yield a zone of specular reflection on both the epithelial (anterior) and endothelial (posterior) faces of the parallelepiped (Figure 10.7). By focusing carefully with the joystick, the examiner can bring the endothelial cells, in the form of a mosaic pattern, into view. The technique requires some practice, so beginners should not be discouraged if they are unable to see the cells the first several times they make the attempt.

Transillumination

Transillumination, or retroillumination, backlights tissues to be examined. This technique allows ready detection of vacuoles of edema in the corneal epithelium, blood vessels in the cornea, deposits on or other abnormalities of the posterior surface of the cornea (Figure 10.8), and tears or areas of atrophy in the iris. A medium-width beam of light is projected onto a part of the eye that lies deeper than the area

Figure 10.7 Specular reflection can make visible deep corneal guttae (orange-peel-like, dark indentations of the endothelium caused by focal excrescences of Descemet's membrane) in early Fuchs corneal dystrophy.

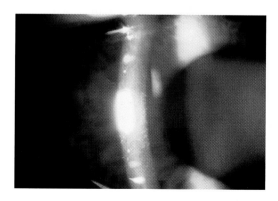

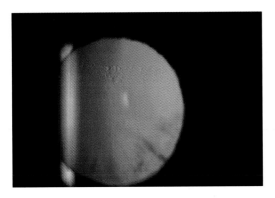

Figure 10.8 Retroillumination from the fundus (the red reflex) clearly backlights the horizontally oriented vesicular abnormalities of the posterior cornea (in the upper portion of the pupillary area), here to demonstrate posterior polymorphous corneal dystrophy.

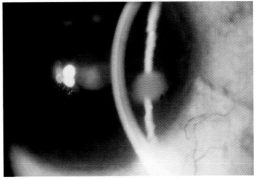

Figure 10.9 Superficial calcium (in Bowman's layer) is made evident by transillumination of the cornea by light reflected from the iris; the corneal parallelepiped is to the left of the ovoid calcium deposit, which is highlighted by the (out of focus) light from the iris.

to be studied, so that the latter can be seen by reflected light while the examiner focuses on the tissues to be examined. For example, to examine the cornea, the light is projected onto the iris while the examiner's view is focused on the cornea. Similarly, the iris may be examined by directing light onto the surface of the lens or the retina (Figure 10.9).

Transillumination from the fundus (retina) is best performed with a dilated pupil and with the viewing and illuminating systems of the slit lamp not parfocal. These systems are generally set to be parfocal; turning the knob near the lower aspect of the illuminating arm of the slit lamp allows the source of illumination to be rotated and decentered nasally or temporally, so that it is no longer parfocal with the viewing portion of the slit lamp. For example, you can focus on the center of the nasal iris while the light beam is at the temporal area of the pupil. This allows transillumination of the iris with a diffuse red glow (red reflex) from the fundus. The technique works best when the light beam enters the pupil from nearly straight ahead (at only a small angle from, and nearly parallel to, the patient's visual axis).

Indirect Lateral Illumination

For indirect lateral illumination, the light is directed just to the side of the lesion to be examined. Some of the light enters the lesion, causing it to glow internally (Figure 10.10). This type of illumination is most useful for translucent lesions such as some corneal opacities or iris nodules.

Sclerotic Scatter

Sclerotic scatter is especially useful for detecting subtle corneal opacities. The less transparent areas become highlighted because they scatter the internally reflected light (Figure 10.11). Like transillumination, sclerotic scatter requires making the illumination arm not parfocal with the viewing arm. A medium-width beam is directed onto the limbus by rotating the illuminating arm temporally, while the examiner views the center of the cornea. The light from the limbus traverses

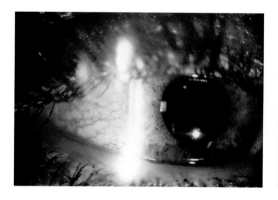

Figure 10.10 Indirect lateral illumination here makes visible 2 immunologically induced (catarrhal) infiltrates to the right of the beam, representing hypersensitivity to bacterial antigens in staphylococcal conjunctivitis.

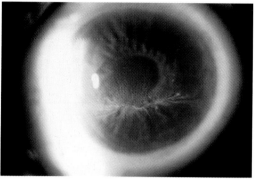

Figure 10.11 Sclerotic scatter produces a diffuse glow of the limbus and a backlighting of any corneal opacities, as with cornea verticillata (whorl-like changes) secondary to epithelial deposition of the oral drug amiodarone, shown here.

the cornea by alternately reflecting off the anterior and posterior corneal surfaces (total internal reflection), so that the cornea functions much as does a fiberoptic cable. The results are that the limbus glows along its entire circumference and the cornea manifests an internal glow as well.

Oscillatory Illumination

Moving the beam (usually an optical section) side to side can sometimes make subtle opacities more evident by allowing them to be viewed alternately by direct and indirect illumination. Sweeping an optical section from limbus to limbus repeatedly can reveal subtle degrees of corneal thinning, as in mild keratoconus. The thickness of the optical section can be seen to vary slightly as the thinner areas are passed over.

■ Special Techniques

Certain accessory instruments and attachments to the slit lamp allow examinations that cannot be performed with the slit lamp alone. Instructions in the use of the slit lamp for measurement of structures or abnormalities are detailed in this section. Uses of the slit lamp for gonioscopy, Hruby-lens and other fundus examinations, tonometry, photography, and laser therapy are mentioned only briefly here, either because they are covered in more detail elsewhere in this manual or because further discussion is beyond the scope of this manual.

The Slit Lamp as a Measuring Device

The dimensions of ocular structures or lesions can be measured, and then noted in the record in millimeters or tenths of a millimeter, by matching the length of the slit-lamp beam to the horizontal and vertical extents of the subject of interest.

Most slit lamps have a knob that, when turned, changes the height of the beam; the knob is associated with a millimeter scale (usually above the knob; see [9] and [7] in Figure 10.1). A reasonably accurate linear measurement can be made by varying the height of the beam until it corresponds to the height of a lesion. This is easily accomplished for vertical measurements because the beam of the slit lamp is routinely oriented vertically. Horizontal measurements can be made by rotating the uppermost, cylindrical portion of the part of the slit lamp that contains the il-luminating bulb (in the case of the Haag-Streit 900 instrument), so as to produce a horizontal beam (other slit-lamp models might have slightly different mechanisms for obtaining horizontal beams). Clinical Protocol 10.1 provides instructions for this method of lesion measurement.

Another method for measuring lesions is the use of an ocular that contains a micrometer scale (Figure 10.12). The image of the scale is superimposed upon the examiner's view of the eye, allowing for direct measurement.

An accessory attachment called a *pachymeter* (or pachometer) is available for the Haag-Streit 900 for measuring corneal thickness (Figure 10.13). It uses a beam-splitting device that cuts the (thin) slit-lamp beam into 2 optical sections, one above and one below a horizontal dividing line. These images are focused onto the cor-nea and are brought together by rotating a calibrated metal plate that is mounted on the slit lamp where the Goldmann tonometer is normally mounted. The images are positioned so that the epithelial line of the lower image is aligned with the endothe-lial line of the upper image. Because the beams of light delineating the cornea are moved by a distance equal to the width of the corneal beam, the corneal thickness can be measured. The thickness is read from the scale on the rotatable metal plate. This procedure also requires the use of a special eyepiece to replace the slit lamp's right ocular, and the ocular needs to be set to +1.50 D more than the examiner's refraction. The slit-lamp pachymeter is seldom used now that electronic optical and ultrasonic pachymeters (not attached to slit lamp) are available. The electronic instruments are easier to use and probably more accurate (see Chapter 12).

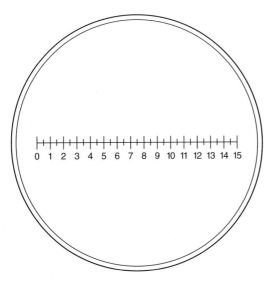

Figure 10.12 An ocular (eyepiece) reticle that is available for taking measurements with the slit lamp displays a 15 mm length, divided into 0.5 mm steps. (Courtesy Haag-Streit USA Inc.)

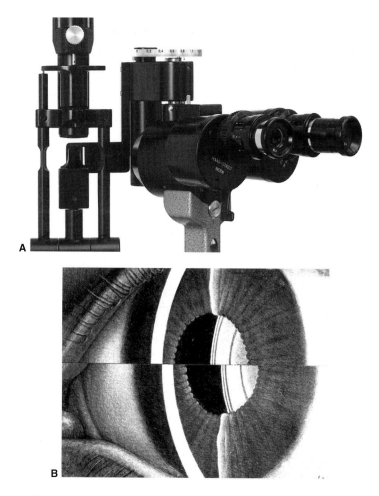

Figure 10.13 **(A)** Pachymeter (or pachometer) for measuring corneal thickness or depth, mounted on slit lamp. **(B)** The split images of an optical section that the pachymeter provides are brought together to measure the corneal thickness. (Courtesy Haag-Streit USA Inc.)

Gonioscopy

Gonioscopy is examination of the angle of the anterior chamber (where the peripheral cornea meets the peripheral iris) by means of a refracting or reflecting contact lens (gonioprism, or goniolens) that is placed against the patient's anesthetized cornea. The goniolens allows light from the slit lamp to enter and exit the angle, which would otherwise not be possible. Some goniolenses also permit visualization of the posterior vitreous and the retina (including the peripheral vitreous, peripheral retina, the macula, and the optic-nerve head), and the choroid. Instructions for performing gonioscopy appear in Chapter 11.

Fundus Examination With the Slit Lamp

Examination of the posterior segment (vitreous and retina) is possible with the slit lamp and 2 kinds of accessory lenses: a Hruby lens and handheld condensing lenses. A Hruby lens is a plano-concave lens that is often attached to the slit lamp.

When swung into position in front of the patient's eye, the Hruby lens allows light from the slit lamp to be focused into the posterior segment of the eye, permitting examination of the fundus. Further detail and instructions for using the Hruby lens with the slit lamp appear in Chapter 13.

High-plus condensing fundus lenses are handheld lenses used for fundus examination by indirect slit-lamp biomicroscopy. The +90 D and +78 D lenses are used most often, but lenses ranging from +60 D to +132 D are available. These lenses function in much the same way as the Hruby lens, although optical differences exist between the 2 types. Clinical Protocol 13.3 provides instructions.

Goldmann Tonometry

A Goldmann tonometer attached to the slit lamp is used to measure intraocular pressure. The procedure requires the use of fluorescein dye and the slit lamp's cobalt-blue filter. Clinical Protocol 12.1 provides instructions.

Slit-Lamp Photography

Some slit lamps have 35 mm still or digital cameras attached, permitting clinical photography. The use of 2 such cameras on a slit lamp makes stereoscopic photography possible. Sometimes a video camera is connected to the slit lamp.

Pitfalls and Pointers

- Remember to set the oculars to your refractive error, or to plano if you use the slit lamp while wearing your glasses; otherwise it can be difficult to obtain a clearly focused view.
- Difficulties occur if the patient is not made reasonably comfortable just prior to, and during, the slit-lamp examination. Proper positioning of the patient is important before beginning the examination. The intensity of the light exposure should be kept at levels that are comfortable for the patient whenever possible.
- It is important to look at the eyelids, other adnexa, and the conjunctiva with relatively dim, diffuse illumination before focusing on the cornea with a parallelepiped or an optical section.
- To take advantage of the full value of the slit lamp, the examiner must become skilled in using all of the methods of illumination and understand when each is best employed.

Suggested Resource

The Eye Exam and Basic Ophthalmic Instruments. This clinical DVD features 3 titles: Fundamentals of Slit-Lamp Biomicroscopy (1993), Goldmann Applanation Tonometry (1988), and Eye Exam: The Essentials (2001). Reviewed for currency 2007. San Francisco: American Academy of Ophthalmology.

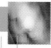

Clinical Protocol 10.1   **Measuring Lesions Linearly With the Slit-Lamp Beam**

1. Set the brightness knob under the slit-lamp table to the first (lowest intensity) setting.

2. Set the brightness lever on the illuminating arm to full brightness.

3. Adjust the slit-lamp beam to slightly thicker than an optical section, using one of the knurled knobs at the bottom of the illuminating arm (Haag-Streit 900).

4. Place the illuminating arm directly in front of the viewing arm so that the slit-lamp beam is parallel to the patient's visual axis.

5. Focus the vertically oriented slit-lamp beam onto the lesion to be measured.

6. Twist the protruding, knurled knob (just below the brightness lever on the Haag-Streit 900) to vary the height of the beam until it equals the height of the lesion.

7. Read the scale (at the base of the bulb housing) that indicates the height of the beam in tenths of a millimeter.

8. Rotate the bulb housing 90° to orient the beam horizontally, and repeat steps 6 and 7 to measure the horizontal dimension of the lesion; the bulb housing may be rotated less than 90° to perform diagonal measurements.

9. Record the measurements in the patient's record.

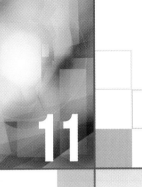

Anterior Segment Examination

11

Whereas the external examination provides an overview of relatively gross abnormalities of the adnexa and some of the more anterior ocular structures, the anterior segment examination consists of a more detailed study of virtually all the tissues of the anterior eye, and some tissues anterior to the mid-vitreous, by means of the slit-lamp biomicroscope.

The examination of the anterior segment should always be thorough, but it need not always be complete. Some evaluations are generally performed only when they are indicated as a result of the history, the external examination, or some other part of the examination. Evaluations in this category include those of the lacrimal gland, of the skin remote from the margins of the eyelids, and of the anterior chamber angle (by gonioscopy).

The components of the slit-lamp biomicroscope and basic principles of its illumination capabilities were detailed in Chapter 10. This chapter describes the order and anatomic components of the biomicroscopic anterior segment examination, including normal anatomic appearance and common or important abnormalities. In a limited way where appropriate, this chapter reinforces how the various types of slit-lamp illumination and procedures are best applied for examining individual anatomic components.

■ Overview of the Anterior Segment Examination

The slit-lamp examination of the anterior segment should proceed from the gross anatomic view to the detailed view. This means that for each anatomic region, examination should begin with relatively low magnification and either diffuse lighting with a broad beam or direct focal illumination, as appropriate. By beginning grossly, the examiner is more likely not to overlook gross abnormalities, or, in other words, not to miss the forest for the trees. When the initial biomicroscopic examination suggests the possibility of an abnormality requiring further investigation, the more specialized slit-lamp illumination techniques and higher magnification can be applied.

The components of the anterior segment examination, listed below, follow an anatomically logical order:

- Lacrimal gland and skin
- Eyelids and eyelashes
- Conjunctiva
- Episclera and sclera
- Tear film

- Cornea
- Anterior chamber
- Iris
- Crystalline lens
- Retrolental space and anterior vitreous

The following text describes the anterior segment examination in terms of structures and findings that are evaluated and provides instructions in various specialized biomicroscopic and other techniques that might be required for complete evaluation.

■ Lacrimal Gland and Skin

Biomicroscopic evaluation of the lacrimal gland and the skin remote from the margins of the eyelids is necessary only if the patient's history or a previous evaluation have suggested the presence of an abnormality needing investigation.

The most anterior portion of the lacrimal gland (the palpebral lobe) is the only portion of this structure that can be examined biomicroscopically. It can be seen by lifting upward (not outward) the temporal aspect of the upper eyelid with a thumb while the patient's ipsilateral eye is directed inferonasally; to examine the palpebral lobe of the lacrimal gland of the patient's right eye, for example, you would ask the patient to look down and to the left.

The normal palpebral lobe of the gland is slightly pink. It can manifest enlargement and inflammation (Figure 11.1), exudate, tumor, or foreign bodies.

To examine the skin remote from the eyelids, employ low magnification and diffuse illumination with white light and a broad beam. Various manifestations of dermatitis may be investigated, including erythema (redness of the skin); eczema, which occurs, for example, with allergic contact or atopic dermatitis and is characterized by varying combinations of redness, tiny papules and vesicles, oozing, flaking, scaling, lichenification (thickening), and sometimes pigmentation (Figure 11.2); urticaria (hives; epidermal edema); angioedema (a deeper urticaria with

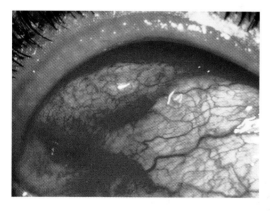

Figure 11.1   Enlarged, inflamed palpebral lobe of the right lacrimal gland.

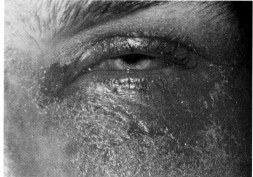

Figure 11.2   Eczematoid (allergic contact) blepharo-conjunctivitis caused by topical ophthalmic medication (atropine).

more involvement of the dermis); vesicular or bullous dermatitis (as occurs with herpes simplex, varicella zoster, or bullous dermatoses such as pemphigus vulgaris or pemphigoid); and other forms of dermatitis (atrophic, exfoliative, pustular, necrotizing, hemorrhagic, seborrheic, discoid).

Dried secretions from the eye can be found on the skin around the eye. Serous transudate and, much less commonly, purulent exudate can originate from the skin itself.

With low magnification, broad beam, and white light the slit lamp can be used to examine ecchymoses (intracutaneous hemorrhages, or "black eyes") or cutaneous tumors. Tumors that may be studied biomicroscopically include actinic keratosis; squamous, basal cell, or sebaceous carcinoma; benign squamous papilloma (skin tag); viral papilloma (verruca, or wart); molluscum contagiosum; cysts; pigmented lesions (nevus, melanoma); vascular lesions; and neurogenic tumors.

Pigmentary abnormalities can also be evaluated biomicroscopically. Pigmentary changes of the skin not caused by tumors include vitiligo (patchy loss of cutaneous pigment), hyperpigmentation secondary to chronic inflammation or trauma, flat nevi, Addison's disease, and argyria (discoloration caused by the deposition of silver-containing compounds).

■ Eyelids and Eyelashes

The eyelid consists of 2 regions or lamellae: anterior and posterior (Figure 11.3). The lamellae are approximately demarcated by a subtle marking called the *gray line* (intermarginal sulcus of von Graefe) that runs horizontally along the margin of the eyelid, posterior to the eyelash follicles and anterior to the meibomian gland orifices. The gray line represents the most superficial portion of the orbicularis oculi muscle (the muscle of Riolan). An incision through (or, more precisely, just behind), the gray line separates the eyelid into its 2 lamellae. The anterior (skin-muscle) lamella

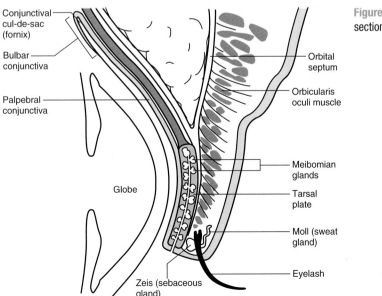

Conjunctival cul-de-sac (fornix)

Bulbar conjunctiva

Palpebral conjunctiva

Globe

Zeis (sebaceous gland)

Orbital septum

Orbicularis oculi muscle

Meibomian glands

Tarsal plate

Moll (sweat gland)

Eyelash

Figure 11.3 Cross-section of the eyelid.

contains the eyelashes and their follicles, the sebaceous glands of Zeis (which empty into the eyelash follicles), and the sweat glands of Moll. The posterior (tarsoconjunctival) lamella contains the sebaceous meibomian glands that lie within the fibrous tarsal plate and open onto the posterior surface of the margin of the eyelid.

Tumors (including nonneoplastic mass lesions) and blepharitis (inflammation of the eyelid) are the most common findings of the eyelids. Low magnification, broad beam, and white light are used for slit-lamp examination of lid tumors and blepharitis.

Tumors

The same tumors that affect the skin (see above) can occur on the skin of the eyelids. Additionally, the eyelids can display tumors that result from abscesses of the glands and lash follicles.

A *hordeolum* is an acute abscess of a sebaceous (Zeis or meibomian) gland of the eyelid. Two variations occur:

- External hordeolum, also known as a *stye*, is an acute inflammation in the area of a Zeis gland of the anterior lamella of the eyelid (Figure 11.4).
- Internal hordeolum, also known as an acute chalazion, is an acute inflammation in the area of a meibomian gland of the posterior lamella of the eyelid (Figure 11.5). Examination of an internal hordeolum requires eversion of the eyelid (see Chapter 9).

A *chalazion* is a subacute or chronic granuloma surrounding lipid that has been extruded into the tissues from a blocked sebaceous gland of the eyelid (Figure 11.6). Hordeola are acute lesions associated with intense inflammation that can be purulent if caused by bacterial infection (usually staphylococcal) or granulomatous if caused merely by extruded lipid. In contrast, chalazia (except for the poorly named acute chalazion) are chronic, nonpurulent granulomas with only low-grade inflammation. Hordeola that do not resolve within a few days show gradually diminishing amounts of inflammation over days to weeks and can evolve into chalazia.

Chalazia that protrude anteriorly (toward the skin of the eyelid) produce a dome-like elevation of the skin with varying amounts of erythema (see Figure 11.6). Chalazia that develop more posteriorly manifest a yellowish mass of lipid and granulomatous inflammation (visible through the palpebral conjunctiva), with

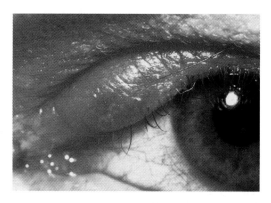

Figure 11.4 External hordeolum (stye).

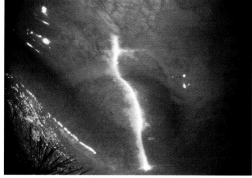

Figure 11.5 Internal hordeolum (acute chalazion).

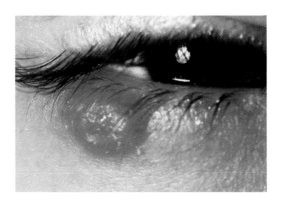

Figure 11.6   Chalazion.

or without polypoid hyperplasia of the palpebral conjunctiva. Very large posterior chalazia can also cause elevation of the skin of the eyelid.

Folliculitis is an acute abscess of an eyelash follicle, rather than a sebaceous gland. Folliculitis is nearly always caused by acute staphylococcal infection and is not a precursor to chalazion, unless a Zeis gland happens also to become obstructed in the course of the infection.

Blepharitis

Blepharitis (inflammation of the eyelid) manifests in a variety of forms, depending on the cause. Anterior, or marginal, blepharitis can be bacterial in origin, or seborrheic, or caused by mites, lice, or dermatitis.

Staphylococcal blepharitis is a common condition typified by the presence of "collarettes"—thin, honey-colored flakes surrounding, and lying among, eyelashes (Figure 11.7). The flakes consist of dried serous and fibrinous extravasation that results from the inflammation that the bacteria cause within the eyelash follicles.

In seborrheic blepharitis, dandruff-like flakes ("scurf") or amorphous accumulations of oily sebaceous material, or both, are found randomly distributed on and among the eyelashes (Figure 11.8). Meibomitis and meibomian dysfunction (see below) are also forms of seborrheic blepharitis but occur in the posterior eyelid.

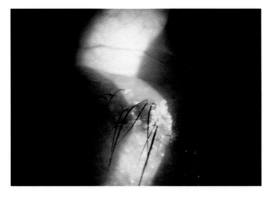

Figure 11.7   Collarette of staphylococcal blepharitis (white flake just inside right edge of slit beam).

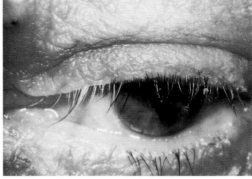

Figure 11.8   Sebaceous material adherent to eyelashes in seborrheic blepharitis (temporal aspect of upper eyelid); note also madarosis (loss of eyelashes) and poliosis (whitening of eyelashes) from prior staphylococcal blepharitis.

Demodectic blepharitis is caused by infestation of the eyelash follicles with a mite, *Demodex folliculorum*, and is especially common in elderly patients (Figure 11.9). This form of "blepharitis" is actually associated with little or no inflammation and is thought generally to be asymptomatic. It is typified by the presence of waxy-appearing, cylindrical cuffs or "sleeves" (hypertrophic follicular epithelium) around the bases of eyelashes (Figure 11.10). Figure 11.11 diagrammatically depicts the difference in appearance between eyelash collarettes, seborrheic eyelash scurf, and eyelash sleeves.

All of the manifestations of dermatitis discussed above in the section "Lacrimal Gland and Skin" can occur on the skin of the eyelids. Accordingly, one can encounter vesicular lesions (herpes simplex, varicella-zoster, impetigo), ulcerative or necrotizing lesions (varicella-zoster, insect or spider bites, anthrax), urticarial or angioedematous lesions (often of allergic origin), polymorphous lesions (erythema multiforme), cellulitis, and so on.

Posterior blepharitis arises from disorders of the meibomian glands. Meibomitis (inflammation of the meibomian glands) can occur in the form of bacterial or, rarely, fungal abscesses or, most commonly, as chalazia. Meibomian dysfunction implies hypersecretion of the glands, often along with abnormally thick and perhaps otherwise biochemically abnormal secretions. The dysfunction is indicated by fullness, excessive secretion, or inspissation of the glands, as well as by irregularity of their orifices (Figure 11.12). It can occur as an isolated problem, but it is especially common in patients who have rosacea.

Angular blepharitis affects mainly the medial or lateral canthal areas of the eyelids, which show eczematoid or ulcerative changes of the skin. The condition develops secondarily in association with some forms of bacterial conjunctivitis (especially that caused by staphylococcus or moraxella).

The following signs are most often associated with long-standing staphylococcal blepharitis but can be seen with other kinds of inflammation of the eyelids:

- Madarosis (loss of eyelashes; see Figure 11.8)
- Poliosis (whitening of eyelashes; see Figure 11.8)

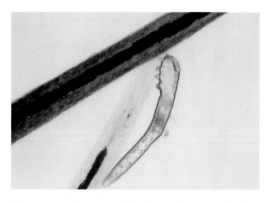

Figure 11.9 *Demodex folliculorum* mite near epilated eyelash from a patient with demodectic blepharitis (unstained, 200×).

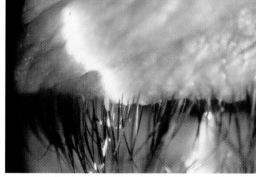

Figure 11.10 Sleeve or cuff in demodectic blepharitis (base of eyelash, just to left of where slit-lamp beam contacts skin of eyelid).

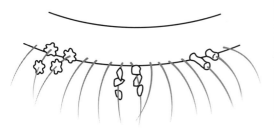

Figure 11.11 Diagrammatic representations of lash collarettes (left), seborrheic material (center), and lash sleeve (right).

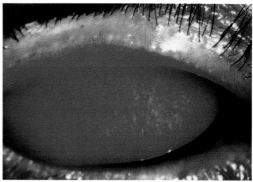

Figure 11.12 Meibomian gland dysfunction in the upper lid of a patient with rosacea; fullness, dilation, and irregularity of various meibomian orifices (near posterior aspect of lid margin) are evident.

- Trichiasis (misdirection of eyelashes, often causing irritation). Trichiasis can occur because the eyelashes grow backwards (because, for example, of scar tissue having distorted the lash follicles) or because the lid margin itself is distorted (as with entropion—a turning posteriorly of the lid margin).

■ Conjunctiva

The conjunctiva is best evaluated in a stepwise, anatomically logical fashion, beginning with the palpebral (tarsal) conjunctiva, then proceeding to the limbal conjunctiva and bulbar conjunctiva.

Palpebral Conjunctiva

The conjunctival aspect of the eyelids (palpebral, or tarsal, conjunctiva) is examined by everting them (see instructions in Chapter 9). The palpebral conjunctiva can be affected by papillae, follicles, granulomas, membranes and pseudomembranes, scarring, and foreign bodies.

Papillae

Papillary conjunctivitis is the term given to any subacute or chronic inflammation of the palpebral conjunctiva that leads to the formation of papillae, which are tiny, dome-shaped nodules that cause the conjunctiva to have a bumpy appearance (Figures 11.13 and 11.14). Each papilla consists of a central core of hyperemic blood vessels that protrude upward, perpendicular to the tarsal plate, surrounded by edema and inflammatory cells and, in some long-standing cases, fibrosis.

Papillae develop because the palpebral (and the limbal) conjunctiva is normally made adherent to underlying tissues by many tiny, vertically oriented, fibrous septa. These septa constrain the tissue from swelling diffusely and evenly, with the result that it swells only in the areas where septa are absent, producing many tiny nodules of swelling (papillae).

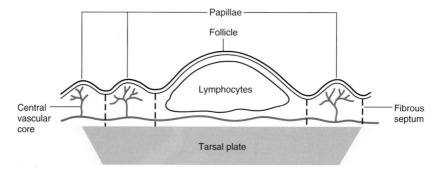

Figure 11.13 Cross-sectional diagrammatic representation of a conjunctival lymphoid follicle and papillae.

Figure 11.14 Diagrammatic representation of the clinical appearance of a conjunctival follicle and papillae.

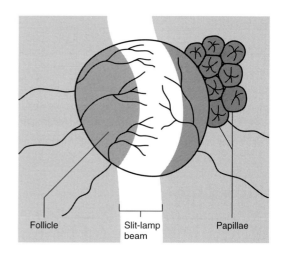

Papillae can be very small (micropapillae), small (referred to as "fine"), medium-sized, or "giant." Micropapillae (less than 0.3 mm in diameter) are of no clinical importance because they are a normal finding. Small (fine) papillae measure 0.3 to 0.6 mm in diameter and are considered to be abnormal (Figure 11.15). However, they are a nonspecific finding, occurring in many different kinds of conjunctival inflammation. They are usually graded on a scale of 1 to 3 (modified as needed with a plus sign), with 3 being the most severe. A moderate reaction could be recorded as *P2 small* (or *fine*) or as *2+ papillary reaction*.

Medium papillae are 0.6 to 1.0 mm in diameter. They are an abnormal finding representing early confluence of small papillae as the latter enlarge and rupture the intervening fibrous septa (Figure 11.16).

Giant papillae are larger than 1.0 mm in diameter and are distinctly abnormal (Figure 11.17). Giant papillary conjunctivitis (GPC) occurs in vernal and atopic conjunctivitis, as a reaction to accumulated deposits on contact lenses or prosthetic eyes, and as a reaction to sutures. Giant papillae represent coalescence of many small or medium papillae and tend to become polygonal as their sides press against one another.

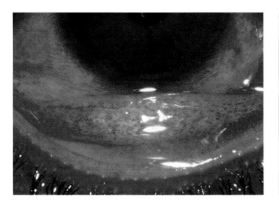

Figure 11.15   Fine papillary reaction of the inferior palpebral conjunctiva.

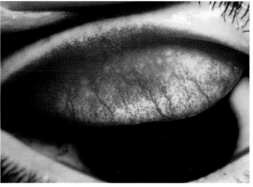

Figure 11.16   Medium-sized papillae of upper palpebral conjunctiva (irregular, pale areas), a reaction to deposits on a soft contact lens. The pallor occurs because the papillae are becoming sufficiently thick and fibrotic as to obscure the vascular cores.

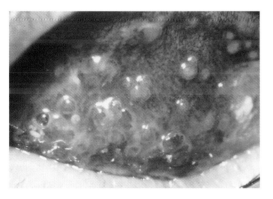

Figure 11.17   Giant papillae of the upper palpebral conjunctiva, a reaction to deposits on an ocular prosthesis.

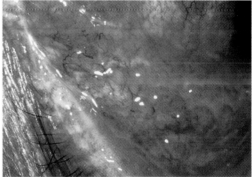

Figure 11.18   Follicular reaction of the lower palpebral conjunctiva, as a reaction to dipivalyl epinephrine eyedrops.

Follicles

The conjunctiva normally contains islands of subepithelial lymphoid tissue. When they enlarge to the extent that they are visible, they are called *follicles*. Follicles are several times larger in diameter than small papillae and consist of masses of lymphocytes, lymphoblasts, and a few macrophages (Figure 11.18). They are like miniature lymph nodes and do not contain central vascular cores as do papillae. Follicles enlarge upward from the conjunctival stroma, causing dome-shaped elevations of the conjunctival surface. The normal blood vessels of the conjunctiva are also pushed upward, so that they seem to course up onto, and over, the surface of each follicle.

Older children and adolescents often have relatively prominent conjunctival follicles (physiologic folliculosis) as a normal finding unassociated with inflammation.

Follicles that occur with conjunctivitis are usually most prominent in the inferior fornix and the inferior palpebral conjunctiva. Follicular reactions can occur in the superior palpebral conjunctiva, but they are always less prominent there than below, except in trachoma.

Pathologic conjunctival follicles constitute a useful clinical finding because they occur in association with only a few specific kinds of conjunctival inflammations, mainly those caused by chlamydia, adenoviruses, herpes simplex (primary infections), molluscum contagiosum, and toxic reactions to certain topical ophthalmic medications.

Granulomas

Granulomatous conjunctivitis is characterized by the presence of 1 or more conjunctival granulomas that are not merely chalazia. The granulomas that occur with conjunctivitis have the same appearance as described above for chalazia, except that the former are more often polypoid (Figure 11.19). A few follicles are often seen in the area of the granuloma when the cause is an infection.

Most cases of granulomatous conjunctivitis are caused by the agent of cat-scratch disease (*Bartonella henselae*). Less common causes include tuberculosis, syphilis, and tularemia, among others. Conjunctival granulomas can develop in patients who have sarcoidosis. Sarcoid granulomas are usually not polypoid; they resemble follicles but have a yellowish center.

Membranes and pseudomembranes

Some kinds of intense conjunctivitis cause transudation of fibrin within, and on the surface of, the conjunctiva (Figure 11.20). The material is seen as a white-to-tan, sometimes rubbery deposition that is adherent to the conjunctiva and that obscures the underlying conjunctival blood vessels.

The layer of fibrin, always with an admixture of neutrophils, is referred to as a *pseudomembrane* if it simply lies on the conjunctival surface, in which case the pseudomembrane may be peeled away without bleeding. A true membrane

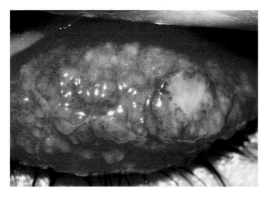

Figure 11.19 Conjunctival granuloma (large, polygonal lesion with central pallor) with adjacent follicles, as a result of cat-scratch disease.

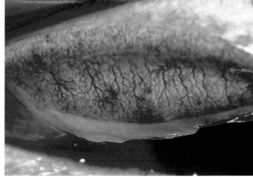

Figure 11.20 Pseudomembranous reaction on upper palpebral conjunctiva in adenoviral conjunctivitis. The pseudomembrane has been partially peeled away, and its edge can be seen folded on itself near the upper border of the tarsal plate (lower part of the photograph).

incorporates the conjunctival epithelium and so cannot be removed without causing bleeding. Otherwise, the difference between a membrane and a pseudomembrane is one of degree, the pseudomembrane indicating a lesser intensity of inflammation.

With the exception of ocular diphtheria, which is said always to cause a true membrane, the causes of this class of conjunctivitis can lead to the formation of either a membrane or pseudomembrane, depending on the severity of the inflammatory response. The main causes are adenovirus, herpes simplex (primary infections), chlamydia (in infants), beta-hemolytic streptococcus, chemical burns, and erythema multiforme.

Scarring

Conjunctival scarring can result from a variety of traumatic or inflammatory processes that affect the conjunctival stroma, where fibroblasts reside.

Conjunctival scarring is seen as white or gray areas of fibrosis. The scarring can be wispy, reticular, linear, stellate, or plaque-like. The more severe degrees of scarring can be associated with contraction of surrounding tissues. Extensive scarring in the inferior conjunctival fornix can lead to foreshortening, or even loss, of the fornix. The same process can occur in the superior fornix, but it is difficult to see unless the upper eyelid is doubly everted. Extreme degrees of scarring can cause a band of fibrous tissue, called a *symblepharon*, to develop between the palpebral conjunctiva and the bulbar conjunctiva; occasionally, these 2 tissues become firmly adherent to each other (Figure 11.21).

Causes of conjunctival scarring include chemical burns and other trauma (including surgery), chalazia, trachoma, membranous conjunctivitis, atopic conjunctivitis, erythema multiforme, ocular cicatricial pemphigoid, and some reactions to ophthalmic or systemic medications.

Foreign bodies

Although foreign bodies can turn up anywhere in the conjunctival sac, they often lodge in the palpebral conjunctiva of the upper eyelid, which should be everted to exclude this possibility. When a patient is being examined for suspected or known foreign body, the lacrimal puncta should also be examined with slit-lamp magnification, because a loose eyelash occasionally becomes trapped in the punctal orifice and rubs the eye. If foreign material is suspected but not found, the conjunctival sac

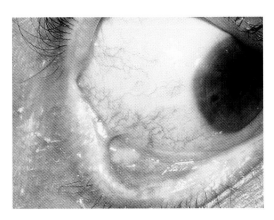

Figure 11.21   Symblepharon (adhesion between the bulbar conjunctiva and the lower eyelid) occurring in ocular cicatricial pemphigoid.

should be swept with a moist cotton swab in an effort to remove any foreign particles or strands of mucus that might contain foreign bodies. Clinical Protocol 11.1 describes the process.

Limbal Conjunctiva

The limbal conjunctiva can be affected by ciliary (limbal) flush, papillae and Horner-Trantas dots, and limbal follicles.

Ciliary (limbal) flush

The anterior ciliary blood vessels form a perilimbal plexus within the conjunctiva and episclera. When hyperemic, these vessels can be seen to extend outward from the limbus for 1 to 2 mm in a radial pattern. Hyperemia of this plexus is seen as a red to violaceous, circumcorneal ring of dilated blood vessels (Figure 11.22). It indicates corneal, episcleral, scleral, or intraocular inflammation.

Limbal papillae and Horner-Trantas dots

The limbal, like the palpebral, conjunctiva has anchoring fibrous septa, so papillae (including giant papillae) can form in the limbal conjunctiva (Figure 11.23). Limbal papillae have the same structure and appearance as palpebral ones, but they do not develop flat tops as do some of the palpebral giant papillae. In extreme cases, limbal giant papillae take on the appearance of a gelatinous mass overlying the entire limbal area.

In some cases of chronic allergic conjunctivitis, focal masses of eosinophils appear on the surfaces of the limbal papillae (see Figure 11.23). These cellular accumulations, called *Horner-Trantas dots*, are yellow-white and usually about 1 to 2 mm in diameter but can be larger. Limbal papillae usually indicate vernal or atopic conjunctivitis.

Limbal follicles

Follicles sometimes develop in the limbal area, but they are not common. They have the same appearance as follicles elsewhere. They are most likely to occur with

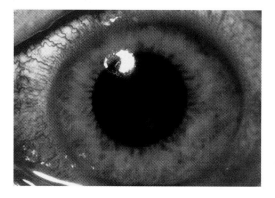

Figure 11.22   Ciliary flush (best seen here along the superior limbus); closely spaced radial vessels extend about 1 mm peripherally from the cornea.

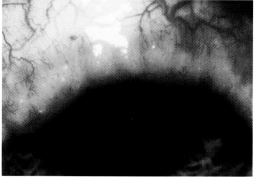

Figure 11.23   Limbal papillae with several Horner-Trantas dots (small white dots), in allergic (vernal) conjunctivitis.

chlamydial infections or toxic follicular reactions to topical ophthalmic medications. Limbal follicles are common in trachoma; with healing they leave round, often depressed, limbal scars known as *Herbert's pits*. Nontrachomatous follicles do not undergo necrosis and so do not form Herbert's pits.

Bulbar Conjunctiva

Although both the bulbar and the palpebral conjunctiva can exude secretions and discharge, pathology is more apparent in the more extensive bulbar tissue. In addition to secretions, the bulbar conjunctiva can manifest chemosis, lymphangiectasia and lymphedema, telangiectasia, hyperemia, epithelial defects and ulcers, and a variety of less common abnormalities.

Secretions and discharge

The characteristics of conjunctival secretions are many and variable and can be diagnostically valuable to the examiner.

Watery discharge on the conjunctiva is actually a secretion rather than a discharge (exudate) because it represents reflex tear flow from the lacrimal gland. The term *tearing* is used when the excess tears merely accumulate within the conjunctival sac; the term *epiphora* is used if the tears spill over the margin of the eyelid onto the face.

Tearing and epiphora can be caused by any irritation of the ocular surface, for example, inflammatory disease or foreign bodies. Other causes include cold wind, yawning, sneezing, gagging, irritating fumes, or lacrimal-outflow obstruction. The last usually manifests epiphora.

Mucoid discharge, too, is a secretion, of the conjunctival goblet cells. These cells normally secrete mucus (mucin) continuously, but in such small amounts as to be unnoticeable.

Serous discharge consists of proteinaceous fluid that is more viscous than aqueous tears. In its pure form, serous discharge is acellular, occurring in mild inflammations of the conjunctiva, although inflammatory cells can be present with more intense inflammations (seromucopurulent, seropurulent discharge), as can blood.

Conjunctival mucus is seen as a nearly clear, sticky material on the ocular surface (Figure 11.24). It most often appears in the form of strands that are several millimeters to centimeters long, although amorphous globs can also be seen. The

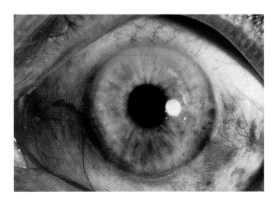

Figure 11.24 Mucous secretion in keratoconjunctivitis sicca, here stained with rose-bengal dye (curvilinear strand nasal to limbus). Note also the rose-bengal staining of the conjunctiva and cornea in the interpalpebral area of exposure (typical of the dry eye).

Figure 11.25   Mucopurulent discharge in bacterial conjunctivitis.

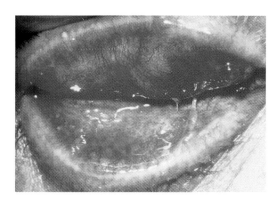

mucus is most often found in the inferior conjunctival fornix or in the area of the semilunar fold and caruncle.

Mucus is a nonspecific finding, its excessive production being brought about by practically any irritation of the ocular surface. Mucus is regularly found in ocular allergies and in dry eyes.

Mucopurulent discharge (mucopus) consists of neutrophils mixed with mucus and so represents a combination of a secretion and a discharge. An old term for mucopurulent is *catarrhal*, meaning that a discharge is less than fully purulent. The term is still used at times, usually in the form of "catarrhal conjunctivitis," which is a synonym for relatively mild (usually bacterial or allergic) conjunctivitis.

Mucopus has the same appearance as mucus, except that the neutrophils give the mucus a white appearance (Figure 11.25). Mucopus tends to accumulate during sleep and so is likely to be most noticeable early in the morning; if the patient cleanses it from the eye at that time, the mucopus might be difficult to detect at the time of an examination later in the day, as this kind of discharge is often scant. In this situation, the examiner may conclude that some mucopus has been present if the patient has a history of the eyelids having been sealed shut upon awakening in the mornings (an indication of the presence of neutrophils).

Mucopurulent discharge is most common with simple bacterial conjunctivitis or the more severe forms of allergic conjunctivitis. It is also found in conjunction with any membranous or pseudomembranous conjunctivitis and with many other external diseases.

Truly purulent discharge consists entirely, or mainly, of neutrophils and is usually copious (Figure 11.26). If wiped away, it often reappears within 5 or 10 minutes. Purulent discharge is usually white, but the color can be altered by microbial pigments (yellow in the case of *Staphylococcus aureus* or greenish-white with pseudomonas). Purulence occurs most often with gonococcal or meningococcal conjunctivitis, bacterial or fungal corneal ulcers, and abscesses.

Chemosis

Chemosis is edema of, or beneath, the conjunctiva (Figure 11.27). It appears as a thickening and ballooning of the tissue. Because the bulbar conjunctiva lacks anchoring septa, the swelling can be diffuse, but it is most prominent in the area of the palpebral fissure where the pressure of the eyelids does not restrict the swelling.

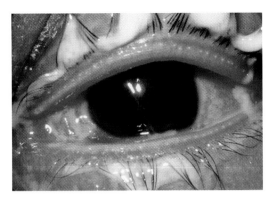

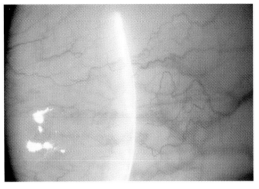

Figure 11.26   Purulent discharge, also known as blennorrhea (flow of pus), in gonococcal conjunctivitis.

Figure 11.27   Chemosis (conjunctival edema) in acute hay fever conjunctivitis.

The color of the edematous conjunctiva can be normal, or it sometimes takes on a slightly yellowish hue.

Chemosis is most often caused by allergy, although it can be caused by a variety of inflammatory conditions, including conjunctivitis, episcleritis, scleritis, uveitis, endophthalmitis, and orbital cellulitis.

Lymphangiectasia and lymphedema

One or more lymphatic channels of the conjunctiva can become dilated (lymphangiectasia), producing the appearance of a clear, slightly elevated, tube-like structure. It is often sacculated, resembling a segment of intestine. Blood is occasionally seen in lymphangiectasis, usually after trauma or inflammation. Lymphangiectasia is often idiopathic, but it is sometimes related to trauma.

Lymphedema of the conjunctiva results from obstruction of lymphatic outflow, leading to a straw-colored, chemosis-like change. The problem is generally caused by scarring or, rarely, tumor in the orbit.

Telangiectasia

Telangiectasia is permanent dilation of small blood vessels. It can occur in the palpebral conjunctiva or in the skin of the eyelids, but it is perhaps most common in the bulbar conjunctiva. The cause is often unknown, but it can be congenital or secondary to chronic inflammation, hypertension, atherosclerosis, orbital vascular abnormalities, rosacea, blood dyscrasias, or hemoglobinopathy (sickle-cell disease). The condition can occur in at least 4 rare diseases, namely, ataxia telangiectasia, Fabry disease, Sturge-Weber syndrome, and Osler-Weber-Rendu disease.

Hyperemia

Increased blood flow with associated dilation of blood vessels (hyperemia) in the conjunctiva produces more or less diffuse redness that is usually most prominent peripherally, tending to fade as the limbus is approached (Figure 11.28). This is because the conjunctival blood supply is most prominent in, and enters from, the peripheral bulbar conjunctiva. This blood supply is distinct from the one that produces a ciliary flush.

Figure 11.28 Hyperemia of the bulbar conjunctiva in bacterial conjunctivitis.

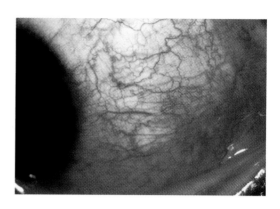

Papillae do not develop in the bulbar conjunctiva because of the absence of fibrous septa. Conjunctival hyperemia is an entirely nonspecific finding that can occur with practically any ocular inflammation, dryness, environmental irritants, and the like.

Epithelial defects and ulcers

Absence or disruption of a portion of the conjunctival epithelium is referred to as an *epithelial defect* or *erosion*. The term *ulcer* implies some loss of conjunctival stroma as well. Epithelial defects and ulcers are detected by the absence of normal conjunctival luster, and by an actual depression in a particular area, often surrounded by some hyperemia. Staining with fluorescein (discussed later in this chapter) can also make evident a defect or ulcer. Defects and ulcers have many causes but are especially common after trauma, including chemical burns.

Other Conjunctival Abnormalities

A detailed discussion of other possible abnormalities of the bulbar conjunctiva is beyond the scope of this book, but such discussions can be found in Section 8, *External Disease and Cornea*, of the Basic and Clinical Science Course of the American Academy of Ophthalmology and many other textbooks. A list of the most important additional abnormalities is presented below. A few of these abnormalities tend to occur only in certain locations, but many of them can occur in either bulbar or palpebral conjunctiva.

- Follicles, granulomas, and membranous reactions (uncommon in bulbar conjunctiva)
- Scarring
- Pigmentations and deposits (accumulation or deposition of melanin, drugs, or systemic or topical heavy metals)
- Dermoid tumors (choristomas, or benign congenital tumors)
- Concretions (epithelial inclusion cysts, rare in bulbar conjunctiva)
- Pinguecula (yellowish, often slightly elevated limbal lesion resulting from ultraviolet exposure)
- Pterygium (triangular fibrovascular bulbar conjunctival growth, extending onto the cornea, associated with pinguecula)

- Phlyctenules (or phlyctens, white or yellow-white round-to-ovoid subepithelial infiltrates often associated with staphylococcal blepharitis or conjunctivitis, or with systemic tuberculosis)
- Keratinization (dry, lackluster, pearly gray alteration of the conjunctival or corneal epithelial surface, sometimes covered with superficial foamy sebaceous matter)
- Tumors, including cysts, papillomas, squamous neoplasia (referred to as conjunctival, or corneal, intraepithelial neoplasia, or CIN), squamous carcinoma, sebaceous carcinoma (secondarily affecting the conjunctiva), nevi, melanomas, lymphomas or benign lymphoid hyperplasia, and angiomas

◾ Episclera and Sclera

Most episcleral and scleral abnormalities are easily observed even with a penlight. A number of differences help the clinician distinguish between conjunctival and scleral or episcleral signs. The episclera and sclera have a blood supply deeper than and separate from that of the conjunctiva. Blood vessels in the conjunctiva are generally finer and less tortuous than the deeper vessels. Furthermore, conjunctival hyperemia has a red appearance, whereas deeper (episcleral and scleral) hyperemia is often violaceous. Conjunctival vessels can be moved by massaging the conjunctiva through the eyelid or directly with a cotton swab; the deeper vessels do not move with such maneuvers. Finally, topical vasoconstricting agents affect conjunctival vessels much more than the deeper vessels.

Episcleritis

Episcleritis is an immunologically mediated inflammation of the tissue that lies between the deep conjunctival stroma and the sclera (Figure 11.29). It is typically benign, short-lived, and not associated with tenderness, ciliary pain, or flare and cell in the anterior chamber. It is diagnosed by the aforementioned features. Thought most often to be idiopathic, episcleritis can also occur with meibomian-gland dysfunction, with or without rosacea.

Episcleritis occurs in 3 forms, depending on the distribution and extent of the deep hyperemia, and on whether or not edema (causing a nodular elevation) is present: diffuse (involving much, or all, of the episclera); sectoral; and nodular (see Figure 11.29).

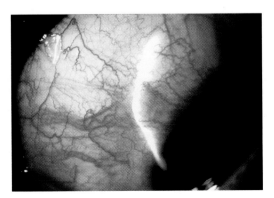

Figure 11.29   Nodular episcleritis; lesion is nodular but superficial to the sclera; this is also an example of sectoral episcleritis, in that it affects only the superonasal aspect of the left eye.

Scleritis

Scleritis is an immunologically mediated inflammation of the sclera itself (always associated with secondary inflammation of the episclera). Deep hyperemia is again seen, along with tenderness, ciliary pain (or, at least, photophobia), and, often, flare and cell in the anterior chamber. Scleritis is likely to have a more prolonged course than episcleritis and can cause damage in the form of scleral thinning (which creates a bluish appearance to the sclera) and complications from uveitis (including glaucoma).

Unlike episcleritis, scleritis is associated with, and is caused by, detectable systemic disease in about one-half of afflicted patients. The most common causes are autoimmune collagen-vascular (connective tissue) diseases, granulomatous diseases such as syphilis or tuberculosis, or gout or hyperuricemia. Roughly 50% of cases are idiopathic, occurring in patients who are otherwise apparently healthy.

Posterior scleritis can occur but will not be discussed in this chapter on the anterior segment examination. Anterior scleritis can be diffuse, sectoral (Figure 11.30), nodular (Figure 11.31), or necrotizing. Necrotizing scleritis with inflammation (ischemic scleritis) occurs in patients who have systemic autoimmune vasculitis and is characterized by severe inflammation and scleral necrosis (Figure 11.32). The affected area often appears to be ischemic in that there are foci of blanched, avascular tissue in or around other nearby areas of severe hyperemia. Conjunctival necrosis can also occur.

Necrotizing scleritis without inflammation (scleromalacia perforans, Figure 11.33) occurs almost exclusively in patients who have chronic rheumatoid disease over the course of many years. There is little or no noticeable, or symptomatic, scleritis, yet the sclera gradually thins so as to produce bulging areas of scleral thinning. Because these areas of thinning are lined with uveal tissue, they have a bluish appearance and are referred to as *staphylomas* (referring to the grape-like appearance).

The inflammation of scleritis can involve secondarily the corneal stroma, producing cellular infiltrate, with or without vascularization (sclerokeratitis).

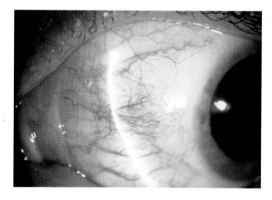

Figure 11.30   Sectoral scleritis (affecting only the nasal aspect of the left eye).

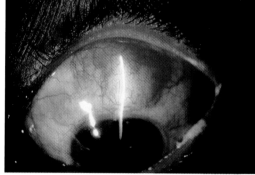

Figure 11.31   Nodular scleritis; note also the thinning of the sclera (bluish area nasal to the nodule) from prior episodes of scleritis.

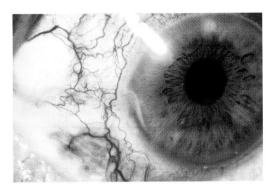

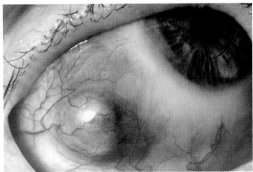

Figure 11.32 Nodular and necrotizing (ischemic) scleritis with inflammation occurring in severe rheumatoid disease with ocular and systemic vasculitis. Note areas of avascularity and bluish area of scleral thinning and necrosis (lower part of photograph).

Figure 11.33 Necrotizing scleritis without (evident) inflammation (scleromalacia perforans) resulting from long-standing rheumatoid disease. Note bluish, nodular staphyloma in the presence of a relatively uninflamed eye.

Pigmentations

A branch of a long ciliary nerve, often accompanied by an anterior ciliary artery, sometimes loops up into or through the sclera, often along with some uveal pigment, producing a blue-black spot in the superficial sclera 3 to 4 mm from the limbus. This anomaly is known as *Axenfeld's nerve loop*.

Congenital melanosis oculi (ocular melanocytosis) is an anomaly that produces deep, slate-gray patches of scleral and episcleral pigmentation, nearly always unilaterally. Associated findings can include ipsilateral hyperpigmentation of the iris, the fundus, and the periocular skin (nevus of Ota; oculodermal melanocytosis).

A blue nevus is one located deep in the conjunctiva or in the episclera that has a dark-blue color. Brown or brown-black pigmentation is produced by pigmented tumors of the uveal tract (for example, ciliary body melanomas), which occasionally erode into the sclera or episclera and can be associated with dilated episcleral vessels, referred to as *sentinel vessels*.

Involutional Hyaline Plaques

Involutional hyaline and calcific plaques of the sclera are sometimes seen in elderly patients. The plaques develop in the areas of insertion of the medial and lateral (rarely the inferior) rectus muscles. They have a gray-brown or yellow-brown translucent appearance (Figure 11.34).

Figure 11.34 Involutional hyaline scleral plaque.

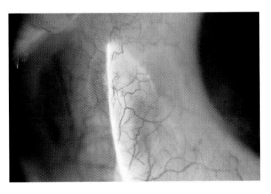

■ Tear Film

The tear film has 3 main components—oil, water, and mucin—and 2 layers. The oil, which originates from the sebaceous glands of the eyelids, forms the most superficial layer of the tear film and serves to retard evaporation of the watery component. The second layer of the tear film consists mainly of a mixture of water and mucin. The concentration of mucin is least under the oily layer and is greatest at the ocular surface. This deep area of concentrated mucin is sometimes referred to as a *third layer of the tear film*.

The aqueous portion of the tear film originates from the main lacrimal gland and the conjunctival accessory lacrimal glands. Mucin is produced by the conjunctival goblet cells and serves to stabilize the tear film and to make the hydrophobic epithelial surface wettable.

Closure of the eyelids (blinking) spreads the tear film over the ocular surface. Evaporation then begins, causing progressive thinning of the tear film. When it becomes so thin that its surface tension can no longer maintain an intact film, it breaks up in focal areas, producing momentary dry spots. These stimulate another blink, and the cycle begins again.

Schirmer testing is used to evaluate tear production and is usually performed as part of the external examination (see Chapter 9). In the anterior segment examination, the tear film is evaluated with the slit lamp for its overall wetness, presence of meniscus, and breakup time, as well as a few minor abnormalities.

Overall Wetness

The general presence or absence of moisture on the ocular surface can be evaluated with diffuse illumination, looking for the normally glistening character of the tear film, in contrast to the matte appearance of the severely dry eye.

Tear Meniscus

When viewed in cross-section with a thin slit-lamp beam (optical section), the tear film forms a roughly triangular meniscus, or "lake," between the margin of the lower eyelid and the place where the eyelid margin apposes the globe (Figure 11.35). Absence of, or a smaller than usual, meniscus is indicative of tear deficiency. A higher than normal meniscus occurs with conditions of tearing or epiphora. The best way to become familiar with the appearance of a normal meniscus is to observe it in a number of patients whose tear films are normal.

Tear Film Breakup Time

The tear film breaks up between blinks. Applying fluorescein dye to the ocular surface and measuring the time between the last blink and the appearance of the first dry spot provides information about the adequacy of the supply of tears, because dry eyes have thinner tear films that break up faster. Clinical Protocol 11.2 provides instructions for measuring tear film breakup time.

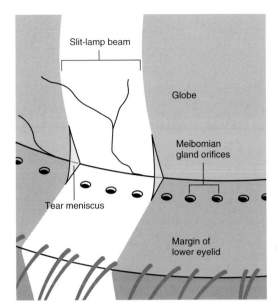

Slit-lamp beam

Globe

Meibomian
gland orifices

Tear meniscus

Margin of
lower eyelid

Figure 11.35 Normally the tear film forms a roughly triangular meniscus along the posterior margin of the eyelid; this is reduced or absent in the dry eye, and increased (higher and more convex) in the wet eye.

Other Tear Film Abnormalities

Various kinds of debris can be seen on or in the tear film. The most common examples are particles of mascara or other cosmetics, airborne foreign bodies, or clumps of mucus. Soapy deposits are formed first when excessive sebaceous oil produces a thicker than normal oily layer of tear film; this can be inferred by noting swirls of multicolored oil on the surface of the tear film ("oil-slick" sign). Still more sebaceous material results in the formation of a partial emulsion of oil and aqueous tears, leading to the accumulation of foamy material that has a yellow-white, bubbly appearance known as *meibomian foam*.

■ Cornea

The cornea consists of 5 layers, listed here from anterior to posterior:

- Epithelium and epithelial basement membrane (the most superficial layers of the cornea)
- Bowman's layer (most superficial part of the corneal stroma)
- Stroma (multiple lamellae of collagen fibers, accounting for 90% of the cornea's thickness)
- Descemet's membrane (collagenous basement membrane of the corneal endothelium)
- Endothelium (a single layer of endothelial cells that act as metabolic pumps regulating corneal water content)

Abnormalities that might be found in these 5 layers are discussed in detail on the next page.

Diffuse illumination and sclerotic scatter (see Chapter 10) are useful screening techniques for beginning the slit-lamp examination of the cornea and for detecting areas that require closer scrutiny. Such areas are then examined with a small to medium-sized parallelepiped (corneal prism) and with the thin, optical section. The latter is especially useful for accurately determining the level of any abnormality.

Epithelium

Epithelial defects and ulcers of the cornea look much the same as do such lesions of the conjunctiva. They are best seen with the aid of stains (discussed later in this chapter). Epithelial filaments are teardrop-shaped tags of partially detached epithelium and mucus. They occur in dry eyes and in various inflammatory conditions.

Fingerprint and map lines are curvilinear, translucent or slightly opaque abnormalities within, or immediately subjacent to, the epithelium, having the appearance of a fingerprint or a map of an island (Figure 11.36). They occur in primary anterior-membrane corneal dystrophy (also known as *epithelial basement-membrane* or *map-dot-fingerprint dystrophy*) and sometimes following trauma.

Intraepithelial cysts can range from microcysts a fraction of a millimeter in diameter to macrocysts of 1 mm or more. They can be clear (as in Meesmann's corneal dystrophy) or opaque and white to tan if filled with cellular debris (as in the dots of map-dot-fingerprint dystrophy).

Punctate epithelial keratitis (PEK) and punctate epithelial erosions (PEEs) occur in a large variety of corneal inflammations and surface disturbances. PEK is the result of small foci of inflammation, usually with lymphocytes, within the epithelium. The examiner sees fine or coarse multiple, gray-to-white intraepithelial dots that might or might not stain with fluorescein or rose-bengal dyes. PEEs, on the other hand, are not visible without such staining (Figure 11.37).

Epithelial edema occurs when stromal edema secondarily involves the epithelium, so it is associated with stromal thickening (discussed below). Early epithelial edema manifests itself by the appearance of many tiny, clear bubbles of fluid (bedewing) within the epithelium. Retroillumination and indirect lateral illumination are useful for detecting slight amounts of bedewing. Bedewing also causes a breakup

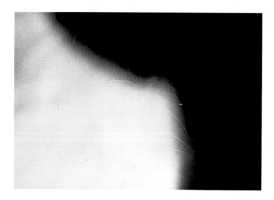

Figure 11.36 Fingerprint lines representing anterior-membrane corneal dystrophy (strips of excessive epithelial basement-membrane collagen beneath, or within, the corneal epithelium).

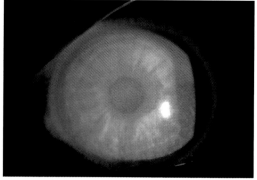

Figure 11.37 Punctate epithelial erosions (PEE) as shown by punctate staining with fluorescein, in this case caused by the toxic effects of neomycin eyedrops.

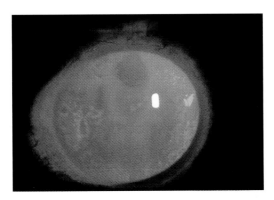

Figure 11.38   Corneal edema in postoperative endothelial dysfunction, made evident by staining the tear film with fluorescein. Mild epithelial edema (bedewing) is seen in the superonasal and superotemporal areas, and bullous keratopathy is seen at 12 o'clock, 3 to 5 o'clock, and 8 to 10 o'clock.

of the fluorescein-stained tear film, which is best seen with diffuse, blue illumination. More severe edema leads to the formation of bullae (bullous keratopathy), in which areas of epithelium detach from the underlying tissue, creating an obviously bumpy epithelial surface (Figure 11.38).

The term *cornea verticillata* describes the verticillate (whorl-like) sliding pattern of normally clear epithelial cells that becomes visible as a result of extensive PEK, depositions of certain medications, or in the rare metabolic disorder Fabry disease.

Patients who are not Caucasian often have circumcorneal melanin pigmentation of the limbus (racial melanosis). Some of this pigment can extend in a swirling pattern into the cornea in an area of trauma or inflammation, where it is known as *striate melanokeratosis*.

Brown, curvilinear deposits of iron are sometimes seen in the basal layer of the corneal epithelium. A horizontally oriented iron line (Hudson-Stähli line) develops normally, and more prominently with advancing age, roughly at the junction of the upper two-thirds and lower one-third of the cornea. The other iron lines of the cornea appear around surface irregularities such as keratoconus (Fleischer ring), a filtering bleb (Ferry line), or the head of a pterygium (Stocker line).

Bowman's Layer

Although sometimes referred to as *Bowman's membrane*, Bowman's layer is not a true or separate membrane but a superficial area of modified stroma in which the collagen fibers are slightly more irregular than those that lie deeper. As a result, Bowman's layer is normally slightly more relucent (reflective of light) than the stroma when it is viewed with the slit lamp; clinically, this gives the layer a subtly granular appearance.

Superficial corneal vascularization, usually with fibrosis, is called *pannus* (cloth) if it extends more than 1.5 mm into the cornea, or micropannus if not (Figure 11.39). This kind of vascularization develops at the level of superficial Bowman's layer. The vessels tend to branch dichotomously. Superficial corneal vascularization occurs as a response to superficial necrosis or hypoxia and so is seen in association with many different pathologic processes.

Calcium deposits in the cornea are found at the level of Bowman's layer, sometimes secondarily involving the epithelium. The deposits usually begin just inside

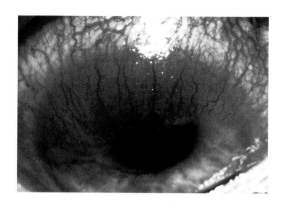

Figure 11.39 Extensive pannus occurring with hypersensitivity to preservative in contact lens solution.

the nasal and temporal limbus in the interpalpebral zone of exposure and, in many cases, eventually extend across the entire cornea (calcific band-shaped keratopathy, or BSK).

The deposits are white and, at first, finely granular. Later, the flecks of calcium become confluent, forming solid plaques. The calcium tends not to accumulate around corneal nerves that are coursing through Bowman's layer to the epithelium, so that the plaques typically have small clear areas ("Swiss-cheese holes"). Calcium deposits develop most often as a degenerative change or as a result of hypercalcemia.

Any disturbance of Bowman's layer can cause fibrosis (scarring). Fibrosis of Bowman's layer occurs spontaneously in Reis-Bücklers corneal dystrophy, a hereditary disorder. Focal scars in this layer are also typical of keratoconus. Corneal scarring occurs in the stroma just as it does in Bowman's layer.

Corneal scars are gray-white and are permanent, although they often become somewhat less dense and opaque with time. Corneal scars are graded as to severity. The least severe is the nebula (or nebulous scar), a faint haze that can be seen only with magnification and that interferes little, if any, with vision. The most severe scar is called a *leukoma*. A leukoma is white, visible without magnification, and interferes with vision if in the visual axis. The intermediate kind of scar is the macula. A macular scar can also be seen without magnification but appears as a gray area instead of being white. Macular scars have variable effects on vision.

An especially nebulous form of corneal scarring is that seen after laser in situ keratomileusis (LASIK) refractive surgery. It is seen often with some difficulty if not specifically looked for, as a subtle, thin, circular ring of scarring in Bowman's layer and stroma.

Stroma

The stroma accounts for 90% of the corneal thickness. It consists of multiple lamellae of collagen fibers surrounded by proteoglycan ground substance. Scattered keratocytes (modified fibroblasts) are also present. The normal, regular arrangement of the collagen fibers is necessary for maintenance of corneal transparency. Any disturbance of the regularity results in some loss of corneal transparency.

Vogt's limbal girdle is an elastotic stromal change that appears just inside the limbus with age. It is seen as a yellow-white line, concentric with the limbus, extending from about 2 o'clock to 4 o'clock and 8 o'clock to 10 o'clock.

Inflammatory cells can infiltrate the cornea in response to infection or sterile, immunologically mediated diseases. The infiltrate can be purulent (neutrophils), nonpurulent (lymphocytes), or granulomatous (epithelioid cells and multinucleated giant cells).

Catarrhal (or marginal) infiltrates are a particular kind of sterile, neutrophilic infiltration (Figure 11.40). They are similar to phlyctenules but typically occur inside the limbus, are more apt to be multiple, and are followed by less scarring and vascularization. Whereas phlyctenules are type-IV (cell-mediated) lesions, catarrhal infiltrates are type-III (antigen-antibody–mediated) infiltrates. They represent a hypersensitivity reaction to coexisting active bacterial conjunctivitis.

Stromal vascularization is deeper than pannus. Stromal vessels are usually relatively straight and roughly parallel, like the bristles of a broom, and they show less branching than do superficial vessels. Stromal vascularization is also known as *interstitial vascularization*. The term *interstitial keratitis* (IK) is often used to describe such vessel ingrowth associated with stromal inflammation (Figure 11.41).

Like its superficial counterpart, stromal vascularization is indicative of stromal necrosis or hypoxia and has many possible causes. It is especially common with purulent keratitis or may occur in association with tuberculosis or congenital syphilis. After a disease process has become inactive, the vessels sometimes appear to become devoid of blood; these are called *ghost vessels* and are seen as clear tubules coursing through the stroma.

Normal corneal thickness is 0.54 to 0.56 mm (540 to 560 μm), but edematous corneas often have thicknesses of 0.7 mm or more. Increased thickness of the stroma is not always visually detectable if the edema is mild, but corneal thickness can be measured with a pachymeter (or pachometer), described in Chapter 10.

Corneal thickness is nearly proportional to corneal water content and so is useful for determining whether or not corneal edema is present. Early stromal edema can often be detected biomicroscopically by noticing fine, undulating striae in the deep stroma and Descemet's membrane (deep striate keratopathy, or DSK), caused as the cornea expands posteriorly with thickening. After looking for DSK with a slit-lamp beam of any width, an examiner can try to ascertain whether the thin, optical-section beam is thicker than normal. This method of detecting corneal

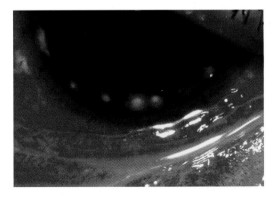

Figure 11.40   Catarrhal infiltrates (antigen-antibody–mediated reactions to microbial antigens) in staphylococcal conjunctivitis.

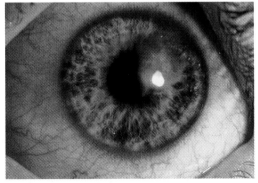

Figure 11.41   Interstitial keratitis: cellular infiltration, vascularization, and edema of the corneal stroma in congenital syphilis.

edema is usually possible only when the edema is substantial and the examiner has gained experience in evaluating corneal thickness by having examined a number of patients with normal corneal thickness.

The methods above are useful for detecting edema of the corneal stroma. Stromal edema eventually extends into the corneal epithelium, producing vesicular, or even bullous, foci of edema on the corneal surface. Instilling fluorescein onto the eye helps the examiner appreciate epithelial edema because the dye will pool around the bases of elevated blebs of edema (so-called *negative staining*). In addition to stromal thickening, stromal edema causes the stroma to become more relucent and silvery and to lose some of its transparency, the cornea taking on a steamy appearance.

Corneal edema in the presence of very high intraocular pressure (as with acute angle-closure glaucoma) displays extensive epithelial edema (which also displays a steamy appearance) and normal (or nearly normal) corneal thickness; the stroma is compressed by the high pressure, forcing much of the fluid into the epithelium. Corneal edema generally indicates dysfunction of the corneal endothelium, usually from dystrophy, inflammation, or trauma.

Stromal thinning occurs in the ectatic corneal dystrophies (eg, keratoconus, keratoglobus, and pellucid marginal degeneration), with necrosis (as with infectious corneal ulcers), or as a result of the production of collagenase, causing keratolysis (a "melting" of the stroma that occurs with certain infections or autoimmune diseases). Stromal thinning is sometimes so extreme that little remains in a particular area other than Descemet's membrane, which then tends to bulge forward (a descemetocele).

Corneal metabolic deposits are numerous and can occur with local (corneal) or systemic diseases. Lipid can appear in the form of the well-known corneal arcus (formerly called *arcus senilis*). The most commonly seen metabolic deposits occur in the 3 classic stromal corneal dystrophies: macular dystrophy (glycosaminoglycan), lattice dystrophy (amyloid), and granular dystrophy (protein of uncertain character).

Corneal nerves are seen as thin, white, dichotomously branching lines in the anterior two-thirds of the corneal stroma. Similar lines seen in the posterior one-third of the stroma are likely to be ghost vessels rather than corneal nerves. Corneal nerves can sometimes become enlarged and more prominent than usual, most commonly from age, keratoconus, and neurofibromatosis.

The very deepest (pre-Descemet's) area of the stroma occasionally shows cornea farinata, tiny gray-white dots of lipoprotein best seen with indirect lateral illumination. Similar changes have been reported to occur with keratoconus and ichthyosis.

Descemet's Membrane

Descemet's membrane, the collagenous basement membrane of the endothelium, is best examined using direct focal illumination and retroillumination. Descemet's membrane wrinkles when the cornea is edematous or if ocular hypotony is present. Trauma (including birth injuries from forceps), necrosis, ectatic corneal dystrophies (keratoconus, keratoglobus), and congenital glaucoma can cause the membrane to rupture. When this occurs, sudden and severe corneal edema (acute corneal hydrops) might ensue and persists until the defect heals (several weeks to months).

Excessive production of Descemet's membrane collagen can be caused by trauma, corneal dystrophy, or inflammation. Healed ruptures leave behind 1 or more thickened ridges of the membrane, referred to as *Haab's striae* in the specific case of congenital glaucoma.

Focal areas of thickening (guttae) occur in the early stages of Fuchs corneal dystrophy, a condition called *cornea guttata*. The appearance may be likened to beaten metal or the pits in the skin of an orange. A few corneal guttae are normally found with aging in the corneal periphery and are called *Hassall-Henle bodies*.

Descemet's membrane normally terminates beneath the opaque limbus, so that the ridge-like termination (Schwalbe's ring) is not visible without gonioscopy (see "Gonioscopy" later in this chapter). Schwalbe's ring can be displaced anteriorly into the peripheral cornea as the congenital anomaly called *posterior embryotoxon*. The clinical appearance is of an arcuate band of thickened Descemet's membrane just inside the limbus (usually nasally or temporally).

Kayser-Fleischer ring is a deposition of copper in peripheral Descemet's membrane. It is usually beige to yellow-brown but can have tints of red, green, or gold. It occurs with Wilson's hepatolenticular degeneration.

Endothelium

The endothelium, the most posterior layer of the cornea, consists of a single layer of endothelial cells that act as metabolic pumps to regulate normal corneal water content. The hydrophilic corneal stroma becomes edematous whenever endothelial function is inadequate. The endothelium is best examined by specular reflection, which allows for visualization of individual endothelial cells (see Chapter 10).

Endothelial cells normally have hexagonal shapes and are roughly uniform in size. The cells have very little ability to regenerate, so as cells die adjacent ones enlarge to fill the gaps. This results in cells that are larger than normal (polymegathism), cells that vary greatly in size (polymegethism), and cells that have varying and abnormal shapes (pleomorphism). Figure 11.42 depicts endothelial cell polymegathism and pleomorphism.

Pigment from the iris, sometimes seen as brown "dust" on the endothelium, can be observed with diffuse, direct illumination. In pigment dispersion syndrome

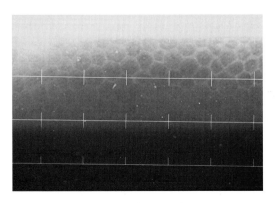

Figure 11.42 Specular microscopy of living corneal endothelium (white dots and flecks are artifacts). Note normal, hexagonal shapes, mild polymegathism (larger cells), and pleomorphism.

and pigmentary glaucoma, the pigmentation usually takes the form of a vertically oriented spindle just below the center of the cornea (Krukenberg's spindle).

Keratic precipitates (KPs) are accumulations of inflammatory cells on the corneal endothelium that occur with intraocular inflammation. KPs can be fine, medium, or large in size and variable in shape. Large KPs usually occur with granulomatous inflammation and can be larger than 1 mm; they have a greasy, yellowish appearance and are called *mutton-fat KPs*. Other KPs are usually white. They can be punctate, round, or stellate. KPs are seen most often on the inferior or central cornea. Following inactivation of inflammation, KPs can disappear, become hyalinized (clear), or become pigmented. In the case of corneal transplant rejection, a line of lymphocytic KPs can sometimes be seen to advance across the endothelium (Khodadoust rejection line).

◼ Anterior Chamber

The anterior chamber is the area between the iris (and anterior surface of the crystalline lens) and the corneal endothelium. It is filled with aqueous humor.

Anterior Chamber Depth

Evaluating the depth of the anterior chamber is important in assessing a patient's risk of or predisposition to angle-closure glaucoma. The depth of the chamber can be evaluated by locating an optical section slit-lamp beam, at an angle of 60°, onto the peripheral cornea (just inside the limbus). The chamber is considered to be shallow if the distance between the corneal endothelium and the surface of the iris is less than one-fourth the thickness of the cornea.

This test is useful before instilling cycloplegic drops to ensure the patient is not predisposed to angle-closure glaucoma, but it is only a screening test and is not a substitute for gonioscopy when glaucoma is suspected. Gonioscopy is discussed in greater detail later in this chapter.

Flare and Cell

Intraocular inflammation produces increased protein, and the appearance of inflammatory cells, in the anterior chamber. The anterior chamber is normally optically empty, meaning that it appears nearly black as the slit-lamp beam passes through it. However, the beam of light becomes progressively more visible as the protein content of aqueous humor increases. This visibility of the beam is called *flare*. When inflammatory cells are present, they are seen in the slit-lamp beam as white dots, rising and falling in the convection currents of the anterior chamber and aqueous humor (rising near the warmer iris and falling near the cooler cornea). Together, these slit-lamp findings are referred to as *flare and cell* and have the appearance of dust particles within a projector's haze of light. Clinical Protocol 11.3 describes the steps in evaluating and recording flare and cell. White inflammatory cells should be differentiated from pigment (brown) or erythrocytes (red).

Blood and Other Foreign Matter

Blood in the anterior chamber, usually from trauma, is called *hyphema*. If the amount of blood is sufficient, it settles inferiorly, forming a flat-topped layer of blood in the anterior chamber (Figure 11.43). At times the entire chamber is filled with blood. The blood is red if fresh, black if old. Black blood filling the chamber is called "8-ball hemorrhage."

Purulent (neutrophilic) exudates can occur in the anterior chamber, usually in conjunction with corneal or intraocular infections, or with Behçet's disease. As with blood, layering of the white to yellow-white purulent material can occur and is called a *hypopyon* (Figure 11.44).

Severe intraocular inflammation is often associated with a hypopyon or with the presence of fibrin in the anterior chamber, seen as strands or clumps of hazy yellow-white or gray-white material.

Lens material and vitreous

Fragments of lens material or vitreous humor are sometimes seen in the anterior chamber after trauma or cataract surgery. Lens material consists of white clumps that are several times larger than inflammatory cells. Vitreous can be present as a single strand, usually extending through the pupil to the site of a corneal or scleral wound, or vitreous can fill the entire anterior chamber. The material is clear, but large amounts are seen to contain some fine, gray strands.

Foreign bodies and cysts

The anterior chamber sometimes contains foreign bodies, including artificial lens implants. Traumatic implantation of epithelial cells into the anterior chamber can result in the formation of a cyst as the cells proliferate; such an epithelial implantation cyst is at first small (less than 1 mm in diameter), round, and white (pearl cyst). Larger cysts are relatively clear and can fill a large part of the anterior chamber, indenting and pushing the iris posteriorly.

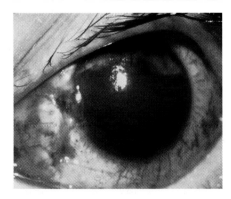

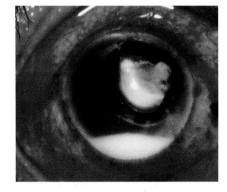

Figure 11.43   Large traumatic hyphema (blood in anterior chamber).

Figure 11.44   Hypopyon with bacterial keratitis.

■ Iris

Direct focal illumination is used most often for examining the iris. Indirect illumination is useful for evaluating the interior of lesions that are not transparent. Transillumination can reveal areas of partial or full-thickness iris atrophy or other defects of the iris. Sequelae of inflammation, *synechiae* are fibrous adhesions between the iris and the cornea (anterior synechiae) or between the iris and the crystalline lens (posterior synechiae). Posterior synechiae sometimes involve the entire circumference of the pupillary margin (seclusio pupillae), preventing aqueous humor from reaching the anterior chamber; glaucoma results, and the accumulation of aqueous behind the iris causes it to bow forward (iris bombé). Iris bombé also can occur when the entire pupil becomes covered by a fibrous membrane (occlusio pupillae).

Nodules

Inflammatory nodules are usually granulomas. They appear with some cases of intense intraocular inflammation. They can be white, yellow, or pigmented. Nodules at the pupillary margin are called *Koeppe nodules*, whereas those on the surface of the iris are called *Busacca nodules*.

Neovascularization

Rubeosis iridis is neovascularization of the iris, usually caused by retinal ischemia. The abnormal vessels are fine, irregular, and plentiful. They appear on the surface of the iris, first in the area of the pupillary margin and peripherally at the root of the iris. The condition often leads to the formation of extensive peripheral anterior synechiae and secondary angle-closure glaucoma.

Rubeosis iridis is to be differentiated from hyperemia of otherwise normal iris vessels. Hyperemia is manifested by the presence of 1 or more individual cord-like vessels coursing in iris crypts somewhere between the pupillary margin and the peripheral iris. Rubeotic vessels are seen more as tight masses of very fine, tangled vessels.

Cysts and Tumors

"Iris" cysts are usually epithelial implantation cysts of the anterior chamber (discussed above). Most tumors of the iris are nevi or melanomas. They are variably pigmented, ranging from tan to brown-black in color (Figure 11.45). They usually cause thickening of the iris, and they can be associated with a dragging onto the front surface of the iris of the dark brown or black pigment epithelium of the posterior surface of the iris (ectropion uveae).

Persistent Pupillary Membrane Remnants

A membrane is normally present over the pupil during embryonic development. It generally disappears, but remnants sometimes persist. They are usually not extensive, but it is not uncommon to see a few spider-web–like strands of this tissue that originate from the iris near the pupillary margin; the other ends can be freely

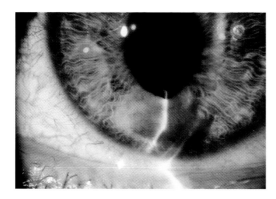

Figure 11.45 Pigmented lesion (melanoma) of iris.

floating or attached elsewhere to the iris, to the anterior lens capsule, or even to the cornea. Stellate deposits of brown pigment are often found on the anterior lens capsule (epicapsular stars) as part of this condition.

Other Abnormalities

Corectopia (displaced pupil) can be caused by congenital anomalies, degenerative conditions, or contracting anterior synechiae. Iris atrophy also occurs in congenital anomalies and degenerative problems, and following inflammation or trauma. If the atrophy is incomplete, one sees a red glow in the area of thinning when the iris is retroilluminated. Actual holes in the iris develop in areas of complete atrophy, which can lead to the impression that several pupils are present (pseudopolycoria).

The term *heterochromia* refers to a difference in iris color of the 2 eyes of a patient. Causes include congenital anomaly, iris atrophy (which renders a blue iris darker blue, or a brown iris lighter brown or even blue), or hyperpigmentation (as from a diffuse melanoma of the iris).

Iridodonesis is a quivering of the iris that can be seen with movements of the eye in patients who are aphakic (lacking a crystalline lens) or who have subluxated or luxated lenses. The condition occurs because of the lack of support of the iris by the lens and its zonular attachments.

Crystalline Lens

The lens is an encapsulated structure that contains several lamellae, or layers, that are formed during different periods of development and life (Figure 11.46). The outer layer is called the *capsule*. The next layer, the *cortex*, continues to grow throughout life. For practical purposes, clinicians often refer to the layers of the lens central to the anterior and posterior cortex as the *nucleus*.

The lens is best examined after pupillary dilation, usually with the optical section. Diffuse direct illumination and retroillumination are useful for evaluating the posterior capsular and subcapsular area. Beginning anteriorly, the slit-lamp beam passes through the anterior capsule, anterior cortex, anterior adult nucleus, anterior infantile nucleus, anterior fetal nucleus, anterior erect fetal Y suture, posterior

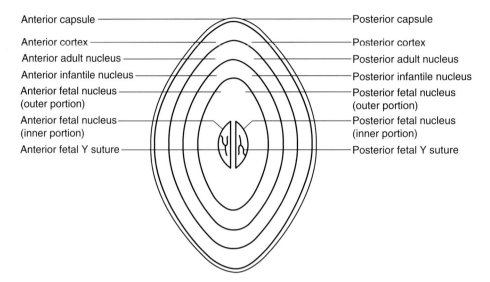

Anterior capsule — — Posterior capsule
Anterior cortex — — Posterior cortex
Anterior adult nucleus — — Posterior adult nucleus
Anterior infantile nucleus — — Posterior infantile nucleus
Anterior fetal nucleus — — Posterior fetal nucleus
(outer portion) (outer portion)
Anterior fetal nucleus — — Posterior fetal nucleus
(inner portion) (inner portion)
Anterior fetal Y suture — — Posterior fetal Y suture

Figure 11.46 Diagrammatic representation of the main layers and nuclei of the crystalline lens as can be seen with the optical section of the slit lamp.

inverted fetal Y suture, posterior fetal nucleus, posterior infantile nucleus, posterior adult nucleus, posterior cortex, and posterior lens capsule.

Cataract

A cataract is an opacity of the lens. It might or might not be visually important, depending on the location and severity. Except in the rare instance in which a cataract might be causing a threat to the eye (eg, lens-induced glaucoma or uveitis), the mere presence of a cataract is not a justification for recommendation of cataract surgery. To do so is unethical unless the patient cannot function adequately according to his or her own visual needs. In fact, patients should nearly always be reassured that cataract surgery is not necessary or advisable until such time as they, themselves, decide that they want it in order to see better.

A cataract can involve the lens capsule (capsular cataract), the lens itself (lenticular cataract), or both (capsulolenticular cataract). Lenticular cataracts can be cortical, nuclear or epinuclear, or subcapsular.

Capsular cataracts

Capsular cataracts are usually superficial, sharply demarcated white areas and are most commonly congenital. They can also develop secondary to inflammation and fibrosis (organization of fibrin). The posterior capsule sometimes manifests a small white dot inferonasal to the visual axis (Mittendorf's dot); this is a remnant of the lenticular attachment of the embryonic hyaloid artery.

Cortical cataracts

Cortical cataracts develop in the anterior and posterior cortex and are mostly associated with age and diabetes mellitus. In the age-related type, fluid accumulates among the lens fibrils, producing lamellar separation. This is seen as roughly

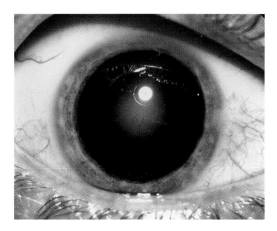

Figure 11.47 Nuclear and early cortical (age-related) cataract. The superficial, radially oriented white dots represent early cortical spokes; the central, hazy, round change represents nuclear sclerosis.

parallel, relucent lines (resembling linear air pockets in an ice cube). These areas then opacify, producing radially oriented cortical spokes (Figure 11.47). Flocculent, snowflake-like opacities can also develop, especially in diabetic patients who have ketoacidosis (the rare, true diabetic cataract); these opacities are sometimes reversible with treatment of the ketoacidosis.

Glaukomflecken are gray-white anterior cortical dots that appear after episodes of very high intraocular pressure. They usually indicate prior acute angle-closure glaucoma.

Nuclear cataracts

Nuclear cataract is the most common, and classic, age-related cataract. It may be thought of as resulting from the compression of the more central portion of the lens by the ongoing formation throughout life of new, more peripherally located cortical lens fibers; although various biochemical changes are also present. This so-called *nuclear sclerosis* first appears as a whitening of the normally silvery nuclear (subcortical) area, followed by progressively more severe changes to yellow-white, yellow, yellow-brown, and finally brown (brunescent) discolorations (see Figure 11.47). Nuclear cataracts are apt to progress slowly, often requiring years to affect vision.

Subcapsular cataracts

Subcapsular cataracts are usually found in the central posterior subcapsular area of the lens and appear as silvery and granular, bubbly opacifications in the visual axis. The patient might see well as long as a few clear areas remain, but the vision drops rapidly as soon as those clear areas opacify. Posterior subcapsular cataract develops, along with nuclear sclerosis, in some cases of age-related cataract, but it can be due to corticosteroid therapy (topical or systemic) or to prior uveitis.

Congenital cataracts

Congenital cataracts can affect the polar areas of the cortex (anterior or posterior), the Y sutures, the fetal or embryonic nuclei, or the capsule (usually anterior). The lamellar (also called *zonular*) form of congenital cataract is common. It shows opacification of the periphery of a particular zone (for example, the fetal nucleus)

Figure 11.48 Lamellar (or zonular) cataract, affecting mainly 1 layer of the lens (anterior infantile nucleus), although some punctate opacities are also seen in the area of the fetal Y sutures.

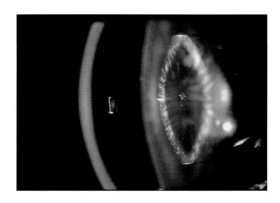

of the lens, yet the interior of the zone is clear (Figure 11.48). These cataracts are often associated with "riders," horseshoe-shaped opacities that cap the zonular opacity; riders are located in a slightly more peripheral level of the lens than is the zonular opacity itself.

Soemmering ring

Soemmering ring is a ring of opacified equatorial (peripheral) lens material, enclosed in lens capsule. It can result from trauma causing rupture of the lens capsule and consequent resorption of most of the lens material, or from incomplete extracapsular cataract extraction.

Pseudophakia and aphakia

Patients who have had cataract extraction with implantation of an artificial intraocular lens implant are said to have *pseudophakia*. The implant is nearly always positioned posteriorly behind the iris, although implants in the anterior chamber are occasionally seen. It is important in pseudophakia to ascertain whether or not the posterior lens capsule is present and whether or not it is clear or opaque. Laser capsulotomy might be indicated if the posterior capsule has become opaque. *Aphakia* is the absence of the lens (and its capsule) and is seen in patients who have had intracapsular (complete) cataract extraction, which is now rarely performed.

Subluxation and Luxation

The crystalline lens is held in its normal position by multiple fine fibrils, the zonule (zonular fibers) of Zinn. The fibers can be disrupted by trauma or systemic disease (most notably Marfan syndrome or homocystinuria), resulting in partial or complete dislocation of the lens from its normal position. In the case of subluxation, the edge of the lens might be visible in the pupil. Complete dislocation (luxation) allows the lens to be displaced into the vitreous or, rarely, into the anterior chamber.

Other Conditions

Peters' anomaly, a congenital anomaly, manifests a corneal leukoma that is often attached to a cataractous lens by way of a fibrous band that extends across the anterior chamber. The band is sometimes attached to the iris instead of the lens. Pseudoexfoliation (or exfoliation) syndrome causes deposits of basement-membrane–like fibrillogranular material to accumulate on various intraocular tissues, but most prominently the anterior lens capsule, where it appears as a disk of fine, gray-white flecks centrally or paracentrally. The condition is associated with small areas of iris atrophy near the pupillary margin (seen by retroillumination), hyperpigmentation of the iris and trabecular meshwork, glaucoma, and fragility of the zonular fibers. The last accounts for an increased risk of zonular rupture during extracapsular cataract extraction (including phacoemulsification).

Retrolental Space and Anterior Vitreous

Evidence of inflammation can be seen with the slit-lamp examination of the retrolental space and anterior vitreous, just as it can be seen in the anterior chamber. Flare and cell in the anterior chamber alone are typical of the form of uveitis known as *iritis*. If flare and cell are found also in the retrolental space or anterior vitreous, the condition is called *iridocyclitis*. Uveitis of the posterior segment can also manifest flare and cell in the anterior chamber, retrolental space, and anterior vitreous, but the most prominent inflammation is more posterior. Table 11.1 summarizes the grading scheme for anterior chamber flare; Table 11.2 includes the scheme for anterior chamber cells.

Table 11.1 The SUN Working Group Grading System for Anterior Chamber Flare

Grade	Description
0	None
1+	Faint
2+	Moderate (iris and lens details clear)
3+	Marked (iris and lens details hazy)
4+	Intense (fibrin or plasmoid aqueous)

The Standardization of Uveitis Nomenclature (SUN) Working Group. Standardization of nomenclature for reporting clinical data: results of the First International Workshop. *Am J Ophthalmol.* 2005;140:509–516: Table 4. Copyright 2005, reprinted with permission from Elsevier.

Table 11.2 The SUN Working Group Grading System for Anterior Chamber Cells

Grade	Cells in Field (high-intensity 1 × 1-mm slit beam)
0	<1
0.5+	1–5
1+	6–15
2+	16–25
3+	26–50
4+	>50

The Standardization of Uveitis Nomenclature (SUN) Working Group. Standardization of nomenclature for reporting clinical data: results of the First International Workshop. *Am J Ophthalmol.* 2005;140:509–516: Table 3. Copyright 2005, reprinted with permission from Elsevier.

■ Gonioscopy

Gonioscopy is examination of the angle of the anterior chamber (the structures between the peripheral iris and cornea including, especially, the trabecular meshwork, through which aqueous exits the eye). Gonioscopy might not be performed during routine anterior segment examinations. However, it is especially important in the evaluation of glaucoma (for differentiating angle-closure and open-angle types, for example). It is also used in studying tumors of the iris and other abnormalities in the area of the angle. Additionally, gonioscopy can afford views of the posterior iris and of the ciliary body and processes.

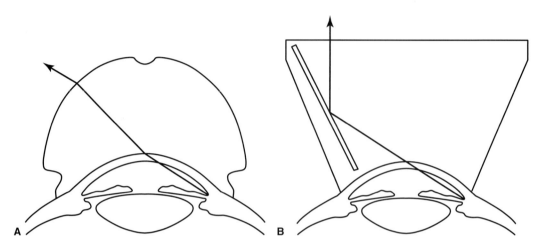

Figure 11.49   Main methods of gonioscopy. **(A)** With the Koeppe lens (direct gonioscopy), light rays from the angle are refracted to the eyes of the examiner. **(B)** With the Goldmann lens (indirect gonioscopy—more often used), light from the angle is reflected to the examiner by means of a mirror. (Redrawn by permission from Kolker AE, Hetherington J, eds. *Becker-Shaffer's Diagnosis and Therapy of the Glaucomas*, 6th ed. St Louis: CV Mosby Co; 1989.)

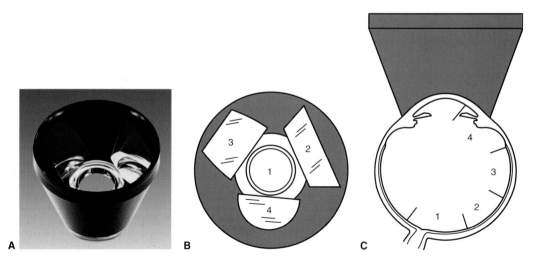

Figure 11.50   **(A)** Goldmann 3-mirror contact gonioscopy lens. **(B, C)** The lens's 3 mirrors are at different angles, allowing for examination of different parts of the internal eye; mirror 4 permits examination of the angle of the anterior chamber and the area of the ciliary body; mirror 3 is used for viewing the peripheral fundus; mirror 2 is for the mid-peripheral fundus; and lens 1 (not a mirror) affords a view of the posterior pole of the fundus. (Part A courtesy Haag-Streit AG, Bern, Switzerland.)

The anatomy and optical properties of the anterior segment of the eye prevent direct visualization of the angle without the use of special (gonioscopy) lenses. These lenses, also called *gonioprisms*, either refract light into the angle (Koeppe lens) or reflect light into the angle (Goldmann lens), thereby illuminating it and permitting it to be seen (Figure 11.49). The Goldmann 3-mirror contact lens, probably the most commonly used type of lens, may be used to view the chamber angle or the fundus (Figure 11.50).

Gonioscopy should usually be performed after refraction and undilated examination of the fundus, because viscous methylcellulose or hydroxyethylcellulose is used to cushion the contact lens when it is applied to the cornea; this gel-like material remains on the eye for several minutes after gonioscopy, and it can obscure the patient's vision and impede the ability of the examiner to see into the patient's eye. Gonioscopy is usually performed prior to pupillary dilation, but repeating the procedure after dilation can provide additional information (the effect of dilation on the angle and a better ability to see the ciliary-body area). Clinical Protocol 11.4 provides instructions for performing gonioscopy.

Figure 11.51 shows a composite drawing of the anatomy of the angle. The trabecular meshwork (or trabeculum) is bounded superiorly by Schwalbe's line

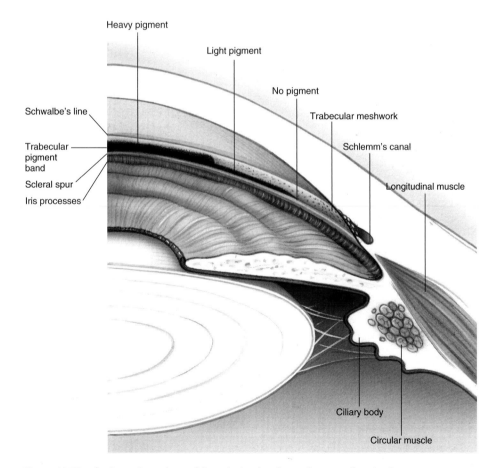

Figure 11.51   Gonioscopic anatomy of the anterior chamber and surrounding structures.

(the peripheral termination of Descemet's membrane) and inferiorly by the scleral spur (into which the longitudinal muscles of the ciliary body insert). Schwalbe's line appears as a thin, opaque, white, linear ridge. The scleral spur is also white and opaque. Between the 2 structures, the trabecular meshwork appears grayish and somewhat translucent. The meshwork can show varying degrees of pigmentation (from none to heavy). If pigmentation is light or absent, a slightly darker-gray line can sometimes be seen in the lower area of the trabecular meshwork. This is Schlemm's canal, a tubule into which aqueous enters after passing through the trabeculum, and from which it then enters the vascular circulation. Posterior to the scleral spur are often a few normal blood vessels and normal iris processes (fine filaments extending from the iris to the lower trabecular meshwork). Still more posterior is an area known as the *angle recess*; this represents a dipping of the peripheral iris as it inserts into the ciliary body.

The angle may be described in the patient's record by noting the most posterior structure that can be seen. For example, if only Schwalbe's line can be seen, the angle is very narrow, but if the scleral spur can be seen, the angle is open. Usually, however, the width of the angle is graded, most often by the Shaffer method, as described in Table 11.3 and shown in Figure 11.52. The Spaeth grading system adds information about the configuration and insertion of the peripheral iris (Figure 11.53).

Table 11.3   Shaffer Method for Grading Anterior Chamber Angles

Grade	Description
Grade IV	The angle between the iris and the surface of the trabecular meshwork is 45° (normal).
Grade III	The angle between the iris and the surface of the trabecular meshwork is greater than 20° but less than 45° (normal).
Grade II	The angle between the iris and the surface of the trabecular meshwork is 20°. Angle closure possible.
Grade I	The angle between the iris and the surface of the trabecular meshwork is 10°. Angle closure probable in time.
Slit	The angle between the iris and the surface of the trabecular meshwork is less than 10°. Angle closure very likely.
Grade 0	The iris is against the trabecular meshwork. Angle closure is present.

Figure 11.52   Shaffer grading of anterior chamber angles: narrow angle (0° to 20°), open angle (20° to 45°).

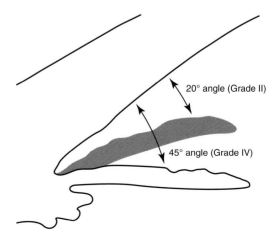

20° angle (Grade II)

45° angle (Grade IV)

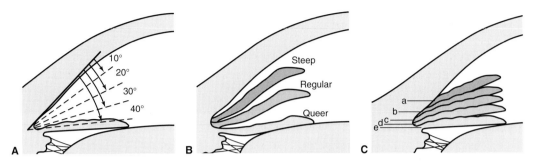

Figure 11.53   Spaeth's gonioscopic classification of the angle of the anterior chamber, based on 3 variables: **(A)** Angular width of the angle recess; **(B)** configuration of the peripheral iris; **(C)** insertion of the iris root (a = highest insertion, e = lowest insertion). (Redrawn by permission from Shields MB. *Textbook of Glaucoma*, 3rd ed. Baltimore: Williams & Wilkins; 1992.)

■ Stains

Stains (dyes) instilled into the tear film can facilitate examination of the ocular surface by highlighting, and making more evident, certain pathologic changes. The most commonly used stains are fluorescein, rose-bengal red (usually referred to simply as *rose bengal*), and lissamine green.

Fluorescein

Fluorescein is available as an eyedrop mixed with a topical anesthetic (Fluress) or as fluorescein-impregnated paper strips. The strips are moistened with a drop of saline solution, artificial tear, or topical ophthalmic anesthetic and then touched to the inside of the lower lid.

Fluorescein does not stain corneal or conjunctival epithelium but readily enters and stains the stroma in areas in which epithelium is absent (or even in areas in which epithelial cells have loose intercellular junctions). Accordingly, fluorescein is very useful for detecting areas of epithelial deficiency that occur, for example, in cases of corneal abrasion, recurrent corneal erosion, or herpes simplex epithelial (dendritic) keratitis.

Fluorescein staining is best seen using diffuse slit-lamp illumination with the cobalt-blue filter; the blue light causes the dye to fluoresce a bright green color. The pattern and morphology of staining have diagnostic value (Figure 11.54).

Fluorescein is useful for detecting corneal perforations or wound leaks (Seidel test). Fluorescein is instilled into the tear film, which is observed with diffuse, blue illumination. Any leak of aqueous humor onto the ocular surface can be detected by noting a trickle of clear, nonstained fluid into the green tear film. Fluorescein is also used for measuring intraocular pressure with the Goldmann tonometer (see Chapter 12). Clinical Protocol 11.2 describes use of the dye for measuring tear film breakup time.

Flare and cell in the anterior chamber should be graded prior to instilling fluorescein, as the dye can enter the chamber and produce a green, false flare. Fluorescein is nonirritating and may be instilled without topical anesthetic.

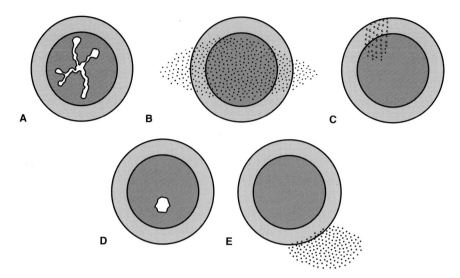

Figure 11.54 Typical patterns of staining with fluorescein or rose bengal and their diagnostic importance. **(A)** Dendritiform staining (dichotomously branching lesions, often with terminally bulbous swellings)—typical of herpes simplex keratitis. **(B)** Staining in the interpalpebral zone of exposure in the dry eye (usually more so with rose bengal than with fluorescein) in keratoconjunctivitis sicca. **(C)** Linear punctate staining in the superior cornea (caused by a foreign body entrapped in the upper palpebral conjunctiva). **(D)** Corneal abrasion or erosion (gross epithelial defect), usually just below the center of the cornea. **(E)** Eyedrop-induced allergy or toxicity (staining on the inferonasal bulbar conjunctiva of the right eye), where drugs gravitate on their way to the lacrimal-outflow system.

Rose Bengal

Rose bengal is available as a 1% eyedrop or as an impregnated paper strip. The strip is used the same way as are fluorescein strips. Unlike fluorescein, rose bengal stains abnormal and devitalized epithelial cells. Therefore, it is useful for conditions such as the dry eye (keratoconjunctivitis sicca) in which epithelial cells are present but abnormal. Rose bengal also stains mucus and keratin.

Rose-bengal staining is best observed using diffuse slit-lamp illumination with the green (red-free) filter (see Figure 10.4). Stained areas are red with either green or white light. Rose bengal (at least the 1% solution) is somewhat irritating and should not be used without first instilling a topical anesthetic agent.

Lissamine Green

Lissamine green is available as a 1% solution or in impregnated paper strips. Like rose bengal it stains devitalized epithelial cells and so is helpful for evaluating dry eyes. Abnormal cells stain blue. Examination may be done with white or blue light. Lissamine green is less irritating than rose bengal.

Pitfalls and Pointers

- Resist any tendency to limit the anterior segment examination to a cursory scanning of the cornea and anterior chamber, using only a single kind of illumination. Examine other important tissues (eyelids, conjunctiva, etc) and use various methods of illumination that can provide valuable information.

• It is often useful to examine the anterior segment (at least that portion posterior to the iris) after, as well as before, pupillary dilation. Otherwise, abnormalities of the lens, retrolental space, and anterior vitreous might be missed or inadequately evaluated.

Suggested Resources

Alward WLM, Longmuir RA. *Color Atlas of Gonioscopy.* 2nd ed. San Francisco: American Academy of Ophthalmology; 2008.

Bacterial Keratitis [Preferred Practice Pattern]. San Francisco: American Academy of Ophthalmology; 2008.

Blepharitis [Preferred Practice Pattern]. San Francisco: American Academy of Ophthalmology; 2008.

Conjunctivitis [Preferred Practice Pattern]. San Francisco: American Academy of Ophthalmology; 2008.

Dry Eye Syndrome [Preferred Practice Pattern]. San Francisco: American Academy of Ophthalmology; 2008.

External Disease and Cornea. Basic and Clinical Science Course, Section 8. San Francisco: American Academy of Ophthalmology; published annually.

Glaucoma. Basic and Clinical Science Course, Section 10. San Francisco: American Academy of Ophthalmology; published annually.

Lens and Cataract. Basic and Clinical Science Course, Section 11. San Francisco: American Academy of Ophthalmology; published annually.

Orbit, Eyelids, and Lacrimal System. Basic and Clinical Science Course, Section 7. San Francisco: American Academy of Ophthalmology; published annually.

Clinical Protocol 11.1

Sweeping the Conjunctival Sac for Foreign Bodies

1. With the patient seated or lying supine, instill a few drops of topical anesthetic. If the patient is seated, the neck should be extended with the back of the head resting on a headrest.

2. Separate the eyelids with your thumb and index finger of 1 hand or with an eyelid speculum.

3. Moisten a cotton swab with topical anesthetic, or sterile saline solution, or artificial tears. A dry swab is apt to leave cotton fibers on the eye.

4. Wipe away any visible strands of mucus by twirling the swab so as to allow the mucus to coil around it; the strands will adhere readily to the swab but will often break if an attempt is made merely to pull them away from the eye. The strands are most often found at the inner or outer canthal areas or in the lower fornix.

5. Sweep the cotton swab across the upper and lower conjunctival fornices to remove any remaining debris.

6. As an additional measure, the conjunctival sac may be irrigated with any sterile, isotonic solution.

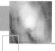

Clinical Protocol 11.2 — Measuring Tear Film Breakup Time

1. Stain the patient's tear film by touching a moistened, fluorescein-impregnated paper strip to the lower palpebral conjunctiva. Fluorescein eyedrops are not used because they add volume to the tear film.
2. Position the patient at the slit lamp and adjust the instrument for diffuse illumination through the cobalt-blue filter.
3. Ask the patient to look straight ahead and to blink.
4. While observing the eye through the slit-lamp oculars, count to yourself the number of seconds that elapse between the blink and the appearance of the first dry spot. The dry spot will appear blue-black (because of the dark blue illumination) when the green-stained tear film pulls away from the area of breakup.
5. Repeat the test 1 or more times for each eye, because a single measurement might be falsely high or low. The normal breakup time (BUT) is at least 10 seconds.

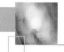

Clinical Protocol 11.3 — Evaluating Flare and Cell

1. Set the slit lamp for a 1 × 1 mm beam with the illumination at full brightness.
2. Situate the patient comfortably at the slit lamp and direct the beam at an angle of 45° to 60° onto the midperipheral temporal cornea and the nasal iris.
3. Estimate the intensity of gray-white flare, using the dark pupil as background for viewing, and grade its intensity (see Table 11.1).
4. Without changing the slit-lamp settings, examine for the presence of cells (white dots rising and falling in the anterior chamber) and grade the presence of cells (see Table 11.2).

Clinical Protocol 11.4 — Performing Gonioscopy

1. Clean the goniolens with mild soap and water, rinse well, and dry with a tissue or soft cloth.
2. Instill topical anesthetic onto 1 of the patient's eyes.
3. Assume standard patient and examiner positions at the slit-lamp biomicroscope (see Chapter 10).
4. Set the slit-lamp magnification to 10×.
5. Put in the concave part of the goniolens a small amount of gonioscopy gel, such as methylcellulose, taking care to avoid creating any air bubbles, which interfere with good visualization. (Make a habit of storing the bottle of gel upside down so air `bubbles do not accumulate near the tip of the bottle.)
6. Instruct the patient to look up. Spread the patient's lids apart with your thumb and forefinger (see Figure 1 in Clinical Protocol 13.5).

Clinical Protocol 11.4 *(continued)*

7. Hold the goniolens between the thumb and forefinger of your other hand, and place the lower edge of the lens on the patient's exposed lower globe. Angle the lens onto the globe from below (see Figure 2 in Clinical Protocol 13.5).

8. Instruct the patient to look straight ahead. Release the patient's lids, allowing the goniolens to hold the lids apart. Switch hands, if necessary, to hold the contact lens in your hand closer to the eye being examined (eg, your left hand for the patient's right eye), so your arm does not interfere with using the slit lamp.

9. Remove any air bubbles caught between the goniolens and the cornea by slightly tilting the lens to allow them to float out. Allow the contact lens to sit gently on the cornea, avoiding unnecessary pressure on the lens by your fingers that are keeping the lens steady.

10. Use the joystick to focus the slit lamp toward the patient and direct a broad, dim beam onto the semilunar-shaped mirror of the Goldmann goniolens or directly into the Koeppe goniolens.

    a. Remember that with a Goldmann lens you are viewing the chamber angle by means of a mirror, so you are seeing the inferior angle if, for example, the mirror is at the 12-o'clock position, and you are viewing the 10-o'clock angle if the mirror is at the 4-o'clock position. To see all areas of the angle, simply rotate the goniolens on the ocular surface.

    b. First obtain an overview of the angle with the broad, dim beam. Ascertain the most posterior angle structure visible without tilting the goniolens; this affords an idea of whether the angle is narrow, realizing that some more posterior structures might be seen by tilting, or pushing on, the goniolens.

11. If you are having difficulty locating Schwalbe's line, narrow the beam to an optical section (medium brightness). The thin beam produces 2 curvilinear lines that represent the anterior and posterior surfaces of the cornea; Schwalbe's line is located where the 2 corneal lines of light meet at the anterior aspect of the anterior chamber angle.

12. Grade the width of the angle (see Table 11.2 and Figures 11.52 and 11.53). Remove the goniolens from the patient's eye and record the angle width in the patient's record. Record also any other notable features of the angle (pigment, synechiae, neovascularization, etc). A simple diagram in the patient's record is useful if the angle is not uniform; draw a circle and write down the grade of angle width at 12, 3, 6, and 9 o'clock.

13. Repeat steps 1 to 12 for the other eye.

14. Wash and dry the goniolens as in step 1 after the examination of both eyes is complete.

12

Tonometry

Tonometry is the measurement of intraocular pressure (IOP). It is performed as part of a thorough ocular examination to help detect ocular hypertension and glaucoma and to diagnose ocular hypotony (low IOP) in conditions such as iritis, retinal detachment, postoperative wound leaks, and occult perforations of the globe. Recent studies have highlighted the effect of central corneal thickness (CCT) on IOP measurement.

This chapter discusses measurement conventions and population means associated with IOP and CCT. In addition, it presents the variety of devices and methods currently available and provides instruction in measuring IOP.

■ IOP Measurement Conventions and Population Means

By convention, IOP is measured in millimeters of mercury (mm Hg). Intraocular pressure, like many biologic parameters, varies in the population as a whole. In large epidemiologic studies, mean IOP is 16 mm Hg, with a standard deviation of 3 mm Hg. Variables such as the time of day, age, and genetic factors influence IOP. Although there is no strict cutoff between normal and abnormal intraocular pressures, most people have IOPs between 10 and 21 mm Hg.

■ Types of Tonometers

Several types of ophthalmic instruments are used to perform tonometry. The instruments can be categorized into 2 groups based on the way they determine IOP. *Applanation tonometers* measure the force needed to flatten, or applanate, a small area of the central cornea. The greater the force needed to applanate a known area of the cornea, the higher the IOP; *indentation tonometers* measure the amount of indentation of the cornea produced by a known weight.

Applanation Tonometers

Some of the most common types of applanation tonometers and their characteristics are listed below.

- The *Goldmann applanation tonometer* is the most common tonometer. Usually mounted on the standard slit-lamp biomicroscope, it measures the IOP of a seated patient with high accuracy in most clinical situations. Measurements are less precise for edematous and scarred corneas.

- The *Perkins tonometer* is a handheld, portable applanating device. The technique for use, mechanism of action, and relative accuracy are similar to those of the slit-lamp–mounted Goldmann tonometer, and it can be used with either a seated or supine patient. Its portability makes this device useful at the bedside or in the operating room. Because it is not mounted to a stable device, however, the steadiness of both the patient and the examiner are harder to control. Nevertheless, with some practice, the Perkins tonometer is a useful instrument.

- The *pneumatic tonometer*, or *pneumatonometer*, is an electronic pressure-sensing device that consists of a gas-filled chamber covered with a Silastic diaphragm. The gas in the chamber escapes through an exhaust vent. As the diaphragm touches the cornea, the gas vent is reduced in size and the pressure in the chamber rises. The instrument supplies a measurement reading directly in mm Hg. The pneumatic tonometer is portable, can be used with a seated or supine patient, and is especially useful in the presence of corneal scars or corneal edema.

- The *Tonopen*, like many similar portable electronic applanating devices, contains a strain gauge and produces an electrical signal as the tip of the instrument applanates the cornea. This device uses disposable sterile rubber covers for the applanating tip, can be used with a seated or supine patient, and is useful in the presence of corneal scars or edema. Some studies have found that the instrument underestimates IOP in the higher ranges. Although the Tonopen is easier to learn than Goldmann tonometry, its accuracy is not quite as high.

- The *noncontact (air-puff) tonometer* determines IOP by measuring the time necessary for a given force of air to flatten a given area of the cornea. Because the instrument does not contact the patient's cornea, no anesthetic drops are needed. Readings obtained with these instruments correlate well with those obtained by Goldmann applanation tonometry except at high and low extremes of intraocular pressure.

Indentation Tonometers

The *Schiøtz tonometer* is an inexpensive, portable, and easy-to-use instrument. The patient must be supine for Schiøtz indentation tonometry. A drawback of this technique is that it assumes that the patient's scleral rigidity is normal and that the corneal curvature approaches that of a standard, which limits accuracy in conditions such as high myopia, prior ocular surgery, and corneal edema. Furthermore, the accuracy of Schiøtz indentation tonometry can be reduced by incorrect technique, inadequate cleaning (the instrument is difficult to clean both adequately and quickly), and improper calibration. The application of a relatively heavy weight to the eye also causes a rise in IOP. Because of a number of practical and theoretical problems, the Schiøtz tonometer is now used much less frequently than in past years.

Although not a device in the usual sense, the examiner's fingertips may be used to indent the globe and roughly estimate intraocular pressure. This is called a *tactile tension*. Estimating IOP by digital pressure on the globe may be used with uncooperative patients or in the absence of instrumentation, but it can sometimes be inaccurate even in very experienced hands. In general, digital estimation of IOP is useful only for detecting large differences between the patient's eyes.

■ Goldmann Applanation Tonometry

The Goldmann applanation tonometer consists of 4 principal operative parts, described below and illustrated in Figure 12.1.

- The *tonometer tip*, the part of the instrument that contacts the patient's cornea, contains a *biprism* (2 beam-splitting prisms) that converts a circular area of contact between the tonometer tip and the patient's cornea into 2 semicircles. By properly aligning the semicircles, the examiner can determine the area of corneal applanation and measure the intraocular pressure with great accuracy.
- A metal *rod* connects the tonometer tip to the instrument's housing.
- The tonometer *housing* contains a mechanism that can deliver a measured force, controlled by the force adjustment knob on the housing, to the tonometer tip.
- The *force adjustment knob* on the housing is used to vary the amount of force needed to applanate the cornea. The scale reading on the knob is multiplied by 10 to express IOP in mm Hg.

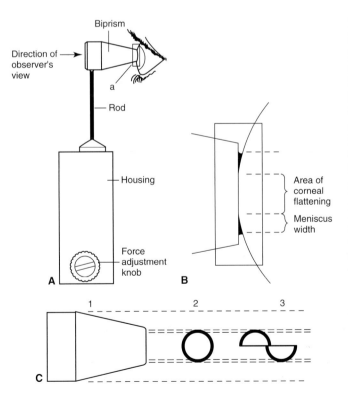

Figure 12.1 Goldmann applanation tonometer and principles of use. **(A)** Main features of the instrument, shown in contact with the patient's cornea. **(B)** Enlarged area from part A shows tear-film meniscus created by contact of biprism and cornea. **(C)** The view through the biprism (1) reveals circular meniscus (2), which is converted by prisms into 2 semicircles (3). (Redrawn with permission from Shields MB, *Textbook of Glaucoma.* 3rd ed. Baltimore: Williams & Wilkins; 1992.)

Clinical Protocol 12.1 provides instructions for measuring intraocular pressure with the Goldmann applanation tonometer.

Disinfection of the Applanating Tip

Disinfecting the applanating tonometer tip is critical in preventing the inadvertent spread of ocular pathogens such as adenovirus and herpes simplex virus type 1. Additionally, such measures eliminate the potential spread of other pathogens, such as hepatitis B and human immunodeficiency virus (HIV). Clinical Protocol 12.2 provides specific instructions for disinfecting the applanating tonometer tip.

■ Schiøtz Indentation Tonometry

The Schiøtz indentation tonometer is a handheld instrument made primarily of metal parts. The principal parts of the instrument are described below and illustrated in Figure 12.2.

- A curved metal *foot plate* is designed for placement upon the patient's cornea.
- A metal *plunger* moves up and down inside a cylinder and rests upon the patient's cornea in the center of the foot plate.
- The instrument's *frame* is held between the examiner's thumb and forefinger by the handles.
- A variety of *weights* are available to place upon the tonometer to provide the indentation force. The 5.5 g weight is used first.
- A numbered *scale* on the tip of the instrument shows the measurement of indentation by way of an *indicator needle*, which is moved by a *hammer* in response to the amount of corneal indentation produced by the weight. The

Figure 12.2 Parts of the Schiøtz tonometer.

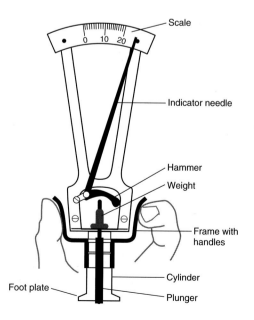

scale reading on the instrument must be converted to mm Hg using a printed Schiøtz conversion table, which is supplied with the instrument.

Clinical Protocol 12.3 provides instructions for performing Schiøtz tonometry.

Disinfection of the Schiøtz Tonometer

As with the applanating tonometer tip, disinfection of the Schiøtz tonometer should occur after every use to prevent the spread of pathogenic organisms. Clinical Protocol 12.4 provides instructions for disinfection of the tonometer tip.

■ Corneal Pachymetry

Corneal pachymetry is the measurement of corneal thickness. It has been used in the evaluation of corneal thickness abnormalities, including thinning disorders such as keratoconus and thickening disorders such as Fuchs endothelial dystrophy. More recently it has been recognized as an important factor in glaucoma management in corneas that may otherwise be without pathology.

There are 2 main methods of pachymetry: optical and ultrasound. Optical methods of pachymetry use light waves to determine corneal thickness and are advantageous in that they do not require corneal contact. Ultrasonic techniques use sound waves to determine corneal thickness via a transducer in a probe tip that touches the cornea. Currently, ultrasound pachymetry is considered the gold standard as it has been shown to be more accurate with significantly less variability than optical methods. It also has the advantage of greater portability and ease of use, and has thus become the predominant method of determining corneal thickness. Clinical Protocol 12.5 provides instructions for performing corneal pachymetry.

Corneal thickness varies according to location, and it is commonly measured in microns (μm). The cornea is thickest peripherally and thinnest centrally. It is central corneal thickness (CCT) that has the greatest application for glaucoma management, and it is this value that will be discussed at length here. Population studies have shown a wide range of normal with mean values for CCT between 537 and 554 μm.

Pachymetry as a means of measuring CCT is an important component of the ocular examination in patients with ocular hypertension and glaucoma, because of its effect on IOP measurement. Tonometry is affected by CCT when using all modern methods for IOP measurement, including the Goldmann tonometer, Perkins tonometer, pneumatonometer, Tonopen, and noncontact tonometer. The gold standard for measuring IOP is the Goldmann tonometer, and it is most accurate with a CCT of 520 μm. As stated above, however, CCT varies considerably even among normal corneas. Since applanation tonometry estimates IOP by the amount of force it takes to flatten the central cornea, a deviation from 520 μm may affect the accuracy of the measurement. A high CCT may give an artificially high IOP, and a thin CCT may give an artificially low reading.

Several correction factors have been suggested for the effect of CCT on IOP measurement. Some have suggested 0.5 mm Hg correction for every 10 micron difference from 542 μm. Others recommend a correction of 3.0 mm Hg for every

50 µm of difference from 550 µm. But the relationship between CCT and IOP is not linear and such correction factors are only rough estimates at best. In addition, the biomechanical properties of corneas, the relative stiffness or pliability, can vary among individuals and affect IOP measurement. There is currently no validated correction factor for the effect of CCT on IOP measurement and any correction should be used with caution and in the context of the overall clinical picture. CCT is important to take into account in a general sense, however. For example, a patient with a very thin CCT with progressive optic nerve damage from glaucoma, despite IOP that appears reasonably well controlled, may be one in which IOP is being underestimated, and the patient may benefit from further IOP lowering. Conversely, in an ocular hypertensive patient with a very thick CCT, the high IOP may actually be lower than what is measured, and the patient can be considered at lower risk for developing glaucoma than if the CCT were thin. It has been estimated that 30% to 57% of elevated IOP in ocular hypertensives may actually be artifacts.

The Ocular Hypertension Treatment Study (OHTS) found CCT to be a strong predictive factor for the development of glaucoma in ocular hypertensive patients. Patients with CCT of less than 555 µm had a significantly greater risk of developing primary open angle glaucoma. CCT is thus now considered an important and essential part of the evaluation of ocular hypertensive patients in establishing their risk for developing glaucoma.

Pitfalls and Pointers

- Prolonged gonioscopy can alter IOP; during the comprehensive ocular examination, tonometry should precede gonioscopy.
- If using the fingers to hold a patient's eyelids open during tonometry, avoid exerting pressure on the globe, which can increase IOP and lead to a falsely high measurement.
- Avoid performing tonometry on patients with infected eyes whenever possible.
- Try to be brief and precise in tonometric testing; excessive repositioning of the tonometer on the patient's cornea can occasionally disrupt the corneal epithelium.
- A patient's tight collar or breath holding can sometimes falsely elevate the IOP; be sure your patients loosen any clothing that is restrictive about the neck before undergoing tonometry, and instruct them to avoid holding their breath during IOP measurement.
- The accuracy of Goldmann applanation tonometry is limited in patients with corneas that are irregular (such as in keratoconus), scarred following trauma, or edematous. The pneumatic tonometer and the Tonopen are generally considered more accurate in these clinical situations.
- Central corneal pachymetry should be performed in patients with ocular hypertension and glaucoma because IOP readings are affected by the patient's central corneal thickness. The actual IOP is underestimated by applanation tonometry in patients with thin central corneas (eg, after refractive surgery); applanation tonometry overestimates the actual IOP in patients with thicker corneas.

Suggested Resources

Allingham RR, Damji KF, Freedman S, et al, eds. The glaucoma suspect: when to treat? In: *Shields' Textbook of Glaucoma*, 5th ed. Philadelphia: Lippincott Williams & Wilkins, 2005:191–196.

Dueker DK, Singh K, Lin SC, et al. Corneal thickness measurement in the management of primary open-angle glaucoma. A report by the American Academy of Ophthalmology. *Ophthalmology.* 2007;114:1779–1787.

Glaucoma. Basic and Clinical Science Course, Section 10. San Francisco: American Academy of Ophthalmology; published annually.

Kass MA, Heuer DK, Higginbotham EJ, et al. The Ocular Hypertension Treatment Study: a randomized trial determines that topical ocular hypotensive medication delays or prevents the onset of primary open-angle glaucoma. *Arch Ophthalmol.* 2002;120:701–713.

Lewis RA. Goldmann applanation tonometry. In: *Eye Exam & Basic Ophthalmic Instruments* [DVD]. San Francisco: American Academy of Ophthalmology; 1988 [reviewed for currency: 2004].

Primary Angle Closure [Preferred Practice Pattern]. San Francisco: American Academy of Ophthalmology; 2005.

Primary Open-Angle Glaucoma [Preferred Practice Pattern]. San Francisco: American Academy of Ophthalmology; 2006.

Primary Open-Angle Glaucoma Suspect [Preferred Practice Pattern]. San Francisco: American Academy of Ophthalmology; 2008.

Clinical Protocol 12.1 **Performing Goldmann Applanation Tonometry**

1. Insert a clean tonometer tip in the biprism holder. The 180° marking on the tonometer tip should be aligned with the white line on the biprism holder.

2. Instill a topical anesthetic drop and fluorescein dye into each of the patient's eyes. Many clinics use a single solution containing both the anesthetic and the dye (Fluress) for this test.

3. Seat the patient at the slit lamp with the patient's forehead firmly against the headrest and chin comfortably on the chin rest. The patient's eye should be aligned with the black band on the headrest column. Instruct the patient to look straight ahead and to open the eyelids widely. The examiner should be seated facing the patient, behind the slit-lamp oculars.

4. Position the cobalt filter in front of the slit-lamp illumination device. The cobalt-blue light causes the fluorescein dye on the patient's eye to fluoresce a bright yellow-green.

5. Set the magnification of the slit lamp at low power, with the light beam at high intensity and shining on the tonometer tip at a wide angle (about 60°).

6. Looking from the side, use the slit-lamp control handle to align the tonometer tip with the patient's right cornea. Adjust the numbers on the tonometer force adjustment knob to read anywhere between 1 and 2 (10 and 20 mm Hg).

(continued)

Clinical Protocol 12.1 *(continued)*

7. Instruct the patient to focus on your right ear, blink once (to spread the fluorescein dye), and then try to avoid blinking, squeezing, or holding his or her breath. If it is necessary to hold the patient's lids open, secure them against the bony orbit; do not apply pressure to the globe.

8. Using the slit-lamp control handle, gently move the biprism forward until it just touches the cornea. Looking through the slit-lamp oculars, confirm that the biprism has just touched the cornea: the spot of fluorescein will break into 2 semicircles, 1 above and 1 below a horizontal line. Raise and lower the slit-lamp biomicroscope with the control handle until the semicircles are equal in size. The semicircles can be viewed monocularly through only one of the slit-lamp oculars; in most slit lamps the semicircles are viewed through the left ocular.

   a. If the patient has a large amount of corneal astigmatism, the semicircles seen by the examiner through the instrument ocular will look elliptical rather than circular. An error will be introduced into the pressure determination. In this situation, rotate the tonometer tip so that the dividing line between the semicircles is 45° to the major axis of the ellipse.

9. Slowly and gently turn the force adjustment knob in the direction required to move the semicircles until their inner edges just touch and do not overlap (Figure 1A).

   a. If the semicircles are separated, as in Figure 1B, the pressure reading will be too low; if the semicircles overlap, as in Figure 1C, the pressure reading will be too high.

   b. If there is too much fluorescein or if the examiner is applying pressure to the globe while holding the patient's eye open, the semicircles will appear thick, and an inaccurate pressure reading will result. A small pulsatile motion of the semicircles might be apparent, synchronous with the patient's pulse.

10. With the slit-lamp control handle, pull the tonometer biprism away from the patient's eye. Note the reading on the numbered dial of the force adjustment knob. Multiply the number by 10 to obtain the intraocular pressure in mm Hg, and record the pressure in the patient's medical record.

11. Repeat the procedure for the left eye.

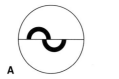   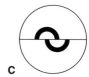

A   B   C

Figure 1 Adjustments for monocular view of fluorescein spots through the slit-lamp oculars. **(A)** Correct position. **(B)** Incorrect position. **(C)** Incorrect position.

Clinical Protocol 12.2 **Disinfecting the Applanating Tip**

1. Remove the tonometer tip from the holder after each use.

2. Disinfect by one of the following methods:

   a. Swab the tip with an alcohol swab or a cotton-tipped applicator that has been soaked in isopropyl alcohol.

   b. Soak the tonometer tip in a 10% solution of sodium hypochlorite (household bleach) *or* 3% hydrogen peroxide or isopropyl alcohol for 10 minutes.

3. Rinse the tonometer tip with water and dry with tissue or gauze to remove residual disinfecting solution, which could damage the corneal epithelium.

Clinical Protocol 12.3 **Performing Schiøtz Indentation Tonometry**

1. Check for proper calibration of the instrument by positioning the tonometer foot plate with the weighted plunger in place on the smooth convex surface (testing plate) provided within the instrument case. If calibration does not register 0 on full depression, a factory recalibration is necessary.

2. Instill a drop of topical anesthetic onto each of the patient's eyes.

3. Place a 5.5 g weight on the Schiøtz tonometer.

4. Position the patient lying on his or her back or tilted back in the examination chair and fixating on the ceiling.

5. Using your nondominant hand, gently spread the eyelids of the right eye open with the fingertips, being careful not to apply any pressure to the globe or orbit.

6. Grasp the handles of the tonometer with the thumb and index finger of your dominant hand and align the scale so it faces you.

7. Maintaining the instrument in a vertical orientation, gently lower it onto the patient's cornea until the foot plate is resting on the cornea. You may balance your thumb on the bridge of the patient's nose and your other fingers on the patient's forehead to steady your hand.

8. Read the scale and lift the instrument straight up and off the patient's eye.

9. Using the calibration table that comes with the instrument, determine the intraocular pressure in mm Hg and record your results in the patient's medical record. Note that the lower the scale reading, the higher the intraocular pressure on the calibration table.

10. If the scale reading is less than 4 (indicating an elevated intraocular pressure), add the 7.5 g weight and repeat the measurement. At very high intraocular pressure, the Schiøtz tonometer is more accurate with a larger weight in position.

11. Repeat steps 5 to 10 for the left eye.

Clinical Protocol 12.4  **Disinfecting the Schiøtz Tonometer**

1. Remove the plunger from the cylinder by removing the weight and unscrewing the bolt around the plunger.

2. Wipe the foot plate and the plunger with alcohol or acetone. A pipe cleaner is helpful for thoroughly cleaning the plunger bore in the body of the instrument.

3. After cleaning, rinse the foot plate and plunger with water, wipe dry with a clean, dry tissue or allow to air dry, and reassemble the instrument. Take care not to touch the foot plate or the plunger tip with the fingertips.

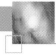 **Performing Corneal Pachymetry**

1. Disinfect the tip of the pachymeter probe with an alcohol swab and dry it with a tissue.

2. Instill a drop of topical anesthetic into each of the patient's eyes.

3. Instruct the patient to look straight ahead and to open the eyelids widely.

4. Gently touch the center of the cornea with the probe tip oriented perpendicular to the cornea. The instrument will beep when a measurement has been made.

Posterior Segment Examination

13

Examination of the eye posterior to the ciliary body and lens is important in assessing overall ocular health and in diagnosing and monitoring specific optic nerve, retinal, neurologic, and systemic disorders. Ophthalmoscopy is the examination of the posterior segment of the eye, performed with the use of an instrument called an ophthalmoscope. The posterior segment can also be viewed with the slit-lamp biomicroscope if special lenses are used. The posterior segment examination, or the fundus examination, is usually performed with the patient's pupils pharmacologically dilated and therefore follows pupillary examination. The bright lights that are used also mean that ophthalmoscopy should succeed visual acuity measurement since intense light can cause temporary loss of acuity from afterimages and retinal bleaching.

This chapter introduces the anatomic features and landmarks of the posterior segment and the diverse instruments and methods used to examine them. To examine the posterior segment effectively requires considerable skill and experience. Although this chapter presents instruction in many specific aspects of ophthalmoscopy and indirect biomicroscopy, the ophthalmology resident best gains proficiency through hands-on instruction and practice and by keeping a careful record of the findings, usually in the form of a detailed drawing.

■ Anatomic Landmarks

The term *ocular fundus* refers to the inner back surface of the eyeball. The structures of the ocular fundus consist of the optic nerve, retina, retinal pigment epithelium, choroid, and sclera. The area called the *posterior pole* is a roughly defined area that includes the optic disc and the macula (Figure 13.1).

The optic nerve exits the eye through the posterior sclera, with its center just above the horizontal meridian. The *optic disc*, or *optic nerve head*, is slightly vertically oval and normally has a pink color. The central depression of the normal optic disc is called the physiologic *optic cup*. The dimensions of the optic disc are approximately 1.5 mm horizontally and 1.75 mm vertically, with slight sex and racial differences. For purposes of estimating distances and measuring lesion sizes during ophthalmoscopy, the size of the optic disc (1 disc diameter = about 1.5 mm) can be used as a reference. The dimensions and relative location of a fundus lesion can then be estimated using disc diameters (DD). Any optical effects that the patient's refractive error might cause will apply to the fundus lesion and the optic disc.

The retinal nerve fiber layer contains ganglion cell axons that run toward the optic disc, with the temporal fibers following an arcuate course around the fovea.

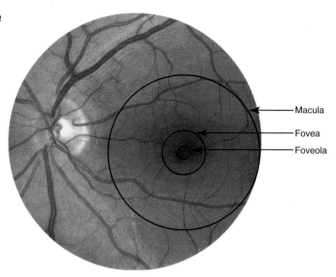

Figure 13.1 Features of the posterior pole.

Macula
Fovea
Foveola

The retinal nerve fiber layer is seen as bright striations and is most easily visible where it is thickest, at the vertical poles of the optic disc. While individual nerve fibers are too small to see by ophthalmoscopy, bundles of nerve fibers are normally visible at the inferotemporal and superotemporal arcades.

The *macula* does not have sharp borders. It occupies the area enclosed by the major temporal blood vessels approximately 5.5 mm in diameter (about 18° in visual angle). The *fovea* is the central area of the macula where there is progressive thinning of the inner retinal layers. It measures approximately 1.5 mm (5°) in diameter, centered 4 mm temporal and 0.8 mm inferior to the center of the optic disc. A circular or slightly oval light reflex around the fovea delineates where the retinal sloping begins. In the *foveal avascular zone*, which normally varies from 0.4 to 0.5 mm (400 to 500 μm), the retina is critically dependent on the choriocapillaris, the inner layer of the choroid, for its metabolic requirements. The *foveola*, the central foveal area that lies just within the capillary-free foveal avascular zone, contains a central point where light is reflected most brightly; this foveolar light reflex approximately corresponds to the anatomic spot called the *umbo*. Table 13.1 correlates the clinical appearance of these anatomic regions with their histologic features.

The *equator* is the largest circumference of latitude of the eye, located midway between the corneal apex and the fovea. Because the equator is not an anatomic structure, its position is described by reference to other structures. Externally, the equator of a normal eye lies about 13 mm from the limbus, about twice as far as the rectus muscle insertions. These topographic zones are illustrated in Figure 13.2. Ophthalmoscopically, the equator is about 4 DD posterior to the *ora serrata*, the scalloped perimeter of the retina, and is just anterior to the ampullae of the vortex veins. The retina peripheral to the equator constitutes nearly one-third of the entire retinal surface area.

For diagnostic localization, the fundus can be conveniently divided into quadrants by horizontal and vertical lines centered on the fovea. The long ciliary vessels lie along the horizontal 3 o'clock (0°) and 9 o'clock (180°) lines and are visible between the equator and the *pars plana*. Short ciliary vessels and nerves are located

Table 13.1   Anatomic Features of the Posterior Pole

Term	Clinical Description	Histologic Definition
Macula	Ill-defined area about 5.5 mm in diameter, centered 4 mm temporal and 0.8 mm inferior to the center of the optic disc; the zone within the temporal vascular arcades might be darker	Central retinal area containing 2 or more ganglion cell layers and xanthophyll pigment (macula lutea), often associated with heavily pigmented retinal pigment epithelial cells
Fovea centralis	A central retinal depression approximately 1.5 mm (1 disc diameter) in diameter, surrounded by an oval, halo-like light reflex	A depression in the inner retina, where the retina slopes from its thickest dimension toward its thinnest
Foveola	The central foveal area approximately 0.35 mm in diameter that lies just within the angiographic capillary-free zone	The central floor of the fovea where the inner nuclear layer and the ganglion cell layer are absent and all photoreceptors are cones
Umbo	The point underneath the dot-like light reflex in the middle of the fovea	Small central concavity (clivus) of the foveola

near the superior and inferior vertical meridians. Figure 13.3 shows the principal landmarks of the posterior segment.

The *ocular media* include the crystalline lens and the vitreous humor. The vitreous gel is not uniform and changes with aging. The central vitreous (Cloquet's canal) is a semifluid funnel that gradually blends with an intermediate zone (Figure 13.4). The vitreous cortex can be optically more dense. The vitreous base extends on both sides of the ora serrata as a Velcro-like attachment with the underlying retina and pars plana.

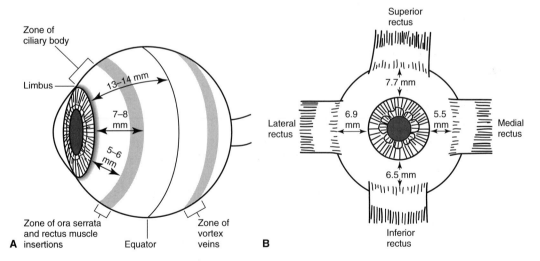

Figure 13.2   Topographic measurements of the globe. **(A)** The sclera is divided according to the eye's inner structures into the zone of the ciliary body (5 to 6 mm from the limbus), the zone of the ora serrata and rectus muscle insertions (a band that extends 8 mm from the limbus), and the equator (about 13 mm from the limbus). The vortex veins exit the globe in various positions; the superior pair is usually 5 to 8 mm posterior to the equator at the 1 o'clock and 11 o'clock positions, and the inferior pair is 5 to 6 mm from the equator at the 5 o'clock and 7 o'clock positions. **(B)** Although not exactly parallel to the limbus, the rectus muscle insertions form a spiral over the ora serrata; as measured from the limbus, the insertions are as follows: medial rectus, 5.5 mm; inferior rectus, 6.5 mm; lateral rectus, 6.9 mm; and superior rectus, 7.7 mm.

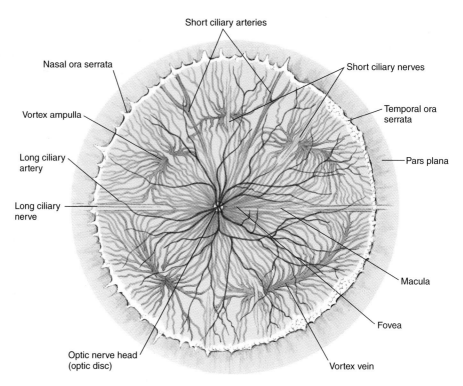

Short ciliary arteries

Nasal ora serrata

Short ciliary nerves

Vortex ampulla

Temporal ora
serrata

Long ciliary
artery

Pars plana

Long ciliary
nerve

Macula

Fovea

Optic nerve head
(optic disc)

Vortex vein

Figure 13.3 Landmarks of the normal posterior segment. (Adapted from Rutnin U, Schepens CL: Fundus appearance in normal eyes. *Am J Ophthalmol.* 1967;64:840–852,1040–1078. Published with permission from Elsevier.)

Figure 13.4 Structure of the normal vitreous body.

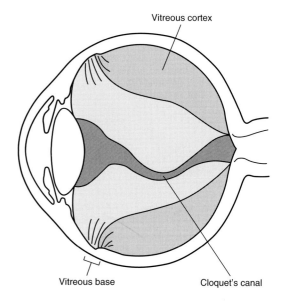

Vitreous cortex

Vitreous base

Cloquet's canal

■ Pupillary Dilation

The pupils should be dilated for an adequate posterior segment examination. A combination of a sympathomimetic drug (phenylephrine) and a parasympatholytic drug (tropicamide) is preferred for pupillary dilation for ophthalmoscopy because of rapid onset and short duration. Having the patient close both eyes for 1 minute after instillation can help slow nasolacrimal drainage and reduce systemic absorption. Systemic absorption of phenylephrine can elevate blood pressure, especially in patients with orthostatic hypotension (who have increased sensitivity to α-adrenergic agonists) or who are taking drugs that potentiate adrenergic effects (eg, reserpine, tricyclic antidepressants, cocaine, and monoamine oxidase inhibitors). The 2.5% concentration of phenylephrine is preferred over the stronger 10% concentration, which has been associated with angina, myocardial infarction, and stroke. Adequate dilation is achieved in about 20 to 45 minutes. Dilation might need to be avoided in a patient who has an iris-supported intraocular lens or a very shallow anterior chamber (to avoid inducing angle-closure glaucoma), or who is under observation by a neurologist or neurosurgeon (eg, for a head injury).

The dilated pupil gradually returns to normal reactivity after 4 to 8 hours. The alpha-antagonist dapiprazole 0.5% can be used to reverse mydriasis partially, but it often causes mild conjunctival hyperemia. Dapiprazole is no longer available in the U.S. Pilocarpine 1% is not typically used for pupillary reconstriction or reversal of cycloplegia after diagnostic dilation because of a possible increased risk of rhegmatogenous retinal detachment and possible ciliary pain.

Infants, especially when premature, are more susceptible to the adverse effects of dilating agents. Phenylephrine 10% should never be used because of the potential to induce hypertension. Concentrations of cyclopentolate greater than 0.5% may lead to feeding intolerance.

Table 13.2 lists commonly used dilating drugs according to their purpose. Table 15.4 in Chapter 15 compares the most commonly used dilating agents. Table 13.3 lists a suggested cycloplegic protocol for infants and children.

Table 13.2   Agents for Pupillary Dilation

Reason for Use	Usual Drugs
Cycloplegic refraction	Cyclopentolate 0.5% or 1%, or cyclopentolate 0.2% and phenylephrine 1% combination
Ophthalmoscopy	Phenylephrine 2.5% and tropicamide 1%
Preoperative dilation	Cyclopentolate 1% and phenylephrine 2.5%
Therapeutic dilation	Scopolamine 0.25%, or homatropine 2% or 5%, or atropine 1%

Table 13.3   Cycloplegic Protocol for Infants and Children

Age	Iris Pigmentation	Drops
Preterm	Light	Cyclopentolate 0.2% and phenylephrine 1% combination
	Dark	Add tropicamide 0.5%
3–12 months	Light	Cyclopentolate 0.5% and phenylephrine 2.5%
	Dark	Add tropicamide 1%
> 12 months	Light	Cyclopentolate 1% and phenylephrine 2.5%
	Dark	Add tropicamide 1%

■ Instrumentation for Examination

Three instruments are available for examining the posterior segment: the indirect ophthalmoscope, the slit-lamp biomicroscope, and the direct ophthalmoscope. All are used in a darkened room. Auxiliary handheld lenses are used with the indirect ophthalmoscope and slit-lamp biomicroscope in order to view the posterior segment. A comparison of properties and uses of all 3 instruments and any lenses used with them is presented in Table 13.4. The magnification and field of view vary among the instruments (Figure 13.5). For indirect ophthalmoscopy, the examiner's

Table 13.4   Comparison of Instruments for Posterior Segment Examination

Technique	Magnification[a]	Field of View	Image	Principal Use
+14 D indirect ophthalmoscopy	4×	40°	Inverted and reversed (real)	Fundus lesion inspection
+20 D indirect ophthalmoscopy	3×	45°	Inverted and reversed (real)	Routine examination
+30 D indirect ophthalmoscopy	2×	50°	Inverted and reversed (real)	Routine examination
+78 D indirect slit-lamp biomicroscopy	10×	30°	Inverted and reversed (real)	Posterior pole observation
+90 D indirect slit-lamp biomicroscopy	7.5×	40°	Inverted and reversed (real)	Posterior pole observation
Hruby lens biomicroscopy	12×	10°	Erect (virtual)	Optic disc and vitreous observation
Goldmann fundus contact lens biomicroscopy	10×	20°	Erect (virtual)	Optic disc and macula inspection
Direct ophthalmoscopy	15×	5°	Erect (virtual)	Optic disc inspection
Fundus camera	2.5×	30°	Erect (virtual)	Photodocumentation

[a] Greater magnification is achievable with the slit-lamp biomicroscope and fundus camera.

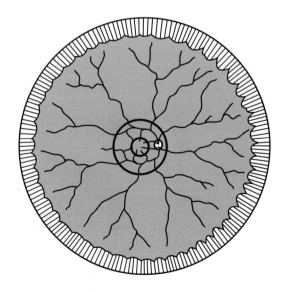

Figure 13.5   Field of view of the posterior segment with ophthalmoscopes and slit lamp with lenses. Outermost edge is the area seen with the indirect ophthalmoscope using a +20 D condensing lens. Inner circle is the area seen with the direct ophthalmoscope. The area that can be seen with the slit lamp and various lenses varies between these 2 dimensions.

magnification is estimated by dividing the power of the patient's eye (about 60 D) by the power of the magnifying lens used (eg, with a +20 D handheld condensing lens used in indirect ophthalmoscopy, the magnification is 60/20 = 3×).

Indirect Ophthalmoscope

The indirect ophthalmoscope consists of a headset with a binocular viewing device that optically reduces the examiner's interpupillary distance and an adjustable lighting system wired to a transformer power source. Portable instruments with rechargeable power packs as well as spectacle-mounted instruments are available.

For indirect ophthalmoscopy, the examiner positions a variety of convex, handheld magnifying ("condensing") diagnostic lenses close to the patient's eye (Figure 13.6). From an arm's-length distance, the examiner tilts his or her head to move the headset's light beam in order to discern an inverted, reversed, magnified image of part of the fundus at the focal point of the condensing lens. Lenses commonly used in indirect ophthalmoscopy range from +14 D to +30 D, affording magnification between about 4× and 2×. The +20 D lens is used for routine examination; the +28 D and +30 D lenses are used to examine patients through a small pupil and to achieve a panoramic overview of the retina; and the +14 D lens is used to view details of the optic disc or individual lesions.

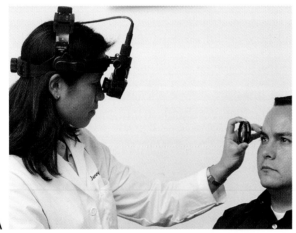

Figure 13.6 **(A)** Examination with an indirect ophthalmoscope. **(B)** Indirect ophthalmoscope: power transformer with rheostat (left), handheld condensing lens and case (center), headset (right).

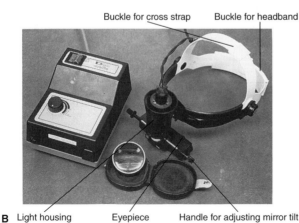

B

The indirect ophthalmoscope provides a stereoscopic, wide field of view (40° to 50°), allows examination of the retinal periphery, and makes it possible to penetrate hazy media. The instrument can also be used as a magnifying loupe to achieve an erect real image by positioning the examiner's eyes about 10 inches from the patient and focusing the condensing lens on the anterior segment.

Slit-Lamp Biomicroscope

Examination of the posterior segment can be performed on patients seated at the slit-lamp biomicroscope (see Chapter 10 for detailed information about this instrument). As with the indirect ophthalmoscope, the slit lamp affords the examiner stereoscopic vision. Handheld plus-diopter condensing lenses can be used, providing the biomicroscopist an inverted and reversed retinal image, a field of view ranging between 30° and 40°, and magnification between 7.5× and 10×. Slit-lamp examination with a high-plus lens is most useful for examining the optic disc and the macula.

Two specialized lenses sometimes used with the slit lamp are the Hruby lens and the fundus contact lens. The concave, high-minus Hruby lens is attached by a swing arm to the biomicroscope and is useful for examining optic disc cupping, macular lesions, and vitreous changes. A handheld fundus contact lens, as well as any gonioscopy lens, is applied on the patient's anesthetized cornea and is most often used to examine the microanatomy of the macula and to evaluate the optic disc and other parts of the posterior pole in patients whose pupils dilate poorly. Fundus contact lenses that have tilted mirrors are available for examining the equatorial and peripheral retina.

Direct Ophthalmoscope

The direct ophthalmoscope is a handheld instrument, sometimes electrical but usually battery-powered. It consists of a handle and a head with a light source, a peephole with a range of built-in dial-up lenses and filters, and a reflecting device to aim light into the patient's eye.

The instrument is used to examine the fundus directly (Figure 13.7). It gives greater magnification (15×) than the indirect ophthalmoscope and provides an erect, virtual image of the retina. The field of view is only about 5°, and stereoscopic vision for the examiner is not possible. Approximately one-half watt of illumination is provided, several times less than the indirect ophthalmoscope and slit lamp. The direct ophthalmoscope is most useful for examining the optic nerve and blood vessels of the posterior pole.

The Panoptic ophthalmoscope, from Welch Allyn, provides a 5 times larger field of view (25°) than the standard direct ophthalmoscope as well as a 26% increase in magnification. It is easier to view the retina through small pupils with the Panoptic ophthalmoscope, and the working distance between practitioner and patient is increased when compared with the standard direct ophthalmoscope.

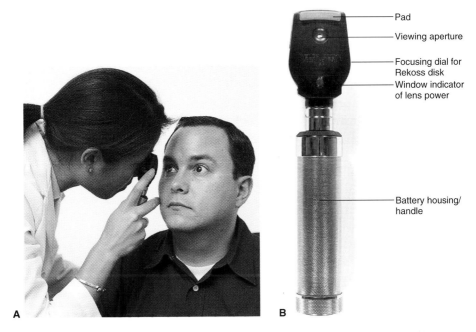

Figure 13.7 **(A)** Examination with a direct ophthalmoscope. **(B)** Direct ophthalmoscope. The dial for selecting the light filter and pattern is on the side of the instrument facing away in this photograph.

■ Indirect Ophthalmoscopy

The indirect ophthalmoscope is widely used for posterior segment examination because of its large field, depth of focus, stereopsis, good illumination, and ease of use with the scleral indentor (a device used to facilitate examination of the retinal periphery). Indirect ophthalmoscopy produces an inverted and reversed real image on the proximal side of a handheld condensing lens, onto which the examiner accommodates. The distance between the image and the observer depends on the examiner's refractive error and correction and on the refractive error of the patient.

Indirect ophthalmoscopy is possible to perform with the patient sitting upright in the examination chair. However, if the examination will take longer than a few minutes or when scleral depression is to be performed, it is easier with the patient supine. A fully reclined examination chair or a padded examination table should provide sufficient height and width for free access around the patient. The examination room should be dimly lit, and the ophthalmologist should be dark-adapted.

Headset Adjustment

The indirect ophthalmoscope headset should be positioned comfortably on the examiner's head. The frame-and-prong buckles or adjustment knobs are set to allow most of the headset's weight to be supported by the top cross-strap rather than the encircling band. The examiner should be able to use the frontalis muscle to raise and lower the headset slightly.

Eyepiece adjustment

The eyepieces should be situated as close as possible to the examiner's eyes, perpendicular to the pupillary plane, without touching the bridge of the nose. A hinged bracket permits the user to adjust the angle of the eyepiece-light housing and simultaneously shift it toward and away from the user's face. Proper positioning will give the housing a slight pantoscopic tilt. A loose eyepiece-light housing will swing freely against the examiner's face, indicating that the screws on the headset bracket must be tightened.

Some examiners do not wear their regular eyeglasses for indirect ophthalmoscopy, because the closer the eyepieces are situated to the examiner's eyes, the larger will be the field of view. A +2 D lens is usually supplied in each of the standard oculars to reduce the amount of accommodation needed to view the image in the condensing lens. For presbyopic examiners who might have trouble accommodating onto the fundus image at one-third m (33 cm), an intermediate or near add will be needed. Myopic and hyperopic examiners should wear corrective lenses or contact the manufacturer to have the eyepiece power changed to match the spherical equivalent of one's spectacle prescription for an arm's-length distance.

Adjust the interpupillary distance of the oculars by shining the oblong light beam onto your thumb held upright on your outstretched arm. Close the left eye, and adjust the right eyepiece bar by sliding it in or out until the illuminated thumb is horizontally centered in the field of the right eye. Repeat this procedure for the other eyepiece. The examiner should now have a comfortable binocular view with the light horizontally centered at an arm's-length working distance.

Light beam adjustment

The light beam is aligned by using the knurled knob that tilts the reflecting mirror on the headset. With both eyes open, adjust the light beam vertically until the light occupies the upper half of the field of view for an arm's-length working distance. This is often done by using one's thumb as a target. While looking through the eyepieces and the condensing lens, point the light beam onto the thumbnail when the knuckle is in the center of the field. A properly illuminated field will provide diffuse illumination of the upper half of the field, and the image of the bulb's filament should be diffused.

The transformer's power is adjusted by incremental or continuous dialing, depending on the instrument. The 4-volt setting on the transformer is the most useful intensity. A lower setting (eg, 2.5 volts) might be needed for children and light-sensitive patients and for examinations longer than 15 minutes. A higher setting (eg, 6 to 15 volts) is used for penetrating through hazy ocular media and for examining the peripheral fundus.

Limiting the duration of indirect ophthalmoscopy helps to minimize the subjective discomfort felt by the patient. A prolonged examination should use a reduced power setting of the headset light and a condensing lens with an ultraviolet filter or yellow coating. Any risk of phototoxicity caused by indirect ophthalmoscopy is also minimized if the examiner avoids repeatedly shining the light onto the fovea.

Choosing and Positioning the Condensing Lens

The lens usually used for a general posterior segment examination with an indirect ophthalmoscope is the +20 D lens. The +30 D and +28 D aspheric lenses have less magnification but are sometimes preferred when a wider field is helpful (eg, with large or diffuse retinal abnormalities), when the pupil does not dilate well, and when viewing the peripheral fundus through an oblique pupil. Lower-power lenses (eg, +14 D) provide more magnification but a narrower field of view and are reserved for examining the optic nerve and individual lesions. Lenses must be kept spotless and free of dust and finger smudges.

Grasp the edge of the indirect lens between the thumb and index finger, with the more convex side toward you (white ring facing the patient). You may hold the lens in your nondominant hand, reserving the dominant hand for scleral depression and drawing the fundus record (see "Scleral Depression" and "The Fundus Record" later in this chapter). The middle finger of the hand holding the lens is used to open the upper or lower eyelid, and the thumb of the opposite hand can be used to hold the other eyelid open (Figure 13.8). Depending on where the examiner is standing, the hand holding the lens can be braced against the patient's upper or lower orbital rim to maintain the proper focal distance and to keep the image centered. Figure 13.9 provides instruction and practice in centering an image in a condensing lens. A +20 D condensing lens gives a 2-inch working distance for an emmetropic eye. Clinical Protocol 13.1 summarizes how to obtain a fundus image with the headset and lens.

Two distracting light reflections corresponding to the images of the ophthalmoscope's bulb on the front and back surfaces of the condensing lens are seen when the lens is held exactly perpendicular to the line of sight. Tilt the lens to spread these reflections apart. Some lenses have an antireflective coating to reduce these bothersome reflections.

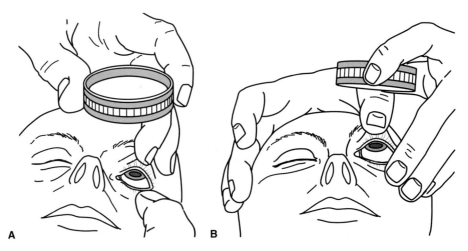

Figure 13.8 Techniques for holding the condensing lens during indirect ophthalmoscopy while holding the patient's eyelids open. **(A)** Elevating upper eyelid with third finger of the hand holding the lens while retracting the lower eyelid with the free hand's thumb. **(B)** Elevating the upper eyelid with the free hand's thumb while retracting the lower eyelid with the third finger of the hand holding the lens.

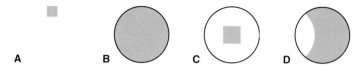

Figure 13.9 Practice and instruction in focusing the condensing lens for indirect ophthalmoscopy. **(A)** A small square, such as this, is the target over which you should hold the lens. **(B)** Center the square in the lens and move the lens toward or away from the page to make the entire image uniformly fill the lens, as in this example. **(C)** If the image in the lens looks like this, you are too far from or too close to the square. **(D)** If the image in the lens looks like this, you are too far sideways.

Changing Position to View Different Fundus Areas

Alignment

During indirect ophthalmoscopy, the examiner maintains a viewing axis through the condensing lens while pivoting around the patient's pupil to examine different portions of the fundus (Figure 13.10). Move your head and tilt the lens while using your rigid third finger as a fulcrum. Keeping the pupil centered in the condensing lens will maintain alignment of the light beam and the view returning to both of the examiner's eyes (Figure 13.11). Some examiners prefer to move their torso and approach the patient from different directions and angles as opposed to examining each portion of the fundus by having the patient look in different directions. Examination of the equatorial and peripheral fundus might require changing the direction of the light beam, switching to a different condensing lens, or tilting the head (Figure 13.12).

Working distance

The ophthalmoscopic examination is performed at arm's length, normally with about 40 to 50 cm between the examiner's headset and the patient's eye. Difficulty

Figure 13.10 For indirect ophthalmoscopy, the examiner maintains a fixed axis with the fulcrum at the patient's pupil when viewing adjacent parts of the fundus. (Redrawn from: The technique of binocular indirect ophthalmoscopy, Benjamin F. Boyd, MD, *Highlights of Ophthalmology*, 1966;9:223, courtesy of Jaypee-Highlights Medical Publishers, Inc.)

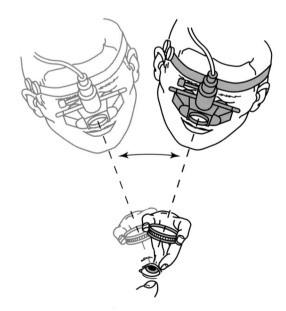

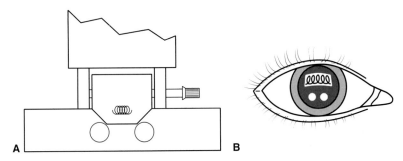

Figure 13.11   **(A)** Indirect ophthalmoscope with the standard eyepiece oculars set 15 mm apart and the light bulb filament reflected in the tilted mirror. **(B)** Examiner's view of the patient's dilated pupil showing the relative positions of the light entering the pupil superiorly and the binocular images produced by the light reflected off the fundus.

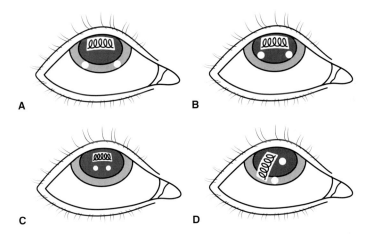

Figure 13.12   Indirect ophthalmoscopy in an eccentric gaze position. When viewing the rotated globe, the pupil appears elliptical rather than round, reducing the effective pupil size. **(A)** Problem viewing the superior periphery with the patient's eye in up gaze because the light and viewing axes are too far apart relative to the pupil. **(B)** Redirecting the light beam brings it closer into alignment with the viewing axis. **(C)** Switching to a higher-power condensing lens (eg, +30 D) reduces the image. **(D)** If B and C maneuvers do not work, tilting your head so that light enters a portion of the patient's pupil will permit viewing by 1 eye.

seeing through a small pupil can be partially overcome by withdrawing to a greater examination distance or by using a higher-power lens.

The working distance between the examiner and the lens does not have to be fixed. The distance can be shortened (lens brought closer to examiner) for greater magnification of fundus details, although the field then becomes narrower and binocularity can be lost more easily. The examiner can shift the lens to estimate grossly the relative height of a lesion. Each 1 cm of up or down displacement needed to focus on the lesion's apex or pit is equivalent to about 1 mm of lesion elevation or excavation, respectively.

Sequence of the Examination

For patients who are about to undergo any type of fundus examination, avoid using any ointment or inducing corneal haze, such as instilling certain topical anesthetics or applying diagnostic contact lenses. Ensure that the patient's pupils are well dilated, and instruct the patient to keep both eyes open. Warn the patient what to expect by explaining that a very bright light will be used that will not be harmful. Having the patient lie down in a relaxed position with the plane of the head exactly horizontal is helpful to begin the examination. This avoids having to hold the lens out in front of you in a fatiguing position and facilitates movement around the patient's head to get optimal views. By convention, the right eye is examined first.

Many examiners begin indirect ophthalmoscopy without the condensing lens by quickly shining the light of the indirect ophthalmoscope into the patient's eye to get a red reflex in order to discern any changes in the anterior eye or media. The condensing lens is then brought into position (Clinical Protocol 13.1). With experience, the examiner automatically finds the proper spot for the lens. The beginner should hold the condensing lens close to the patient's eye, then withdraw it slowly until a focused image is seen. Keep in mind that the fundus image that the examiner sees is completely inverted; that is, it is upside down and reversed.

The examiner begins the examination of the fundus by identifying the optic disc, then shifting the viewing axis from 1 part of the fundus to another, keeping the axis centered at the patient's pupil. Rather than having the patient look in 1 direction and then observing this view of the fundus, the examiner should follow each meridian from the posterior pole to the periphery by changing the viewing axis. This enables each meridian to be examined completely, following retinal vessels from the optic disc to the equator. Smooth body–lens coordination will help obtain a continuous, sweeping picture of an entire meridian of the fundus, from the optic disc to the periphery. The superior or nasal periphery is often examined before the inferior and temporal fundus, because the patient experiences less photophobia in the former regions.

When examining the peripheral fundus, the examiner must change position to see through the tilted pupil. Moving your body around the patient's head or tilting your head will permit the light beam to enter and allow you to see the fundus. If only 1 eye's visual axis is aligned with the reflected image, stereoscopic viewing will not be possible.

After each eye has been examined, suspected abnormalities such as optic disc cupping or pallor are evaluated by rapidly alternating views of the patient's eyes with the indirect ophthalmoscope to compare optic nerves and other fundus details. Finally, scleral depression is performed to examine the peripheral fundus and ora serrata of each eye.

Scleral Depression

Scleral depression, or indentation, is done to examine the area between the equator of the fundus (14 mm from the limbus) and the ora serrata (8 mm from the limbus). Scleral depression brings the region around the ora serrata into view, away from the optical distortions produced by the edges of the condensing lens.

A scleral depressor is used for the examination (Figure 13.13). A commonly used type of scleral depressor, made of metal, consists of a thimble-like section with a short, curved stem attached to the closed cap of the thimble and ending in a T-shaped nib (the depressor tip). This type of depressor can be worn over the index

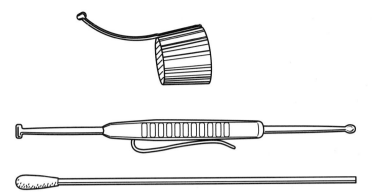

or middle finger of the dominant hand, thereby freeing the fingers to help keep the patient's eyelids open. This depressor can also be held between the thumb and the index and middle fingers. The pencil depressor, another type of instrument also made of metal, has a long, slim handle with a T-shaped or olive-shaped knob on its end. The long handle is grasped, as would be a pencil, between the thumb and first 2 fingers of the dominant hand (ie, the hand not holding the condensing lens). This type of depressor allows ready alignment of the instrument with the viewing axis. A cotton-tipped applicator can also be used in a similar way, although its end is too broad for routine use.

To perform scleral depression, the tip of the scleral depressor is placed on the eyelid just past the tarsus, and the examiner applies gentle pressure to indent the sclera. The amount of pressure on the depressor should not exceed that used for tactile tonometry. Clinical Protocol 13.2 includes instructions for examining the posterior segment with scleral depression.

Scleral depression can be uncomfortable for the patient, and some patients even find the procedure painful, particularly if the examiner does not use careful and responsive movements. Patient cooperation can be encouraged by gradual advancement to the limit of the patient's tolerance. Be especially careful not to allow the depressor tip to slip off the eyelids and onto the cornea.

Sequence of scleral depression

Because the ora serrata is most easily visualized superonasally, this area is often examined first in a circumferential sequence. To begin scleral depression, the examiner stands to the right of the patient. The right hand grasps the scleral depressor. The patient is asked to look inferotemporally. The depressor is applied at the upper tarsal margin of the inner portion of the upper eyelid. The patient is then asked to look straight ahead. As the upper eyelid moves up, the instrument's tip is slid along the globe. The examiner then tilts his or her head to direct the headset's light beam into the patient's pupil and the left hand brings the condensing lens into position, enabling the examiner to observe the superonasal equatorial fundus. Gentle pressure is then exerted with the scleral depressor. The indented fundus should be seen, and the condensing lens is brought slightly closer to the examiner to focus on this mound. The patient is then instructed to look superonasally, and the examiner's fingers help keep the patient's eyelids open. The instrument's tip is then slid anteriorly until the superonasal ora serrata is seen.

This entire sequence is repeated in all principal meridians, always keeping the examiner's visual axis and the scleral depressor in alignment. This entails moving around the patient's head and instructing the patient to look in the appropriate direction each time a new section is examined. After examining the superonasal ora serrata, lift and reposition the depressor superiorly, superotemporally, inferotemporally, inferiorly, and inferonasally to see the entire ora serrata and the posterior one-third of the pars plana (Figure 13.14). The nasal and temporal horizontal meridians are usually examined last because they are often the hardest to examine for the beginning ophthalmologist.

Check with the patient periodically about discomfort. A topical anesthetic eyedrop is used if it becomes necessary to place the depressor directly onto the globe.

Having achieved a circumferential view of the ora serrata and the peripheral fundus, any fundus lesion is reexamined. The examiner locates the lesion on the mound produced by scleral depression and rolls the lesion over the indentation by moving the depressor with fine anteroposterior and sideways movements. Changing the angle of observation of a lesion on the fundus mound will allow the examiner to determine the lesion's relative elevation or depression and will highlight its margins.

Tips on scleral depression

- If the area of indentation cannot be seen, resist the temptation to press harder and instead move the depressor gently into the line of sight, hugging the border of the tarsus.
- Release the pressure on the depressor if the patient begins to squeeze the eyes forcibly.
- Because the pupil appears oval when you are viewing the retinal periphery, you might have to tilt your head slightly to keep both of your eyes focused on the fundus image. Movement of the lens just off direct alignment achieves a prismatic effect that can help you get a more peripheral view.
- At each location, first hold the depressor stationary by pressing lightly onto the globe, indenting it about 2.5 mm. Then shift the depressor's tip laterally (by

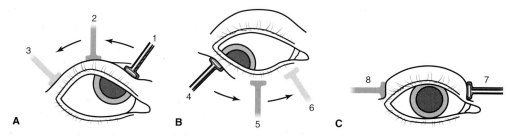

Figure 13.14   Sequence of circumferential scleral indentation through upper and lower eyelids. **(A)** Examination of superior periphery. The depressor tip is first placed superonasally (1), then moved superiorly (2) and superotemporally (3). **(B)** Examination of inferior periphery. The depressor tip is placed inferotemporally (4), then moved inferiorly (5) and inferonasally (6). **(C)** Examination of periphery in horizontal meridians by placing the depressor tip nasally (7) then temporally (8).

half its diameter) and anteroposteriorly. The rolling mound produced by these slight movements can bring out details of fundus lesions and will enhance the contrast around a retinal break.

- The mound produced by scleral depression should be kept in view at all times. Slight movements of the depressor can cause the indented image to disappear from view. To avoid this, always move the depressor in the direction opposite to the direction you want the visibly indented area to go, whether laterally, anteroposteriorly, or obliquely. The axis of observation might also have to shift, in the same direction that the examiner wants the visibly indented area to go. These lateral movements maintain a collinear relationship between the eyepieces of the ophthalmoscope, the condensing lens, and the depressor tip, pivoting at the pupil.

Transillumination

Transscleral illumination can help to differentiate choroidal lesions. A Finnoff transilluminator is placed against the bulbar conjunctiva in the meridian to be examined. The examiner observes this fundus quadrant by indirect ophthalmoscopy. The ophthalmoscope's light is then turned off, and the examiner studies the red glow and assesses the relative light transmitted through the eye wall by the transilluminating light source.

Posterior Segment Examination With the Slit Lamp

This section reviews biomicroscopy with indirect slit lamp, Hruby lens, and contact lens.

Indirect Slit-Lamp Biomicroscopy

High-plus handheld condensing lenses are useful for examining the posterior segment with the slit-lamp biomicroscope. The most commonly used lenses are the +90 D and +78 D lenses, but other lenses are available from +60 D to +132 D. The stereo-magnified view provides a good way to examine the optic disc and posterior pole. Both clear and yellow convex lenses are available; the yellow filter absorbs ultraviolet and short-wavelength visible light of less than 480 nm but substantially distorts the color of the fundus image. Almost all condensing lenses used with the slit lamp are double-aspheric lenses, so it does not matter which side is held toward the patient. Lower-powered (eg, +60 D) lenses afford a more magnified view but are harder to focus. Some lenses have adapters that expand the field or increase magnification.

For indirect slit-lamp biomicroscopy, the condensing lens is held in the same way as for indirect ophthalmoscopy; the fingers can be similarly employed to help keep the patient's eyelids open (Figure 13.15). The slit lamp's light-beam width can be varied, although the image degrades when the beam width is more than 10 mm. The lens power determines the field of view, and the magnification is varied by changing the magnification setting on the slit lamp. A setting of 10× or 16× is

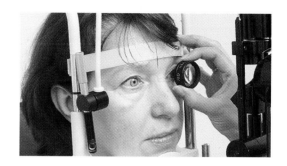

Figure 13.15   Use of a condensing lens to observe the fundus at the slit-lamp biomicroscope.

generally selected to begin the examination; higher magnification will not improve resolution. As with other types of posterior segment examinations, the right eye is usually examined first.

Moving the instrument's viewing and illumination arms makes indirect ophthalmoscopy with the slit lamp a dynamic, creative examination. Light intensity with the slit lamp is often more than with the indirect ophthalmoscope. Consequently, the duration of viewing should be kept below 5 minutes per eye to avoid phototoxicity. Clinical Protocol 13.3 includes instructions for examining the posterior segment with the slit-lamp biomicroscope.

Hruby Lens Biomicroscopy

The Hruby lens is a planoconcave high-minus lens (–55 D or –58.6 D) that neutralizes the optical power of the normal eye (+60 D) and forms an erect, virtual image of the fundus. This preset, noncontact lens is fixed by a movable arm to the slit-lamp biomicroscope (Figure 13.16). It is used to examine the posterior pole and vitreous cavity with the help of a fixation target for the other eye. Clinical Protocol 13.4 provides instructions for examining the posterior segment with the Hruby lens attached to the slit-lamp biomicroscope.

Figure 13.16   Use of the Hruby lens attached to the slit-lamp biomicroscope.

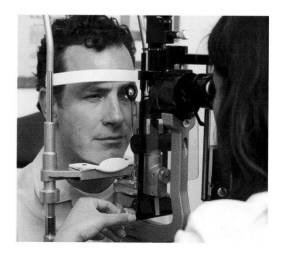

Overview of the examination

The optic nerve is first evaluated for cupping and other changes. The peripapillary retina is then examined for the nerve fibers that enter the optic disc circumferentially. Nerve fibers are most easily seen adjacent to the superotemporal and inferotemporal edges of the optic disc and are more obvious with moderately dark fundus pigmentation. Bright linear reflections are normally seen from closely packed bundles; as the nerve fiber layer thins during optic neuropathies, dark slits are seen. Increasing the light or putting in the red-free filter on the slit-lamp illumination arm can help the examiner to see the nerve fiber layer.

Attention is then turned to the macula. After examination with a 4 mm wide beam, a thin slit is focused onto the fovea. Sideways movement of a narrow slit beam can help to visualize the relative convexity or concavity of a macular lesion. A patient with a suspected macular hole or other lesion is asked whether a thin beam focused directly across the foveola appears complete, has central thinning or break, or has another distortion (Watzke-Allen test). Indirect lateral illumination of the fovea can help identify cystoid macular edema.

The vitreous body is then examined. By this time the examiner should be sufficiently dark-adapted to evaluate the posterior vitreous cavity. Mobility of vitreous strands is assessed by having the patient look up and down and then rapidly return to primary position. In up gaze the gel tends to move downward, in down gaze it moves in the opposite direction, and when the eye comes to rest in the straight-ahead position the undulating fibrils continue to move for about 10 seconds. An angle of greater than 10° between the axis of observation and the line of illumination helps to visualize vitreous opacities. Using the green or blue filter can enhance the visibility of vitreous structures.

Contact Lens Biomicroscopy

Used with the slit-lamp biomicroscope, a fundus contact lens is valuable for examining the posterior pole, particularly if the pupil is small. Contact lens biomicroscopy combines stereopsis, high illumination, and high magnification with the advantages of a slit beam. Clinical Protocol 13.5 includes instructions for examining the posterior segment with a fundus contact lens and the slit-lamp biomicroscope.

Several types of contact lenses are available, including the Goldmann fundus lens (with a power of –64 D) and the Goldmann 3-mirror lens. The central portion of the Goldmann 3-mirror lens enables examination of the central and posterior vitreous and the posterior pole. Angled mirrors help to study vitreoretinal relationships at the equator and in the periphery. Each mirror is tilted differently (59°, 67°, and 73°) to give views of the peripheral retina, the equatorial fundus, and the area around the posterior pole, respectively. Refer to Figure 11.50 and Chapter 11 for detailed information about the Goldmann 3-mirror lens and gonioscopy.

Wide-field (panfunduscopic) indirect contact lenses with a field of view up to 130° are available for fundus examination and for performing laser photocoagulation, although the fundus image is inverted. It is possible to examine the peripheral fundus by applying scleral depression (a special conical holder with an attached scleral depressor is available for use with the Goldmann 3-mirror lens).

■ Direct Ophthalmoscopy

The direct ophthalmoscope gives approximately 15× magnification (depending on the patient's refractive error) and is most useful for examining the optic disc and posterior pole. The rheostat is generally turned to the brightest light, unless the patient is very light sensitive. Some instruments have a sliding polarizing filter for reducing glare. Besides the open light, filters contain different spot sizes, a streak projection, a calibrated grid, a fixation target, and a red-free filter. These illumination options and their uses are listed in Table 13.5. The grids are meant for localizing and determining the size of fundus lesions but are not normally used because it is customary to describe lesions in terms of disc diameters. The slit aperture is not used much because of difficulties in seeing contour clues monocularly.

The monocular direct ophthalmoscope is particularly useful for viewing through a small pupil to determine the shape and contour of the optic nerve. Even with pupillary dilation, the examiner will not be able to see beyond the equator with the direct ophthalmoscope.

Overview of the Examination

Direct ophthalmoscopy is performed with the eye that corresponds to the eye being examined, putting the examiner cheek to jowl with the patient. Even if you have a strong monocular dominance, you must learn to perform direct ophthalmoscopy with the correct eye and in a comfortably balanced position.

The direct ophthalmoscope is focused by twirling the dial for the Rekoss disk (named after Egbert Rekoss, who invented the rotatable disk of concave and convex

Table 13.5   Illumination Openings of the Direct Ophthalmoscope

Aperture	Description	Use
○	Full spot	Viewing through a large pupil
○	Small spot	Viewing through a small pupil
●	Red-free filter	Help in detecting changes in the nerve fiber layer and identifying microaneurysms and other vascular anomalies
▯	Slit	Evaluating retinal contour
⊕	Reticule or grid	Measuring vessel caliber or diameter of a small retinal lesion (marked in 0.2 mm increments)
◉	Fixation target	Identifying central or eccentric fixation

lenses that he added to Hermann von Helmholtz's ophthalmoscope in 1852). The optimal focusing lens on the Rekoss disk depends on the patient's refractive error, the examiner's refractive error (including unintended accommodation), and the examination distance (Table 13.6).

To begin a basic direct-ophthalmoscopic examination, the focusing lens is set at zero (or the examiner's refractive error), and the patient's red reflex is checked from a distance of 2 feet (Figure 13.17A). By focusing the ophthalmoscope on the iris, opacities in the refractive media can be seen as dark shadows. Vitreous floaters are seen as the patient rotates the eye up and down. The technique works best with a dilated pupil. The examiner then approaches the patient's eye without accommodating, perhaps by imagining looking into the distance through a keyhole or by keeping the other eye open to look at a distant wall. The instrument is steadied against the patient's face by resting the ulnar border of the hand holding the instrument against the patient's cheek; the thumb of the free hand raises the upper eyelid (Figure 13.17B). The patient is instructed to stare into the distance. Many lanes and hospital rooms have a target marked on the wall opposite the examining chair or on the ceiling for this purpose.

While holding the patient's eyelids open, the examiner dials the ophthalmoscope's focusing lenses into place to clarify the fundus image. Minus lenses, for

Table 13.6   Focusing the Direct Ophthalmoscope

Direct Ophthalmoscope[a]	Patient's Refractive Error
−30 D	−15 D
−20 D	−12 D
−10 D	−8 D
−5 D	−4 D
0	plano
+5 D	+6 D
+10 D	+15 D

[a] Comparison of the direct ophthalmoscope's refractive power with the patient's spherical equivalent. Assuming the examiner's eye is emmetropic or corrected and the examination distance between the ophthalmoscope and cornea is 20 mm.

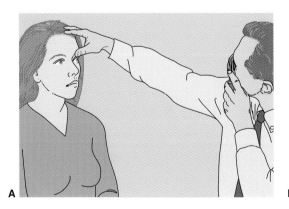
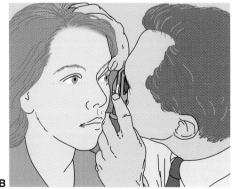

A B

Figure 13.17   Direct ophthalmoscopy. **(A)** Checking the red reflex to detect any opacities in the refractive media. **(B)** Focusing on the optic disc.

example, are used to correct for the patient's myopia and for the examiner's unintended accommodation. With the examiner's eye being emmetropic or corrected, the power of the ophthalmoscope's focusing lens is near the patient's distance refraction for low myopia or hyperopia. Optimal viewing occurs 2 to 3 cm from the patient's eye.

As the patient stares at a distance target, the ophthalmoscope is angled about 15° temporal to fixation so that the patient's optic disc is at or near the first visible field. The light beam must remain centered within the pupil, although slight tilting of the ophthalmoscope can avoid troublesome corneal light reflexes. At this point, the examiner is ready to begin examining the fundus. Clinical Protocol 13.6 describes the steps for evaluating the fundus.

The retinal nerve fiber layer bundles are seen as fine, bright striations fanning off the optic disc. The reflectivity of the inner limiting membrane can make the bundles harder to see in youngsters. The green (ie, red-free) filter enhances the visibility of the retinal nerve fiber layer. Examination should begin where the retinal nerve fiber layer is best visualized, at the inferotemporal region close to the optic disc; the examination then proceeds to the superotemporal region, followed by the superonasal and the inferonasal parts. Except for spindle-shaped slits between bundles, localized defects of the retinal nerve fiber layer do not occur in normal eyes.

■ The Fundus Record

Whether you are performing indirect ophthalmoscopy, slit-lamp examination of the posterior segment, or direct ophthalmoscopy, a record of the examination is kept by means of a fundus drawing and a drawing of the optic discs. The retinal drawing is made inside a circle centered on the fovea that shows the relative positions of the optic disc, major retinal blood vessels, and ora serrata. Standard preprinted fundus charts, or vitreoretinal charts, display 3 concentric circles representing the equator, the ora serrata, and the anterior limit of the pars plana (Figure 13.18). Roman numerals indicate the fundus meridians in clock hours. Labeled horizontal and vertical cross-section schematics are provided for recording changes in the vitreous body. Vitreous changes are recorded on the horizontal and vertical cross-sections of the globe.

A separate chart is used for recording the appearance of the optic disc (Figure 13.19). This chart shows 5 concentric circles, the outermost representing the border of the optic disc. The relative size and shape of the optic cup is drawn within the borders, using the intersecting lines as centering guides and the inner concentric circles to help with area dimensions. The major vessels can be drawn to show their relationship to the borders of the optic cup. Zones of optic disc pallor and areas of nerve fiber layer dropout should be labeled.

Standard color coding for drawing the fundus makes it easier for examiners to read or compare fundus drawings. Table 13.7 lists the colors and the entities they are used to represent; Figure 13.20 shows a sample drawing. The drawing is begun by sketching the fundus posterior to the equator, including the location of the major retinal blood vessels. The features in each meridian are then drawn as the examination proceeds to the fundus periphery (Figure 13.21). Residents should

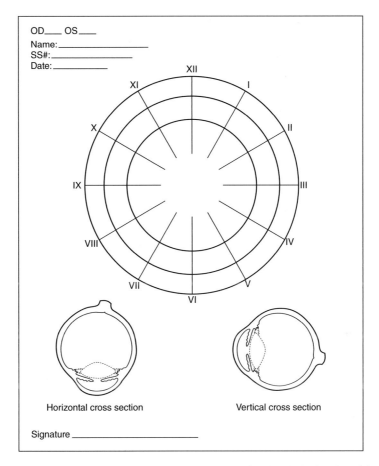

Figure 13.18 Vitreoretinal drawing chart. The inner circle identifies the relative location of the equator, the middle circle represents the ora serrata, and the outer circle locates the ciliary processes (anterior limit of the pars plana). The roman numerals indicate the fundus meridians in clock hours. The labeled horizontal and vertical cross-sections are used for recording changes in the vitreous body.

accurately depict fundus lesions by their color, size, shape, location, elevation, and relationship to retinal and choroidal blood vessels. The spherically shaped fundus cannot be easily mapped in an anatomically correct way on a flat drawing. For example, the equator of the eye always has a larger circumference than the ora serrata, but the opposite is shown on the standard fundus record. As a result, lesions anterior to the equator are exaggerated in size on the fundus record.

Drawing the Indirect Ophthalmoscopic View

The image obtained by the indirect ophthalmoscope is vertically inverted and laterally reversed. The record of the examination is made by correctly drawing all landmarks and abnormalities as if the patient were staring at the examiner with the anterior segment removed. Transposing the image that is seen onto drawing paper that has been rotated 180° will correctly depict the fundus relationships (Figure 13.22).

The technique of fundus drawing during indirect ophthalmoscopy relies on the examiner knowing the relative position from posterior pole to the fundus

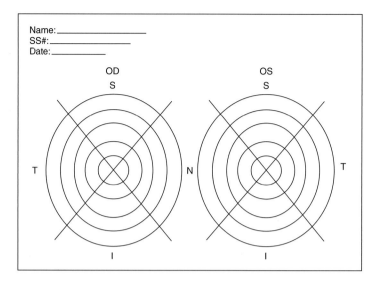

Name:_____
SS#:_____
Date:_____

OD   OS
S   S

T   N   T

I   I

Figure 13.19 Optic disc drawing chart. The concentric circles (actually ovals) and quadrant dividing lines serve as guides when drawing the borders of the optic cup. These circles represent 0.2, 0.4, 0.6, 0.8, and 1.0 cup diameter: disc diameter ratios and outline areas of approximately 4%, 16%, 36%, 64%, and 100%, respectively.

Table 13.7   Color Code for Fundus Drawing

Color	Representations
Red	Retinal arterioles, attached retina[a], retinal hemorrhage, microaneurysms, retinal break or hole
Blue	Retinal venules, detached retina, outline of retinal break or hole
Orange	Elevated neovascularization
Purple	Flat neovascularization
Yellow	Exudate, edema
Green	Vitreous opacity (eg, hemorrhage)
Brown	Pigmentation, detached choroid
Black	Ora serrata, drusen, hyperpigmentation

[a] Or use light red or leave uncolored for attached retina.

periphery. Drawing the inverted, reversed image takes practice. In examining a supine patient, the beginning resident should place the chart on the patient's chest so that the 12-o'clock chart meridian points toward the patient's feet, thereby preparing to make an inverted drawing of an inverted image (see Figure 13.22). Clinical Protocol 13.7 summarizes the steps of making the fundus drawing.

The retinal periphery is examined by moving around the patient, always standing directly opposite the meridian that is being examined. Because more peripheral details are seen at the bottom of the condensing lens, the image is drawn onto the part of the chart closest to the examiner (see Figure 13.22). After making many drawings, the experienced examiner will learn to correct mentally for the inverted image.

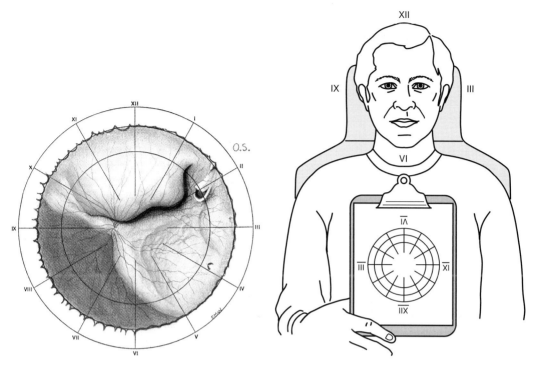

Figure 13.20 Example of a retinal drawing showing bulbous retinal detachment with peripheral exudates (yellow) and large and small horseshoe tears. (Drawing courtesy Fred M. Wilson Sr, MD.)

Figure 13.21 The vitreoretinal drawing chart is inverted on the supine patient's chest so that the examiner can draw the image that is seen in the condensing lens onto the chart.

Drawing the Slit-Lamp Biomicroscopic View

In indirect biomicroscopy with the slit lamp, the image of the posterior pole seen in a face-to-face examination is drawn onto an inverted fundus chart beside the biomicroscope. For the examiner to draw the equatorial and peripheral fundus with indirect slit-lamp biomicroscopy (or with a mirrored contact lens), the paper is turned as the patient's gaze direction changes (or as the contact lens is rotated) so that the meridian being drawn corresponds to the clock hour being examined.

For Hruby lens and contact lens biomicroscopy, the image is drawn as the examiner sees it.

Drawing the Direct Ophthalmoscopic View

An accurate drawing is made of the optic discs. The examiner should note the cup dimensions, the neuroretinal rim area, and other optic nerve and peripapillary changes. Because indirect ophthalmoscopy often underestimates the cup-disc ratio, stereoscopic examination with a +78 D lens, the Hruby lens, or a fundus contact lens is also used to add this information to the drawing.

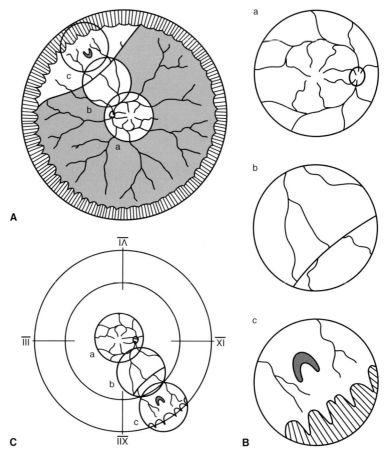

Figure 13.22 Transposing indirect ophthalmoscopic fundus views to a vitreoretinal chart. **(A)** The patient's fundus viewed directly as if the anterior segment were removed. **(B)** Three corresponding views as seen by the examiner (a, b, c). **(C)** Each image is drawn as seen directly onto the inverted chart.

■ Imaging Studies

Many types of imaging studies are useful in evaluating and documenting vitreo-retinal and choroidal findings. These include fundus photography, angiography, ultrasonography, and optical coherence tomography, as discussed below. Radiography, computed tomography (CT), and magnetic resonance imaging (MRI) also contribute information to the diagnosis of ocular abnormalities, but discussion of these techniques is beyond the scope of this manual.

Photography

Photographs help to document abnormalities of the fundus. Magnified photographs are taken of the optic disc and macula, and stereoscopic pairs can be useful. In addition to the standard 30° field, wide-angle images are also available. Clear instructions on the reasons for photography must be given to the ophthalmic photographer so the correct fields and magnifications are selected. Corresponding photographs are usually taken of both eyes for comparison.

Angiography

Fluorescein angiography (FA) is a critical test in the evaluation of retinal and choroidal disease. Sodium fluorescein solution is injected intravenously, and the fluorescent properties of the dye are captured (using the special filters placed within the fundus camera) as it passes through the retinal and choroidal circulations.

The endothelium of the retinal vasculature and the tight junctions of the retinal pigment epithelium (RPE) maintain the inner and outer blood ocular barriers, respectively, and are normally impermeable to the dye. The circulation time, or transit time, of the dye can be measured as it sequentially passes through the retinal arterial, capillary, and venous systems. Retinal vascular occlusive disease can delay the transit time, and retinal microvascular diseases such as diabetic and hypertensive retinopathy can cause abnormal leakage of the dye.

The choroid is more difficult to evaluate with FA due to the normally leaky, fenestrated choriocapillaris that obscures the overlying choroidal vessels. However, various choroidal diseases causing abnormalities of the RPE and leading to subretinal leakage can be identified with FA, including choroidal neovascular membranes, central serous retinopathy, and inflammatory choroidopathies.

Indocyanine green (ICG) angiography is helpful in elucidating choroidal disease because the dye is almost completely bound to protein after intravenous injection and has limited diffusion through the small fenestrations of the choroid. ICG fluoresces in the near infrared range of the light spectrum. Choroidal neovascularization, as with the wet form of age-related macular degeneration, can be more accurately characterized in the presence of blocking lesions such as blood or when the membrane is occult and difficult to identify with FA.

Ultrasonography

Diagnostic ultrasonography, or echography, is a useful technique when media opacification prevents adequate ophthalmoscopy of the posterior segment. Two formats are available: an A-scan is a 1-dimensional display used to characterize tissues, and a B-scan is a 2-dimensional display used for architectural information (Figure 13.23).

B-scan echography is often performed through the eyelids using methylcellulose as a coupling gel (Figure 13.24). Increased resolution is possible by placing the probe directly on the anesthetized globe or by using water-bath immersion. The B-scan image is a cross-sectional display of the globe and orbit. Moving the probe allows the examiner to create a 3-dimensional mental image. The mobility of intraocular abnormalities is noted during imaging. Photographs of the display screen are often taken, but the examiner should record all findings on the vitreoretinal drawing.

A-scan ultrasonography is used to measure the echographic amplitudes of the tissue interfaces along a linear wave front. The horizontal baseline of the graphic display represents distance, and the vertical dimension plots echo intensity.

Ultrasonographic technology is critical in the clinical evaluation of various choroidal tumors, including choroidal melanoma.

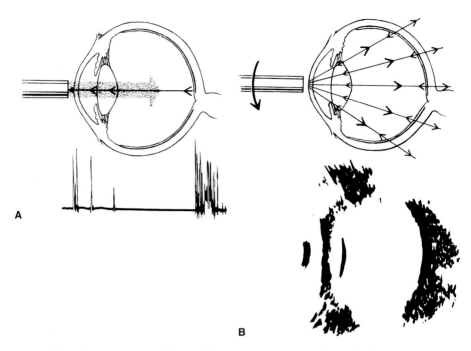

A

B

Figure 13.23   Ultrasonography of the eye. **(A)** In A-scanning, a beam of ultrahigh-frequency sound waves enters the eye (top) and is reflected by ocular tissue interfaces at different amplitudes (bottom). **(B)** In B-scan echography, the transducer moves back and forth in a plane (top), and the display shows the echo pattern for the tissue interfaces as dots (bottom). (Reprinted, with permission, from Michels RG, Wilkinson CP, Rice TA. *Retinal Detachment.* St. Louis: Mosby-Year Book; 1990.)

Figure 13.24   Application of ultrasound probe to the closed eyelids with a cross-sectional image displayed on the screen.

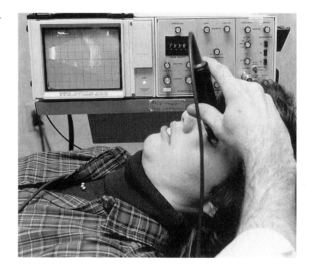

Optical Coherence Tomography

Optical coherence tomography (OCT) is a noninvasive, noncontact imaging technology that uses interferometry and low-coherence laser light to create micrometer-resolution cross-sectional images (tomograms) of the retina. A 2-dimensional image of the backscattered light from the different layers of the retina is produced which appears similar to histopathologic specimens. Newer Fourier-domain, or spectral-domain, technology delivers greater detail with shorter acquisition time than time-domain OCT scanners (Figure 13.25).

OCT is an outstanding tool in evaluating the vitreomacular and retinal-RPE interfaces. It is very useful in diagnosing impending, early, or late macular holes and their response to surgical treatment. OCT imaging has also greatly increased the accuracy in diagnosing and monitoring macular edema due to various diseases such as diabetic retinopathy and retinal venous occlusive disease. A retinal thickness map can be created by determining the distance between the inner and outer retinal boundaries. Macular volume can be assessed and followed over time to determine efficacy of therapy. In addition, OCT can shed light on subretinal diseases such as choroidal neovascularization and its sequelae.

In glaucomatous optic nerve damage, the retinal nerve fiber layer thins as nerve fibers die, and the optic cup increases in size. OCT can measure the absolute thickness of the retinal nerve fiber layer around the optic disc. The measurements can be compared to age-matched normal values and followed serially over time to detect clinical progression of glaucoma. A *scanning laser polarimeter* can also be used to assess the retinal nerve fiber layer. A combination of a scanning laser ophthalmoscope and a polarization modulator and detector, the scanning laser polarimeter takes advantage of the birefringent properties of the retinal nerve fiber layer to measure its relative thickness. A *confocal scanning laser ophthalmoscope* can create a 3-dimensional image of the optic nerve head. While these instruments show great promise, one cannot rely solely on optic nerve head and retinal nerve fiber layer imaging devices to diagnose and follow glaucoma with the instruments that are currently available. Detailed and careful clinical observation and comparison with baseline stereophotographs of the discs remain crucial to the examination of the glaucoma patient.

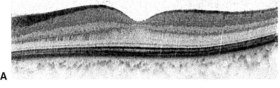

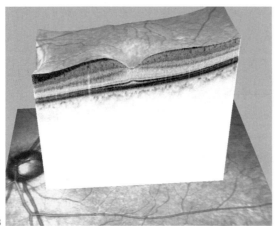

Figure 13.25 Optical coherence tomography of normal macula. **(A)** Cross-sectional image showing foveal depression. The layers of the retina are distinctly apparent above the dark (highly reflective) retinal pigment epithelium. **(B)** 3D reconstructed image of the macula.

■ The Normal Fundus and Its Common Variations

To be comprehensive in performing ophthalmoscopy, the examiner should note a variety of characteristics of every principal structure of the entire posterior segment. Table 13.8 lists the major features that should be recorded during a stepwise examination of the posterior segment. Embryonic remnants and other normal developmental variations should be noted. Various age-related changes are often found, and while most do not require treatment, these too should be drawn or described (Table 13.9).

Optic Disc

The optic disc is described by its color and topography. The nasal half tends to look pinker and slightly less distinct than the temporal rim. *Myelinated nerve fibers* are white, feather-like bundles extending usually in one or more directions from the optic disc. They can also occur separate from the disc. *Hyaline bodies* (improperly but commonly called drusen) of the optic nerve are calcified sphingomyelin concretions that are sometimes found within the optic nerve head. The presence of either myelinated nerve fibers or hyaline bodies should be recorded on the optic disc drawing or described in the chart.

Table 13.8 Major Features of the Posterior Segment

Structure	Characteristics to Note
Optic disc	Cup: cup-disc ratio, cup shape and depth, visibility of lamina cribrosa
	Rim: shape or area, pallor, border demarcation
	Surrounding area: juxtapapillary chorioretinal status, visibility of nerve fiber layer
	Blood vessels: venous pulsations, caliber and patency, hemorrhages and exudates, neovascularization
Retina	Blood vessels: caliber and patency of arterioles and venules; AV crossings; intravascular, perivascular, and extravascular opacities and hemorrhages; integrity of capillary network; neovascularization
Background	Pale areas: composition, size, number
	Red areas: depth; hue; and border
	Dark areas: elevation, size, location
Macula	Light reflex, level, color and opacities
Vitreous	Clarity, uniformity

Table 13.9 Normal Degenerative Changes of the Aging Eye

Location	Alteration
Posterior pole	Loss of foveal light reflex, drusen
Retinal vessels	Narrowing, increased light reflex
Equator	Drusen, reticular pigmentary degeneration
Periphery	Chorioretinal degeneration, paving-stone degeneration
Vitreous humor	Liquefaction, floaters, posterior vitreous detachment

Optic cup

The physiologic optic cup is the slight indentation at the center of the optic disc, through which the major retinal vessels enter and exit the eye. Normal cups occupy 30% to 50% of the area of the optic disc. Genetic variations lead to some normal cups filling almost 70% of the disc's area. Because determining the cup-disc ratio by ophthalmoscopy is often inaccurate, the examiner's job is to be consistently arbitrary (or to get photographs for comparison and to perform biometry). OCT analysis can also be helpful in accurately assessing the nerve for glaucomatous damage. In addition to the cup-disc ratio, other measurements may be recorded.

Normal disc measurements for people of European descent are as follows: disc area, 2.6 mm^2; cup area, 0.7 mm^2; and rim area, 1.9 mm^2. Blacks have 10% larger disc and cup areas, while the optic discs of Asian ethnic groups tend to be somewhat smaller. Asymmetry of the cup-disc ratio of more than 0.2 between the 2 eyes occurs in less than 1% of normal individuals.

Scleral rim

A physiologic scleral rim is seen when the choroid and RPE do not reach the optic disc. Its outer border is formed by the edge of the RPE and the inner border by the scleral canal of the optic nerve. If either of these pigmented layers is thickened, a pigment crescent (conus) is seen. A darkly pigmented area is caused by the RPE extending farther than usual, and a lightly pigmented area is seen if the RPE stops short and exposes the choroid. Other normal variants include slightly blurred disc borders, resulting from a narrowed scleral aperture in hyperopic eyes and from a tilted disc in myopic eyes.

Posterior Pole

The macula has a diameter of about 18°, and its central zone, the fovea, a diameter of 5°. The yellow color of the macula lutea is not visible with white light but can be seen with bright illumination through a red-free interference filter. A healthy nerve fiber layer is slightly opaque with parallel striations in an arcuate pattern above and below the macula. The central point of the foveola often has a reflex that is an inverted image of the light source. Loss of the foveal light reflex is a common age-related change of the posterior pole, along with atrophic spots of the retinal pigment epithelium (RPE). Drusen, which are yellow-white deposits between the RPE and Bruch's membrane, constitute an abnormal change, the dry form of age-related macular degeneration. The wet form causes severe central vision loss due to bleeding and scarring from choroidal neovascular membranes.

Retinal Blood Vessels

Retinal blood vessels radiate from the optic disc, dividing dichotomously into a pattern of branches unique for each individual. While the inner retinal layers are usually supplied by the central retinal artery and its branches, cilioretinal arteries derived from the ciliary circulation are present in about 20% of all eyes and can supply circulation to a portion of the inner retina between the optic nerve and fovea. Congenital tortuosity of the retinal arterioles and venules is sometimes found.

The width of the central retinal artery (or at least the visible blood column, because the vascular wall is normally transparent) is about 0.1 mm.

Retinal venules

Under normal conditions of intraocular pressure and aortic and carotid artery sufficiency, retinal arterial pulsations are not seen, but retinal venous pulsations are common. During systole the retinal arterial pulse pressure is briefly transmitted to the intraocular pressure. When the intraocular pressure exceeds the retinal venous pressure during diastole, the retinal veins collapse. Spontaneous retinal vein pulsations are seen at the optic disc in 80% of normal people. When present, these pulsations indicate that retinal venous pressure (ie, intracranial pressure) is normal.

Retinal arterioles

The caliber and light reflectivity of the retinal arterioles are noted. A chronic rise in blood pressure produces narrowing of the retinal arterioles. In arteriolosclerosis, an age-related process that thickens arteriolar walls, the light reflex takes up more of the arteriolar width because the width of the bright stripe down the center of the blood column is proportional to the thickness of the vessel wall. Vessels with a wide light reflex are said to exhibit *copper-wiring*. When the light reflex is obscured and the fibrotic arteriole is a thin white stripe, they are referred to as silver-wire arterioles.

Vascular crossings

Retinal arteries generally remain at one level and the vein passes underneath; compression of the venule is then seen as nicking in hypertensive individuals. When the vein passes over the artery, a humping effect is seen.

Fundus Background

Physiologic color variations are commonly encountered in the background of the normal fundus. In a lightly pigmented (blond or albinotic) fundus, retinal and choroidal blood vessels are seen on a virtually white background. The fundus of a darkly pigmented person has an even, dark color, especially at the posterior pole. Nonuniform distribution of choroidal melanin, as occurs in some myopic fundi, produces a streaked or tessellated fundus background.

The venous tributaries of the choroid drain into the *vortex ampullae*, of which there are usually 4 (at 1, 5, 7, and 11 o'clock positions) but sometimes more. A circle connecting the vortex ampullae corresponds roughly to the equator of the globe. The long posterior ciliary nerves are broad, yellow lines along the horizontal meridians. The long posterior ciliary arteries are usually inferior to the temporal nerve and superior to the nasal nerve.

Drusen

Drusen are small yellowish excrescences at Bruch's membrane. Drusen are more common at the equator, especially nasally, than in the posterior pole. Macular drusen are more often found in the elderly and can be punctate or geographic.

Pigmentary changes and nevus

Congenital hypertrophy of the retinal pigment epithelium appears as a well-circumscribed, densely black, flat spot; grouped lesions are sometimes called *bear tracks*. Reticular pigmentary degeneration is an age-related degeneration of the retinal pigment epithelium. Also called honeycomb degeneration, it forms a fishnet or honeycomb pattern that is most prominent along the nasal equator.

A choroidal nevus is a dark, minimally elevated lesion that can have associated drusen and does not typically grow.

Peripheral Fundus

The ora serrata is characterized by about 50 ora teeth that point anteriorly and by ora bays that are formed between the teeth. The serrations of the peripheral retina are generally most pronounced nasally, sometimes with meridional ridges or folds, and the ora is smoother temporally. The transition from the deep nasal ora bays to the shallow temporal bays occurs at approximately 5 o'clock and 11 o'clock in the right eye and at 1 o'clock and 7 o'clock in the left eye.

Normal variations of the ora teeth include forked teeth, bridging teeth, giant teeth, and ring-shaped teeth. An enclosed ora bay must be distinguished from a retinal hole. A deep ora bay is sometimes seen nasally at the horizontal meridian. The temporal periphery is the most common site of lattice degeneration and pars plana cysts. The nasal periphery is the most common site of prominent ora teeth and meridional folds, particularly in the superonasal quadrant.

A pigmented zone (demonstrable by transillumination of the globe) is located along the ora serrata. This area of retinochoroidal adhesion is 3 to 4 mm wide in the temporal periphery and 1 mm wide in the nasal periphery and represents the normal fusion of the retina and the retinal pigment epithelium.

Several changes of the fundus periphery can be found (Figure 13.26). One or more *pearls* at the ora serrata might be identified. These ora pearls are drusen that look like shiny white spherules near the ora serrata. They have no clinical importance despite their remarkable appearance.

Cystoid degeneration appears as an area of granular tissue. This belt of agglomerated cysts occurs at the extreme retinal border, especially temporally. Cystoid degeneration can coalesce to form senile retinoschisis, a benign splitting of the retina. *Pars plana cysts* are transparent, elevated cysts measuring 1 or 2 disc diameters. Pars plana cysts are usually multiple, bilateral, and limited to the posterior half of the temporal pars plana. They are difficult to visualize without accurate scleral depression.

White with pressure is a term used to describe a blanched color of a flat area of the peripheral retina during scleral depression. This condition is usually caused by preretinal vitreous opacification. *White without pressure* is a related phenomenon that is visible without scleral indentation.

Chorioretinal degeneration is a stippled pigmentary change that occurs adjacent to the ora serrata. *Paving-stone degeneration*, also known as *peripheral chorioretinal degeneration* and *cobblestone degeneration*, consists of clusters of nummular, atrophic, depigmented spots in the periphery. Because there is loss of the outer retina, the retinal pigment epithelium, and the choriocapillaris, a patch of white sclera is

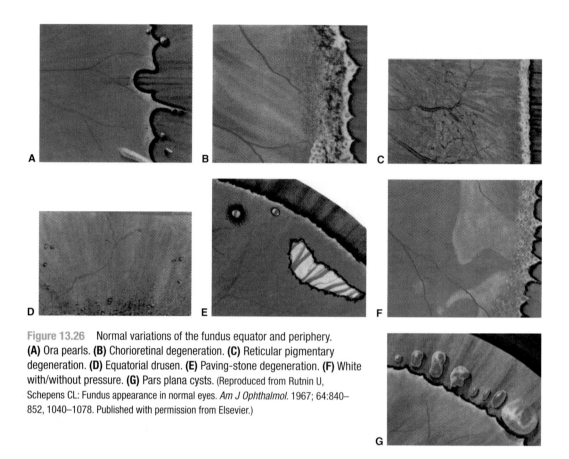

Figure 13.26 Normal variations of the fundus equator and periphery. **(A)** Ora pearls. **(B)** Chorioretinal degeneration. **(C)** Reticular pigmentary degeneration. **(D)** Equatorial drusen. **(E)** Paving-stone degeneration. **(F)** White with/without pressure. **(G)** Pars plana cysts. (Reproduced from Rutnin U, Schepens CL: Fundus appearance in normal eyes. *Am J Ophthalmol.* 1967; 64:840–852, 1040–1078. Published with permission from Elsevier.)

visible, with baring of the choroidal vessels. Clumps of pigment can border the margin of these circumscribed areas. Coalescent patches form an elongated zone with a scalloped margin parallel to the ora serrata. *Lattice degeneration* is a spindle-shaped area of retinal thinning that can have overlying white, sclerotic blood vessels.

Vitreous Humor

Light reflexes off the internal limiting membrane are more apparent in the young and, with reduced illumination, a glimmering halo is seen encircling the macula.

Remnants of the fetal hyaloid artery include an epipapillary membrane or veil, referred to as Bergmeister's papilla. The hyaloid canal passes from the optic nerve head to the lens, and a residual point of attachment often can be seen as a dot on the posterior capsule (Mittendorf's dot).

Neither the anterior nor the posterior limit of the vitreous base can be seen in an eye with a normal vitreous humor. With a posterior vitreous detachment, a white line is sometimes seen on the retina just posterior to the ora serrata and is the posterior limit of the vitreous base. The anterior limit of the vitreous base is infrequently visible as a white line in the middle of the pars plana. The boundary of the vitreous base varies among different individuals but normally extends about 2 mm either side of the ora serrata.

Age-related liquefaction, beginning in the central posterior vitreous, produces optically clear cavities. Liquid vitreous entering the space posterior to the vitreous cortex produces collapse (syneresis). A *posterior vitreous detachment* is a separation between the posterior vitreous cortex and the internal limiting membrane and can cause floaters. The incidence typically increases after age 50. *Asteroid hyalopathy* consists of small white spheres of calcium-phosphate-phospholipid crystals that do not usually impair vision.

Pitfalls and Pointers

- Other imaging problems and their causes are summarized in Table 13.10. Model eyes are available for training and practice, and a teaching mirror shows the beginner exactly what is supposed to be seen. Skill in the art and interpretation of indirect ophthalmoscopy takes daily practice with patients.
- A bright light hurts the patient. A considerate examiner avoids dazzling the patient with an unnecessarily high voltage setting. Beginning the examination at the equator and periphery can give the patient a chance to adapt to the light before the posterior pole is examined. Proper lens position is usually possible using only a small edge of the light beam, thereby shortening the duration of bright flashes to the patient. As the examiner changes position, the light should not be shining unnecessarily into the eye. Allow brief rest periods to let the patient recuperate.
- Often a quick look at the posterior pole is all an examiner will be able to achieve in small children. Turning down the illumination brightness, keeping the child in the parent's lap, and avoiding any touching of the child's face can facilitate indirect ophthalmoscopy. For children who continue to move their eyes, try using only a bright, handheld flashlight, such as a Finnoff transilluminator. While sighting down the light beam that is directed at the child's dilated pupil, interpose a condensing lens to view the posterior pole.
- During scleral depression, inability to see the indented area is often wrongly interpreted as insufficient pressure. As the examiner pushes harder, the patient moves the eye, making it impossible to find the retinal periphery. If the area of scleral depression cannot be seen, the examiner should realign the axis of view or the depressor.
- To avoid confusion in localizing a fundus lesion, recall that a fundus lesion is located in terms of meridians of the clock. Its placement along an

Table 13.10   Common Problems During Indirect Ophthalmoscopy

Problem	Reason
Large portion of the image is dark or distorted	Faulty lateral or vertical lens positioning
Image is too small	Condensing lens too near or too far from the eye
Central reflections obscuring the image	No lens tilt
Irregular reflections and haziness	Dirty lens
Dull image	Light not properly centered in the pupil
Peculiar meshwork of vessels	Looking at conjunctiva
Image suddenly lost	Patient moved eye
Inability to go from 1 fundus area to another	Moving the viewing axis in the wrong direction

anteroposterior meridian is estimated in disc diameters in relation to the ora serrata, equator, and fovea. Keeping the axis of observation fixed with the lens withdrawn, the examiner guesses what portion of the far side of the inside of the eyeball would be illuminated by the light passing through the pupil. The anteroposterior location is then confirmed by placing the scleral depressor on the lesion and looking to see how far back the depressor is from the limbus. The ora serrata is 8 mm behind the limbus, and the equator is usually 12 to 14 mm from the limbus.

- Although the direct ophthalmoscope is simple to use and provides an upright, high-magnification image of the retina, its lack of stereopsis, small field of view, and poor view of the retinal periphery limit its utility. Many ophthalmologists will use slit-lamp biomicroscopy with a +78 D or +90 D handheld condensing lens to examine the macula and disc in lieu of direct ophthalmoscopy, especially when the pupil is dilated.

- Although bradycardia from the oculocardiac reflex is uncommon during routine examination, vasovagal syncope can result from application of a fundus contact lens. The contact lens should be held, but not pushed, against the eye and removed if the patient begins to feel faint.

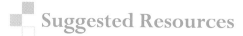

Suggested Resources

Retinal Conditions

Age-Related Macular Degeneration [Preferred Practice Pattern]. San Francisco: American Academy of Ophthalmology; 2008.

Diabetic Retinopathy [Preferred Practice Pattern]. San Francisco: American Academy of Ophthalmology; 2008.

Posterior Vitreous Detachment, Retinal Breaks, and Lattice Degeneration [Preferred Practice Pattern]. San Francisco: American Academy of Ophthalmology; 2008.

Indirect Ophthalmoscopy

Friberg TR. Examination of the retina: Ophthalmoscopy and fundus biomicroscopy. In: Albert DM, Miller JW, Azar DT, Blodi BA, eds. Albert & Jakobiec's *Principles and Practice of Ophthalmology*. 3rd ed. Philadelphia: WB Saunders Co; 2008.

Regillo CD, Benson WE, Edmunds W. *Retinal Detachment: Diagnosis and Management*. 3rd ed. Philadelphia: Lippincott Williams & Wilkins; 1998.

Rubin ML. The optics of indirect ophthalmoscopy. *Surv Ophthalmol.* 1964;9:449–464.

Direct Ophthalmoscopy

Orient JM. *Sapira's Art and Science of Bedside Diagnosis.* 3rd ed. Philadelphia: Lippincott Williams & Wilkins; 2005.

Fluorescein Angiography

Berkow JW, Flower RW, Orth DH, Kelley JS. *Fluorescein and Indocyanine Green Angiography: Technique and Interpretation.* Ophthalmology Monograph 5. 2nd ed. San Francisco: American Academy of Ophthalmology; 1997.

Optical Coherence Tomography

Lin SC, Singh K, Jampel HD, et al. Optic nerve head and retinal nerve fiber layer analysis: a report by the American Academy of Ophthalmology. *Ophthalmology.* 2007;114:1937–1949.

McDonald HR, Williams GA, Scott IU, et al. Laser scanning imaging for macular disease: a report by the American Academy of Ophthalmology. *Ophthalmology.* 2007;114:1221–1228.

Clinical Protocol 13.1   Obtaining a Fundus Image in Indirect Ophthalmoscopy

1. Ask the reclining, well-dilated patient to gaze steadily at a distant target on the ceiling. Having the patient look just above and beyond your shoulder (your right shoulder when examining the patient's right eye) will help to align your view onto the posterior pole. Patients with poor vision are asked to extend an arm and to stare at their outstretched thumb.

2. While standing above the patient, direct the headset's light by tilting your head so that it illuminates the fundus when focused through the condensing lens.

3. Holding the condensing lens in the standard manner, position it just in front of the patient's eye and center the pupil in it.

4. Pull the lens slowly away from the patient's eye by flexing your wrist and by bending the fingers holding the lens (Figure 1) until you see a stereoscopic, focused image of the fundus in midair in front of the condensing lens (Figure 2). For a +20 D condensing lens, the image is seen when the lens is positioned about 5 cm in front of the patient's eye.

5. Accommodate on this image with both eyes, and maintain it by keeping the headset's light in the patient's pupil.

6. If light reflections from the front and back surfaces of the condensing lens are centered (Figure 3A), tilt the lens slightly to move them apart (Figure 3B).

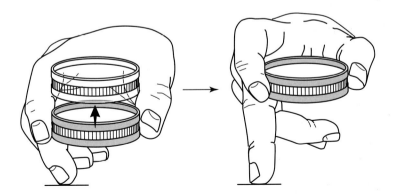

Figure 1 The lens is pulled slowly away from the patient's eye. (Redrawn from: The technique of binocular indirect ophthalmoscopy, Benjamin F. Boyd, MD, *Highlights of Ophthalmology*, 1966;9:213, courtesy of Jaypee-Highlights Medical Publishers, Inc.)

(continued)

7. Shift the field of view by moving your head and the condensing lens along a fixed axis. Use the extended finger of the hand holding the condensing lens as a pivot to keep your viewing axis centered on the patient's pupil (Figure 4).

8. Mentally note that the image of the patient's fundus is inverted and reversed.

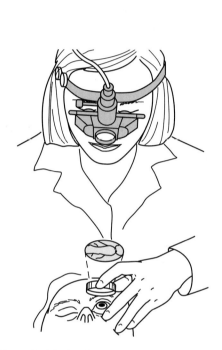

Figure 2 The lens is stopped midair when a stereoscopic, focused image of the fundus is visible.

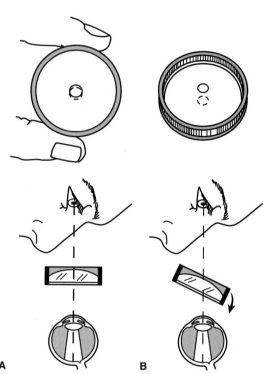

Figure 3 Positions of light reflections on the pupil. If the reflections are centered **(A)**, the examiner tilts the lens slightly **(B)** to move the reflections apart. (Modified from: The technique of binocular indirect ophthalmoscopy, Benjamin F. Boyd, MD, *Highlights of Ophthalmology*, 1966;9:219, courtesy of Jaypee-Highlights Medical Publishers, Inc.)

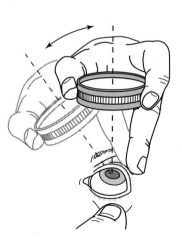

Figure 4 Keeping the viewing axis centered. (Redrawn from: The technique of binocular indirect ophthalmoscopy, Benjamin F. Boyd, MD, *Highlights of Ophthalmology*, 1966;9:222, courtesy of Jaypee-Highlights Medical Publishers, Inc.)

Clinical Protocol 13.2   Performing Scleral Depression

1. While standing opposite the area to be examined, instruct the reclining patient to look toward you. It can also help in positioning to have the patient turn his or her head away from the direction of the zone of regard.

2. Increase the voltage setting on the ophthalmoscope transformer to the highest setting that the patient can tolerate, to compensate for the reduced light entering the eye obliquely through the pupil.

3. With your dominant hand, hold the thimble-style scleral depressor by either inserting your index finger, as with a thimble, or by grasping the outside of the "thimble" between your thumb and index finger, as you would a surgical instrument (Figure 1).

4. Rest the tip of the scleral depressor lightly at the skin crease of the eyelid (Figure 2). Align the shaft of the instrument with your visual axis and keep the depressor nearly parallel to the surface of the patient's eye (Figure 3A).

5. Instruct the patient to move the eyes toward the tip of the scleral depressor (Figure 3B). Often it is only necessary for the patient to resume a straight-ahead, primary position rather than to gaze excessively far in the meridian being examined.

6. Press the depressor gently. This action creates a mound in the fundus (Figure 3C).

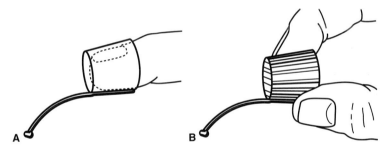

Figure 1   The scleral depressor is held thimble-style **(A)** or as you would hold a surgical instrument **(B)**.

Figure 2   The depressor tip rests lightly at the eyelid skin crease.

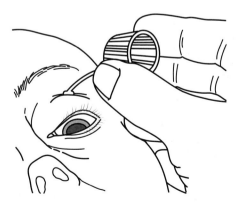

(continued)

7. As for indirect ophthalmoscopy of the posterior pole, keep the ophthalmoscope's light beam in the upper half of the field and first obtain a red reflex, then interpose the condensing lens (Figure 4).

8. While keeping the depressor tangential to the globe and pressing against the equator, a grayish mound should come into view in the lower part of the red reflex, indicating that the depressor tip is aligned with the axis of observation (Figure 5).

9. Modify the lens position to bring the bulging, indented part of the peripheral fundus into clear focus.

10. To view the ora serrata, instruct the patient to look slightly farther in the direction of the tip of the scleral depressor. While keeping the fundus image focused, slide the depressor's tip anteriorly until the ora serrata is seen in the inferior part of the fundus image (Figure 6A).

11. To view the equatorial fundus, instruct the patient to shift gaze toward primary position without moving the scleral depressor (Figure 6B).

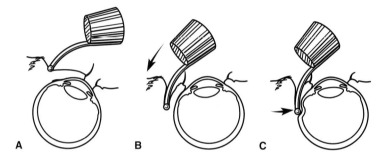

Figure 3   The depressor tip is held nearly parallel to the patient's eye **(A)**. The patient move the eyes toward the tip **(B)** and the examiner gently presses the depressor **(C)**. (Figure 3 from: The technique of binocular indirect ophthalmoscopy, Benjamin F. Boyd, MD, *Highlights of Ophthalmology*, 1966;9:243, courtesy of Jaypee-Highlights Medical Publishers, Inc.)

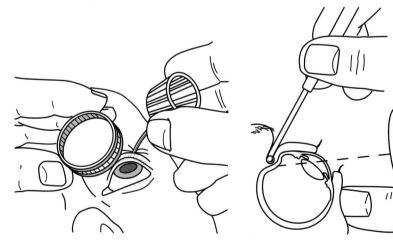

Figure 4   Technique for indirect ophthalmoscopy.

Figure 5   Visualizing a grayish mound to indicate correct alignment of the depressor tip.

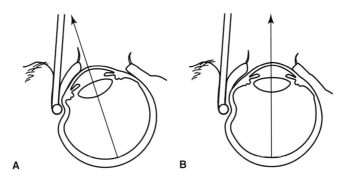

Figure 6   Depressor tip position for visualizing the ora serrata **(A)** and equatorial fundus **(B)**.

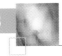

Performing Indirect Slit-Lamp Biomicroscopy

1. Assume standard patient and examiner positions at the slit-lamp biomicroscope (see Chapter 10).

2. Ensure that the patient's pupils are well dilated.

3. Set the slit-lamp magnification to 10× or 16×.

4. Focus and center a slit beam about 4 mm wide onto the corneal surface at the central, nearly coaxial position. Use the brightest (below supramaximal) light intensity that the patient can easily tolerate.

5. Hold the +78 D or +90 D condensing lens stationary between thumb and forefinger, approximately 5 to 10 mm from the patient's cornea, bracing your hand against the headrest frame or the patient's cheek and resting your elbow comfortably on a support. This permits you to see the anterior segment to make sure the pupil is centered in the lens. The third and fourth fingers help open the patient's eyelids.

6. Keeping the slit beam centered on both the condensing lens and the cornea, grasp the slit-lamp joystick with your free hand and pull the slit lamp away from the patient until the patient's red reflex becomes visible, then stop.

7. Move the condensing lens toward you until the red reflex becomes a focused fundus image. The distance between the lens and the patient's cornea will be shorter for higher-powered lenses. If you encounter bothersome light reflection, tilt the condensing lens about 6° and angle the slit beam.

8. Ask the patient to fixate steadily just past your ear. This should bring the optic disc into view. Get the optic disc into the center of the fundus image either by realigning the viewing arm or directing the patient's gaze appropriately.

9. Figure 1 shows a suggested sequence of examination. Beginning at the optic disc (1), proceed temporally across the posterior pole to make a circumferential sweep around the posterior pole (2 through 6), ending at the macula (7). This sequence requires redirecting the patient's gaze in these directions using verbal instructions or a target such as a fixation light or your fingertip. Direct the patient's gaze into primary position using a fixation target after the central fundus examination is complete.

(continued)

Clinical Protocol 13.3 *(continued)*

10. To examine the vitreous cavity, angle the slit beam about 10° to 20° from the axis of observation. Move the condensing lens slightly toward you to examine the vitreous. Having the patient follow a target that moves a few degrees can help you to see strands of the vitreous humor. To help visualize opacities or the Weiss ring of a posterior vitreous detachment, move the slit-lamp joystick and illumination arm to produce alternating direct illumination and retroillumination. Vitreous examination can also be enhanced by a small circular rotation of the condensing lens in one plane.

11. To examine the peripheral vitreous and fundus, reduce the illumination-observation angle and rotate the slit beam to the meridian being observed. Scleral depression can be performed to bring the equatorial fundus into view.

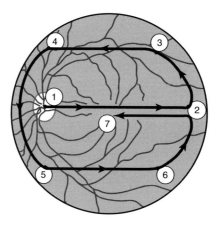

Figure 1 Suggested sequence of examination for slit-lamp biomicroscopy.

 Clinical Protocol 13.4 **Performing Hruby Lens Biomicroscopy**

1. Assume standard patient and examiner positions at the slit-lamp biomicroscope (see Chapter 10).

2. Ensure that the patient's pupils are fully dilated.

3. Set the slit-lamp magnification to 10× or 16×.

4. Focus and center a slit beam about 4 mm wide onto the corneal surface at the central, nearly coaxial position. Use medium-bright light intensity that the patient can easily tolerate.

5. Move the Hruby lens into position as follows:

   a. If attached on the top of the slit lamp, allow the bar to slide toward the headrest and rotate the lens so it clicks in place.

   b. If the lens is on a hinged side arm, put the arm into the groove on the slit-lamp housing, making sure the plano side of the lens faces the patient and the concave side is toward you.

6. Direct the patient's gaze into primary position using the fixation light on the instrument or other target.

7. Push the joystick forward or pull it back to focus the fundus image in the Hruby lens.

Clinical Protocol 13.4 *(continued)*

8. Move the fixation target so that the optic nerve is centered in the field. Redirect the patient's gaze to examine the center of the macula.

9. Move the joystick toward you to refocus the image in the vitreous cavity. Moving the illumination arm at a 10° angle and having the patient look up or down quickly and then refixating will help you to see vitreous strands and opacities.

Clinical Protocol 13.5   Performing Contact Lens Biomicroscopy

1. Instill topical anesthetic onto the eye.

2. Assume standard patient and examiner positions at the slit-lamp biomicroscope (see Chapter 10).

3. Ensure that the patient's pupils are well dilated.

4. Set the slit-lamp magnification to 10× or 16×.

5. Put into the concave part of the contact lens a small amount of gonioscopy gel, such as methylcellulose solution, taking care to avoid creating any air bubbles. Explain to the patient, in a reassuring way, what is to be done.

6. Instruct the patient to look up. Spread the patient's lids apart with your thumb and forefinger.

7. Hold the contact lens between the thumb and index finger and place the lower edge of the contact lens on the patient's exposed lower globe (Figures 1A, 1B).

8. Angle the contact lens onto the globe from below and instruct the patient to look straight ahead (Figures 2A, 2B). Release the patient's lids and allow the contact lens to hold the lids apart. Switch hands, if necessary, to hold the contact lens in your hand closer to the patient's eye (eg, your left hand for the patient's right eye) so your arm does not interfere with using the slit lamp.

9. If any air bubbles are caught between the contact lens and the cornea, slightly tilt the lens to allow them to float out. Allow the contact lens to sit gently on the cornea, avoiding unnecessary pressure on the lens by your fingers that keep the lens steady.

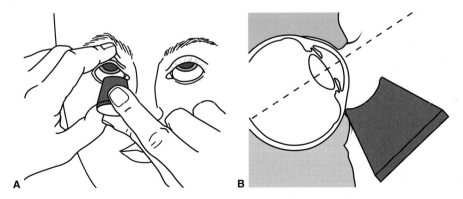

A   **B**

Figure 1   Position of contact lens on the lower globe **(A)**, with side view shown **(B)**.

(continued)

10. Use the joystick to focus the slit lamp toward the patient. Begin with the illumination arm in the coaxial position and examine the posterior pole. Tilt the lens slightly to maneuver light reflections from the lens surface away from the central viewing area.

11. If a 3-mirror lens is used, position the light source on the same side as the side of the eye being examined so that the light beam bounces off the mirror. Begin with the largest, least-angled mirror to examine the area around the posterior pole.

12. To examine the adjacent fundus area, twirl the lens on the eye with a dialing motion for 1 or 2 clock hours. Realign the slit beam to view the new fundus area.

13. After circumferential examination of the fundus with 1 mirror, repeat with the other 2 mirrors to examine the equatorial and peripheral fundus. The lens might need to be rocked or rotated to see all parts of the fundus.

14. Remove the lens by tilting it off the cornea. Clean and disinfect the contact lens before reuse.

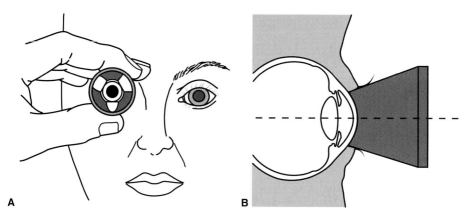

Figure 2   Contact lens in place, with the patient's eyes in straight-ahead position **(A)**, with side view shown **(B)**.

 Clinical Protocol 13.6   **Evaluating the Fundus With the Direct Ophthalmoscope**

1. Find the optic disc by following a retinal blood vessel. The arrows formed by vascular bifurcations point to the optic disc. Depending on the patient's refraction, the entire disc or only a portion of it will be visible in any one view.

2. Examine the peripapillary retina. Use a red-free absorption filter to examine arcuate nerve fiber layer defects that occur in glaucoma and other optic neuropathies.

3. From the optic disc, follow the blood vessels outward to examine the superonasal (1), inferonasal (2), inferotemporal (3), and superotemporal (4) areas around the posterior pole (Figure 1). Note the vascular color, caliber, bifurcations, crossings, and the surrounding background.

4. Use the red-free light to highlight the refractile changes in the vascular wall caused by arteriolosclerosis, especially at points of arteriovenous compression.

Clinical Protocol 13.6 *(continued)*

5. Examine the macula (5) for irregularities. Use a slit beam to detect distortions of the retinal surface. Level differences can be seen by a blurring of a portion of the light stripe; lacking stereopsis, estimating the convexity or concavity of a fundus lesion with the slit beam of the monocular direct ophthalmoscope is difficult.

6. If choroidal or retinal pigment epithelial abnormalities are suspected, direct the ophthalmoscope adjacent to the fundus detail under study. Allow proximal illumination to help you to distinguish between translucent and opaque lesions.

7. Approximate the height of an elevated lesion (eg, choroidal tumor or disc edema) by using the focusing dial.

   a. First focus on flat retina, then refocus on the lesion surface.

   b. Subtract the 2 dioptric values to deduce the level difference (in a phakic or pseudophakic eye, 3 diopters = 1 mm).

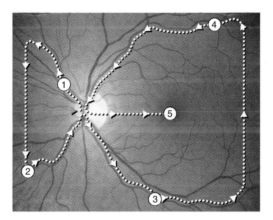

Figure 1   Suggested sequence of examination for fundus evaluation using the direct ophthalmoscope.

Clinical Protocol 13.7   Drawing the Indirect Ophthalmoscopic Fundus

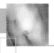

1. Invert the vitreoretinal chart on the patient's chest.

2. View, then draw, an initial landmark, such as the superonasal blood vessels of the posterior pole.

3. Follow the vessels anteriorly and continue to draw their bifurcations and branches in 1 quadrant.

4. Repeat for the remaining quadrants.

5. Using scleral depression, locate the blood vessels already drawn in each meridian and sketch their terminal branches.

6. Draw the ora serrata.

7. Reexamine any fundus lesion and sketch its borders and details in relationship to the blood vessels and other landmarks already drawn.

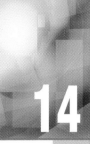

14 Ophthalmic Emergencies

This chapter gives a brief overview of common emergencies encountered by beginning ophthalmology residents on call, including how to evaluate the emergency room patient and how to treat common emergencies; it is not exhaustive in coverage. Opinions differ with regard to certain aspects of therapeutics (such as the management of hyphemas), but the information given should serve as a useful base upon which to build further knowledge as your training progresses. The treatments for most of the conditions listed in this chapter are evolving and, in some cases, controversial; other sources of information must be consulted on an ongoing basis. Some entities covered here are not medically urgent but are often seen in the emergency room.

The diagnosis and management of ophthalmic emergencies require a disciplined, methodical approach to ensure proper care and to avoid mistakes. The need for a quick examination of an emergency patient should not preclude thoroughness. Proper documentation, timely treatment, and meticulous attention to details are necessary for optimal medical care as well as for medicolegal reasons (see Chapter 3). If you are uncertain of how to handle an ophthalmic emergency, you are obligated quickly to seek the help of an experienced ophthalmologist and to obtain appropriate consultations from other medical specialists as the situation demands.

Emergency Equipment and General Evaluation

Ideally, patients arriving through the emergency room should be evaluated in the eye clinic or in an examining room complete with a visual acuity chart, slit lamp, and indirect ophthalmoscope. This will not always be possible, but some portable equipment must be made available for evaluation of emergency patients. To meet this need, prepare a bag containing essential equipment and supplies, including the following:

- Light source (eg, muscle light, small flashlight)
- Direct ophthalmoscope
- Near vision card
- Pinhole occluder
- +2.5 D lens and +20 D lens
- Small toys or other pediatric fixation targets
- Fluorescein strips
- Eyelid retractor

- Small ruler (with millimeters)
- Certain ophthalmic medications such as proparacaine (Ophthaine), timolol maleate (Timoptic) 0.5%, pilocarpine 2%, and tropicamide 1%

Other, less portable equipment, such as an indirect ophthalmoscope and slit lamp with Goldmann tonometer, is usually available in examination rooms, although including a Schiøtz tonometer or Tonopen in the emergency bag is a good idea.

Evaluation of patients with eye injuries or disorders begins with a thorough history. Always inquire about the patient's vision before the injury or disorder. Knowing that a patient presenting with blunt trauma and 20/200 vision also has a history of amblyopia drastically changes the clinical picture. However, never defer treatment of a true ocular emergency (chemical burn, central retinal artery occlusion, or acute angle-closure glaucoma) to take the history. In all emergency cases, the history should be tailored to suit the nature of the disorder. If surgical intervention is a possibility, ask about the patient's last oral intake and withhold further oral intake until a therapeutic decision is made. Also, ask about the last tetanus booster in all cases of penetrating or perforating trauma.

Like the history, the ophthalmic examination is streamlined to accommodate the emergency patient. As the first step, the visual acuity must be determined as soon after presentation as possible, before a condition (corneal opacity, hyphema, lid swelling) evolves to preclude measurement. To assess acuity in the emergency setting, it is useful to have a pinhole occluder on hand to help account for refractive errors, a +2.5 D lens to help account for presbyopia, and a near reading card. If the patient's vision is greatly impaired, color vision using bright red and green bottle caps and light projection to all quadrants should be documented. The pertinent aspects of the external, motility, confrontation visual fields, pupillary, and anterior segment examinations, tonometry, and ophthalmoscopy are then performed in that order. If significant head trauma exists, defer dilation of the pupils to preserve the pupillary reaction for periodic neurologic evaluations. Maneuvers that apply pressure to the globe, such as scleral depression and Schiøtz tonometry, should not be performed on patients with potentially ruptured globes or hyphema.

Pediatric Evaluation

Special techniques are needed for the evaluation of children in the emergency setting. Patience, tact, and sensitivity to the concerns of parents are essential. To avoid prompting crying spells in pediatric patients, try to gather as much information as possible by careful observation without touching the child. Avoid threatening demeanor and gestures—keep a low profile during the evaluation, if possible, moving about slowly and deliberately. Toys and interesting fixation targets can simplify pediatric examinations, and infants might be easier to evaluate if given a pacifier or bottle to quiet them. However, withhold oral intake if surgical repair is contemplated.

Use a papoose board to restrain an uncooperative child during the examination. If the globe is open, however, the papoose board should not be used; it can provoke straining and elevated intraocular pressure, which could lead to extrusion of ocular contents. Alternatively, swaddle a small child or infant tightly (see Chapter 9), or ask a nurse or parent to help restrain an uncooperative child. Consider sedation only as a last resort. If it is necessary, sedate the child under controlled conditions, with strict monitoring and availability of emergency equipment and personnel trained in advanced pediatric life support to avoid complications. You might need to consult an anesthesiologist. If the child is a surgical candidate, some of the evaluations that are particularly difficult to perform may be deferred until the child is under anesthesia.

Examination of the anterior segment and fundus may be facilitated by the use of a pediatric lid speculum and, for small children and infants who cannot be placed at the slit lamp, a portable slit lamp.

■ Ocular Trauma in the Emergency Setting

Patients seen in the emergency room with ocular trauma might have other, nonocular injuries. Priority must be given to treatment of life-threatening conditions, and communication among the various physicians involved is helpful in establishing the best sequence of treating the multiple injuries. A protective eye shield should be taped in place until the patient is stabilized. Attention can then be turned to the ocular trauma. The most common traumatic ocular disorders and their treatments are detailed below.

Corneal Abrasion

Corneal abrasions are epithelial defects due to trauma, such as a fingernail scratch of the eye, contact lens overwear, or ultraviolet burns from welding. Corneal abrasions are generally accompanied by significant pain, foreign-body sensation, tearing, blepharospasm, and sometimes decreased vision. Exclude herpes simplex viral keratitis, which can simulate abrasion. A corneal erosion is a spontaneous epithelial defect that is frequently recurrent and can occur at the site of a prior corneal injury or in association with corneal dystrophy.

The evaluation is made easier by instilling a drop of topical anesthetic, the response to which is often dramatic. If herpes simplex keratitis is suspected, check the corneal sensation before instilling the topical anesthetic; instructions for doing so are in Clinical Protocol 9.1. Vision can then be more accurately assessed and the eye more thoroughly examined at the slit lamp. The diagnosis is facilitated by fluorescein dye, which stains the part of the cornea devoid of epithelium.

It is critical to distinguish between a typical corneal abrasion and a corneal ulcer. Corneal ulcer implies that there is an infection of the cornea associated with an epithelial defect, generally presenting as a white opacity in the cornea, often with a hypopyon. In patients with vertical corneal abrasions, rule out a foreign body embedded in the tarsal conjunctiva of the upper or lower lid by examining the everted lid with the biomicroscope and sweeping the fornices with a moistened cotton swab. Clinical Protocol 9.6 presents complete instructions for lid eversion;

Clinical Protocol 11.1 includes instructions for sweeping the conjunctival sac and fornices. Tarsal conjunctival foreign bodies will cause corneal abrasions in a vertically linear pattern, produced as the foreign body rubs up and down the corneal epithelium with blinking.

Treatment

The treatment of a typical corneal abrasion is as follows:

1. Instill a drop of topical anesthetic onto the affected eye.
2. Rule out a foreign body in the affected eye. Inspect the fornices.
3. Instill a drop of cycloplegic agent (eg, homatropine 5%) to relieve the discomfort caused by ciliary spasm.
4. Apply a patch over the closed lids to reduce discomfort caused by the lids moving against the cornea. This technique is described in Clinical Protocol 14.1.
   a. Allow the patch to remain until reexamination. It is not necessary to patch patients with abrasions smaller than 3 to 4 mm in diameter. Note that the need to patch patients with clean abrasions less than 10 mm in diameter has been called into question.
   b. Never patch an eye if bacterial or fungal infection (eg, conjunctivitis or blepharitis) is present.
   c. Because of the probability of an infection, patients with abrasions related to contact lens wear or vegetation (eg, tree branch) should not be patched.
5. Alternatively, apply a bandage soft contact lens. This is especially good for patients with bilateral abrasions.
6. Remove the patch and reexamine within 24 hours. A patch should not remain more than 24 hours because of the risk of infection. If the patient experiences worsening symptoms while patched, he or she may remove the patch before reevaluation. Discontinue patching if the abrasion is mostly healed. The need for antibiotic drops or ointment at this time is controversial.

For abrasions associated with contact lens wear, remove the contact lens and inspect both it and the cornea for defects with the slit lamp. If the patient wears hard lenses, treat the abrasion as described above for a typical abrasion. If the patient wears soft lenses, you might need to rule out a potential microbial keratitis (eg, pseudomonas) by culturing the cornea and contact lens case if the clinical appearance warrants. If you suspect strongly the presence of microbial keratitis, the patient should be given appropriate antibiotics until the culture results become available.

Corneal Foreign Body

Foreign bodies (metal, dirt, wood, vegetable matter, glass, or even caterpillar hairs) embedded in the cornea can be acquired while striking metal or stone, be blown into the eye by the wind, or occur by many other seemingly innocuous means.

Knowing the nature of the foreign body is important because metallic foreign bodies embedded in the cornea can leave a rust ring, and vegetable foreign bodies such as wood pose a greater risk of microbial keratitis (Figure 14.1). Try to determine the source of the foreign body during history taking and consider the possibility of intraocular foreign body in the presence of a corneal foreign body. The upper and lower eyelids should be everted to exclude the possibility of foreign bodies in the tarsal conjunctiva or the fornices. If there is any suspicion of associated microbial keratitis, the cornea should be scraped, stained, and cultured as for a corneal ulcer.

Treatment

Treatment depends on the nature, location, and depth of the corneal foreign body. Superficial foreign bodies that appear to have penetrated no deeper than the superficial stroma may be removed in the clinic or emergency room, as described in Clinical Protocol 14.2. If the foreign body is very deep or if corneal perforation is suspected, treat the patient in the sterile setting of an operating room equipped to handle corneal perforations. The patient should wear a rigid fenestrated aluminum (Fox) shield until it is time for surgery (Clinical Protocol 14.1).

Eyelid Laceration

All patients with eyelid lacerations should be meticulously evaluated for the possibility of concurrent injuries, such as canalicular lacerations, occult trauma to the globe, orbital wall fracture, extraocular muscle laceration, and embedded foreign body. Inquire about the object causing the laceration, the time and severity of the injury, and any associated symptoms and signs.

Treatment

Any ocular conditions associated with an eyelid laceration (eg, embedded foreign body) should be treated as required. Eyelid lacerations need not be repaired immediately and are best done by a physician experienced in such repairs. The repair may be delayed for 12 to 24 hours, especially if the wound is contaminated or is a result of a human bite. Because of the rich vascular supply of the eyelids, infections are uncommon and debridement should be minimal, if necessary at all. Tissue on pedicles and flaps should not be removed.

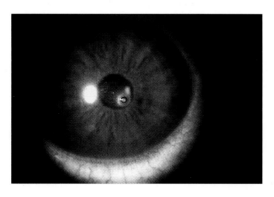

Figure 14.1 A metallic corneal foreign body, surrounded by a visible rust ring and grayish corneal edema.

Blunt Ocular Trauma

Blunt ocular trauma results from a direct blow to the eye by a blunt object. Ophthalmic sequelae include subconjunctival hemorrhage, hyphema (see below), lens dislocation, globe rupture, orbital wall fractures (see below), iridodialysis, angle recession and subsequent glaucoma, iris sphincter rupture, traumatic iritis, posterior segment alterations, and traumatic optic neuropathy.

The first 2 questions to answer when evaluating a patient with blunt trauma are

1. Is the globe ruptured?
2. Is there a hyphema?

Crepitus on palpation supports the diagnosis of an orbital wall or orbital floor fracture. Gently retract the eyelids manually or with an eyelid retractor to expose the globe. Measure the visual acuity, if possible. Inspect the ocular surface for signs of perforation. Check the pupil for traumatic mydriasis with sphincter rupture, miosis associated with traumatic iritis, iridocyclitis, and afferent pupillary defect indicative of traumatic optic neuropathy. Evaluate the anterior segment with the slit lamp, looking for hyphema, traumatic iridocyclitis, and subluxation of the lens. Although acute swelling of the eyelids might preclude it, gonioscopy should be performed at an appropriate time to rule out angle recession, which places the patient at risk for glaucoma in the future. Perform a motility examination. An isolated elevation deficit suggests inferior orbital blowout fracture; mild to moderate generalized limitation of eye movements can accompany orbital edema or hematoma.

Applanation tonometry is difficult if the orbit is swollen and the eyelids are tightly closed (Figure 14.2), and intraocular pressure can be artificially elevated from forced opening of the eyelids to obtain the measurement. A pressure in the low teens or less than 10 mm Hg in a setting of blunt ocular trauma suggests the possibility of a ruptured globe. A thorough fundus examination is required, but scleral depression should be deferred in patients with hyphema or suspected scleral rupture. Typical posterior segment disorders associated with blunt ocular trauma include commotio retinae, retinal hemorrhages, choroidal rupture, vitreous hemorrhage, and traumatic retinal detachment (see below).

Treatment

Treatment of blunt ocular injuries depends on the nature of the findings, as detailed throughout this chapter. The physician may recommend supportive measures such as intermittent ice packs to the orbit for the first 1 to 2 days (if the globe is intact), elevation of the head of the bed, and medical pain management. The patient should avoid anticoagulants and aspirin.

Traumatic Hyphema

Hyphema denotes blood in the anterior chamber (Figure 14.3). The bleeding can occur spontaneously (eg, in patients with iris neovascularization or juvenile xanthogranuloma), after intraocular surgery (eg, cataract surgery, trabeculectomy, and vitrectomy), or after traumatic injury, particularly blunt ocular trauma. Traumatic hyphemas vary in clinical manifestations and potential complications. Ranging in

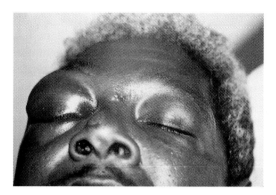

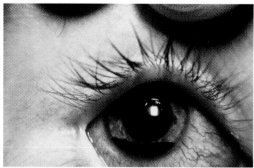

Figure 14.2   Marked orbital swelling after blunt trauma can make the ocular examination difficult or impossible.

Figure 14.3   Hyphema (blood in the anterior chamber). (Photograph courtesy W.K. Kellogg Eye Center, University of Michigan.)

size from microscopic to complete, hyphemas might subside spontaneously or with medical management, or they can require surgical evacuation. Hyphemas may be graded by the height of layered blood (in mm). They are frequently associated with other signs of blunt ocular trauma, including corneal abrasions, traumatic iritis, angle recession, pupillary sphincter rupture, and posterior segment abnormalities.

Intraocular pressure is especially likely to be elevated in large hyphemas, following a rebleed, or in a patient with sickle cell disease. Therefore, the intraocular pressure should be closely monitored in patients with hyphema. If a history of bleeding disorders exists, obtain a laboratory workup that includes CBC, clotting studies, platelet count, and liver function tests. A sickle cell preparation and hemoglobin electrophoresis should be obtained in black patients. Baseline blood urea nitrogen and creatinine should be obtained if aminocaproic acid (Amicar) is to be used for treatment, to monitor the potential toxicity of the medication.

Rebleeding is a major concern after a traumatic hyphema and suggests a poor visual prognosis. It tends to be more severe than the initial bleeding and is more likely to be associated with elevated intraocular pressure. Patients who experience rebleeding might need to be hospitalized. Rebleeding typically occurs 2 to 5 days after initial trauma. Therefore, patients with hyphema should be examined daily for at least the first 5 days from onset and, if managed as outpatients, should be instructed to return immediately for reevaluation if sudden decrease in vision or increase in pain occurs. Patients can develop elevated IOP with potential optic nerve damage. Corneal blood staining can occur, especially if endothelial dysfunction and IOP elevation coexist.

Treatment

The treatment of traumatic hyphema is controversial. Guidelines concerning whether or not to hospitalize and whether or not to prescribe cycloplegics, strict bed rest, or sedation are not strictly established. Generally, a protective eye shield, moderate restriction of physical activity, and elevation of the head of the bed during the first 5 days from onset are reasonable recommendations.

Patients with hyphema should be examined daily for at least the first 5 days. If the intraocular pressure is elevated, glaucoma medications may be started as needed. Topical beta-blockers (eg, timolol maleate) and carbonic anhydrase inhibitors, either in topical form (eg, dorzolamide) or systemic form (eg, acetazolamide, methazolamide), can lower the pressure sufficiently in some patients. Methazolamide is preferable to acetazolamide in patients with possible or proven sickle cell disease or trait to avoid the side effect of metabolic acidosis, which can trigger sickling of red blood cells and exacerbate the intraocular hypertension by blocking the trabecular meshwork. Surgical drainage is indicated in selected cases, including those with prolonged elevations of intraocular pressure or cases that fail to clear with medical management.

Therapeutic attempts to reduce the likelihood of rebleeding include oral and/or topical corticosteroids (prednisone) and oral aminocaproic acid (Amicar); patients should not receive aspirin or other nonsteroidal anti-inflammatory drugs. Patients receiving Amicar should be informed of the possibility of postural hypotension, which might be especially bothersome during the first day of treatment.

Orbital Fracture

Blunt head trauma is often associated with fractures of bones in the orbital and periorbital areas. Fractures affecting the orbital floor but sparing the orbital rim (blowout fractures) are the most common. The thin medial wall of the orbit, the lamina papyracea, is the second most frequently fractured structure. Much greater force is needed to fracture the orbital rim than the thin walls of the orbit. Blowout fractures are caused by objects larger than the diameter of the orbital opening, such as a fist, a dashboard, or a baseball, striking the anterior orbit. Smaller objects tend to rupture the globe.

Symptoms and signs of orbital floor blowout fractures include ecchymosis and edema of the eyelids and cheek, nosebleed, orbital and eyelid emphysema, limitation of up gaze or down gaze (with associated diplopia), enophthalmos or exophthalmos, and loss of sensation in the distribution of the inferior orbital nerve (ipsilateral cheek and upper lip). Limited eye movements can result from restrictive strabismus caused by entrapment of extraocular muscles in patients with orbital wall fractures (most common), from generalized edema and soft tissue injury, from damage to the trochlea, or from damage to the ocular motor nerves. Loss of vision can be caused by optic nerve damage or globe injury.

A thorough evaluation is helpful. Baseline exophthalmometry measurements should be obtained (see Clinical Protocol 9.3). Computed tomography of the orbits and brain should be obtained, especially if surgical repair is contemplated.

Treatment

The physician should consider prescribing nasal decongestants for 1 to 2 weeks and intermittent applications of ice packs for the first day or two. Advise the patient not to blow the nose vigorously, to avoid orbital emphysema. Consider broad-spectrum antibiotic prophylaxis, particularly if sinus infections coexist. Indications for surgical repair of blowout fractures are controversial. General indications include diplopia in the primary or reading position, significant enophthalmos, or a large fracture. The timing of repair is also controversial, but repair is not considered a surgical emergency and usually can safely be delayed for several days.

Globe Laceration

Because some lacerated globes might appear relatively normal, you should maintain a high index of suspicion in cases that have a suggestive history. Symptoms and signs of ocular perforation include significantly decreased vision; hypotony; shallow or flat anterior chamber; altered size, shape, or position of the pupil; visible tracks through the crystalline lens or vitreous, tracing the line of passage of a foreign body; and marked conjunctival chemosis (clear fluid under the conjunctiva) or subconjunctival hemorrhage. Another sign of likely laceration of the globe is total (or large) hyphema with low or normal intraocular pressure; total hyphemas in *intact* globes are nearly always associated with *elevated* pressure.

A Seidel test can detect ocular perforation or a wound leak. In this simple test, a moistened fluorescein strip is applied directly over the suspected site of perforation while the examiner observes the site through the biomicroscope using the cobalt-blue light. If a leak exists, the dye will be diluted by the aqueous and will appear as a green stream within the dark-orange concentrated dye. It is important to recognize the presence of vitreous or uveal tissue on the ocular surface. Do not mistake vitreous for mucus and try to wipe it away vigorously; if in doubt, defer the determination to someone more experienced or until the patient is in the operating room.

Avoid the following actions during the evaluation of a patient with a potentially ruptured globe:

- Applying pressure on the globe during the examination (eg, tonometry, scleral depression, gonioscopy) or by patching.
- Ordering magnetic resonance imaging studies in patients with potential metallic intraocular foreign bodies. Computed tomography (CT) is the proper imaging modality in this setting. A protective aluminum Fox shield should be left in place over the affected globe during the CT scan.

Measure the visual acuity as the first step in the examination, then perform the rest of the examination as described earlier in this chapter. Gently obtain cultures from the cul-de-sac or wound site if needed. Keep the rigid shield over the globe when it is not being examined.

The physician should always consider the possibility of a retained foreign body in any patient with a globe laceration, even if the history does not directly suggest it. Appropriate imaging studies should be obtained in patients with suspected retained foreign bodies. Magnetic resonance imagining is contraindicated if the suspected foreign body is metallic with a magnetic nature, and CT is preferred. Ultrasound can also be helpful. Indicate on the radiology order slip the nature of the trauma and any suspicion of a foreign body; this helps the radiologist design an appropriate imaging study as well as interpret its results. For suspected intraocular foreign bodies, thin cuts (1 to 1.5 mm) may be ordered. In general, contrast dye is not needed when imaging acute traumatic ocular and orbital injuries.

Treatment

In the emergency setting, consider the administration of antiemetics to suppress nausea and vomiting. Sedatives and analgesics may be administered judiciously. Tetanus prophylaxis should be administered if needed. A rigid shield should be placed over the eye. A light patch in addition to the shield is optional and, depending on the circumstances, might even be inadvisable (to avoid undue pressure on the globe). Give appropriate prophylactic parenteral antibiotics. Definitive repair is then performed in the operating room. In cases of massive disrupting injury to the globe, informed consent for possible primary enucleation should be obtained from the patient or the family after thorough explanation and counseling. However, every attempt should be made to preserve the eye if there is even a remote chance of any vision.

Ocular Infections in the Emergency Setting

Ocular infections encountered in the emergency room range from the generally innocuous, such as mild bacterial infections resulting in conjunctivitis or hordeolum, to those that threaten vision, such as infections that produce corneal ulcers and endophthalmitis. This section discusses certain acute ocular infections that are commonly encountered in the emergency setting.

Acute Conjunctivitis

Patients with acute conjunctivitis commonly present to the emergency room physician with red eye, a discharge, and ocular irritation. The specific clinical signs and symptoms of the individual disorders are discussed in Chapter 11. Generally, acute bacterial conjunctivitis is characterized by conjunctival injection and mucopurulent discharge. Viral conjunctivitis usually shows watery or mucoid discharge and, unlike bacterial conjunctivitis, might be associated with ipsilateral preauricular lymphadenopathy.

Treatment

Bacterial conjunctivitis responds to topical antibiotic treatment. An exception is gonococcal conjunctivitis, which requires systemic antibiotics (eg, for neonates, ceftriaxone 25 to 50 mg/kg/day IV or IM in a single dose) supplemented by topical drops. As with chlamydial neonatal conjunctivitis, the mother of an infant with gonococcal conjunctivitis and her sexual partner should also be treated.

Patients with viral conjunctivitis should be considered contagious for the first 10 days after onset and given appropriate instructions to avoid viral spread. Generally, viral conjunctivitis requires only supportive treatment with cold compresses, artificial tears, or topical vasoconstrictors to provide symptomatic relief.

Dendritic Keratitis

Herpes simplex keratitis (HSK) is caused by actively replicating virus, either HSV-1 or HSV-2. Patients typically present with unilateral ocular symptoms, including pain, photophobia, tearing, and decreased vision. Patients may have a herpetic skin lesion and a history of previous episodes.

The clinical signs of epithelial keratitis include preauricular lymphadenopathy, conjunctival injection, mild iritis, decreased corneal sensation, and an epithelial lesion. The epithelial ulcer may be dendritic or geographic. A dendritic ulcer is the classic corneal lesion. This lesion is linear and dichotomously branching, with each branch terminating in a bulb. The borders of the lesion are heaped up with swollen epithelial cells that stain with rose bengal or lissamine green. The center of the lesion is devoid of epithelial cells and stains positively with fluorescein (Figure 14.4). The geographic ulcer is usually a larger, amoeba-shaped corneal ulcer with a dendritic edge. Typically, the underlying corneal stroma has little to no inflammation.

The diagnosis of HSV epithelial keratitis is usually made on clinical findings, making laboratory tests unnecessary; however, viral culture, fluorescent antibody testing, DNA amplification, and Tzanck smear may be useful in securing the diagnosis in atypical and challenging cases.

Treatment

HSV epithelial keratitis is self-limited and often resolves spontaneously. The aim of treatment is to hasten the resolution and minimize corneal scarring. Debridement of the involved epithelium is generally recommended. The infected epithelial cells are poorly adherent to the underlying stroma, and gentle wiping with a cotton swab (following topical anesthesia) is usually sufficient to remove the majority of infected cells without damaging the neighboring healthy epithelium. Acceptable treatment options include both topical and oral antivirals. Topical trifluridine 1% drops every 2 hours or 3% vidarabine ointment 5 times a day are the mainstays of treatment in the United States, while topical acyclovir 3% ointment is the drug of choice in the rest of the world. Topical acyclovir has less epithelial toxicity but is currently unavailable in the United States. Trifluridine is toxic to corneal epithelium, and it should not be used for longer then 1 to 2 weeks. Some authors advocate the use of oral acyclovir 400 mg 5 times a day in place of the topical agents because of this toxicity. There appears to be no advantage to using both in combination. A cycloplegic agent can be added if anterior chamber inflammation is noted. Topical corticosteroids can worsen the infection and should be discontinued at the time of diagnosis. Finally, prophylactic doses of acyclovir (400 mg 2 times a day) can be

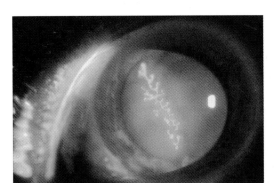

Figure 14.4 Fluorescein staining of herpetic dendritic keratitis. (Reprinted, with permission, from Reidy JJ, Basic and Clinical Science Course, Section 8: *Cornea and External Disease*. San Francisco: American Academy of Ophthalmology, 2009–2010. Photograph courtesy of James Chodosh, MD.)

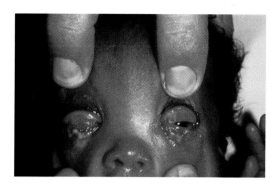

Figure 14.5   Gonococcal conjunctivitis in an infant (ophthalmia neonatorum).

used in patients who have recurrent disease and have been shown to decrease the recurrence rate by approximately 40%.

Ophthalmia Neonatorum

The term *ophthalmia neonatorum* describes a form of conjunctivitis encountered within the first month of life (Figure 14.5). Common causes include *Chlamydia trachomatis, Staphylococcus aureus, Streptococcus pneumoniae, Neisseria gonorrhoeae,* and herpes simplex virus. Affected infants show purulent (gonococcal) or mucopurulent discharge, conjunctival injection, eyelid edema, and chemosis. The mother should be questioned about previous sexually transmitted disease.

Conjunctival scrapings should be obtained for Gram stain, Giemsa stain, and chlamydial immunofluorescent antibody test. Cultures should be obtained in blood and chocolate agar. Viral cultures or fluorescent antibody tests are ordered as indicated.

Treatment

The initial treatment of ophthalmia neonatorum rests on the clinical impression and the results of the Gram and Giemsa stains. A pediatric consultation should sometimes be obtained. In neonates with conjunctivitis caused by *Chlamydia trachomatis*, systemic erythromycin therapy is recommended, since pneumonitis and otitis media can coexist. The recommended oral dosage is 50 mg/kg/day for 2 weeks (divided into 4 daily doses and mixed with the infant's formula), combined with erythromycin or sulfacetamide ointment 4 times daily. The infant's mother and her sexual partner should also be treated. Sexual abuse of a child may be suspected with certain infections and appropriate authorities should be alerted, but only with the approval of the faculty or staff member.

Preseptal and Orbital Cellulitis

Preseptal cellulitis is an infection that involves the soft tissues of the eyelids but does not involve the orbital structures (Figure 14.6). It affects only the eyelids and periorbital tissues anterior to the orbital septum, a fibrous barrier that separates the anterior lids and facial tissues from the orbit itself. Patients present with erythema, swelling, and tenderness of the eyelids and surrounding periorbital area. Preseptal cellulitis does not usually require a diagnostic workup.

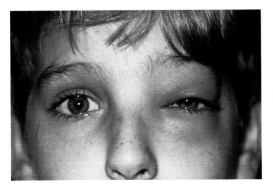

Figure 14.6   Preseptal cellulitis.

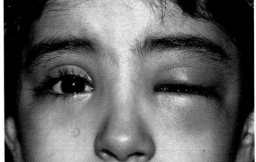

Figure 14.7   Orbital cellulitis.

The presence of proptosis, ophthalmoplegia (limited ocular motility), decreased vision, significant pain on eye movements, or abnormal pupillary reflexes indicates orbital cellulitis, a much more serious infection involving extension of the infection posterior to the orbital septum and into the orbit (Figure 14.7). It results most commonly from spread of infection from adjacent structures, such as the teeth, sinuses, or lacrimal sac. In children, it most commonly arises due to spread from ethmoid sinuses. Additional symptoms and signs include red eye, fever, lethargy, brawny lid swelling, conjunctival congestion, chemosis, and diplopia.

The diagnostic workup of orbital cellulitis includes blood cultures and, if an eyelid wound is present, wound cultures and Gram stains. Computed tomography of the orbit is indicated to exclude a retained foreign body, subperiosteal abscess, intracranial involvement, and contiguous sinus disease.

Treatment

Patients with mild preseptal cellulitis can be treated with oral antibiotics on an outpatient basis. Antibiotics are selected to cover the most likely organisms, which include *Staphylococcus aureus, S epidermidis,* and *Streptococcus pyogenes.* In small children, one must also consider *Haemophilus influenzae.*

The treatment of severe preseptal cellulitis or orbital cellulitis should begin urgently, because patients are at risk for cavernous sinus thrombosis, meningitis, and brain abscesses. The patient should be admitted, and broad-spectrum intravenous antibiotics covering Gram-positive, Gram-negative, and anaerobic organisms should be administered until the precise infectious agent is identified. Topical antibiotic ointment may be added.

Because sinus drainage can be required in severe cases, otolaryngologic evaluation is obtained in patients with mucoceles or sinusitis. If the patient with orbital cellulitis has diabetes mellitus, particularly with ketoacidosis, or is otherwise immunocompromised, mucormycosis, a life-threatening fungal infection, must be seriously considered, since immediate surgical debridement and antifungal therapy would be needed to save the patient's life. Affected patients can show a black eschar in the nose or on the roof of the mouth.

Endophthalmitis

Endophthalmitis denotes infection within the eye including vitreous involvement while sparing the sclera. Panophthalmitis is an infection that involves all coats of the eye. These serious infections can be endogenous (eg, sepsis in a debilitated patient), postoperative or exogenous (eg, after cataract surgery), or post-traumatic. The resident must learn to recognize these disorders because they require immediate treatment if the eye is to be saved. Patients with endophthalmitis typically present with ocular pain, decreased vision, conjunctival injection, anterior chamber inflammation and hypopyon, and vitritis.

The diagnosis rests on clinical grounds and is confirmed with periocular cultures, anterior chamber tap, and vitreous paracentesis and/or biopsy with appropriate cultures and stains. Systemic risk factors for endogenous endophthalmitis include systemic debilitation, indwelling catheters or intravenous drug history, immunodeficiency, cardiac valvular disease and chronic antibiotic use, and an appropriate sepsis work up should be initiated. Acute exogenous endophthalmitis classically presents within 2 to 7 days of intraocular surgery and requires urgent vitreous tap and antibiotic injection to eradicate the infectious agent (typically *Staphylococcus* or *Streptococcus* species). Chronic exogenous endophthalmitis may be caused by bacterial (eg, *Propionibacterium acnes*) or fungal infection.

Treatment

Time is of the essence. Acute exogenous endophthalmitis requires emergent vitreous paracentesis and broad spectrum antibiotic injection (eg, Vancomycin 1.0 Mg/ 0.1 mL and Ceftazidime 2.0 mg/0/1 mL) with or without steroid injection (Dexamethasone 400 μg/0.1 mL). Obtain a consultation with appropriate subspecialists (such as a retinal surgeon) to consider vitrectomy, especially with severe vision loss worse than the counting fingers (CF) level. Unfortunately there is a very high risk of blindness with acute endophthalmitis especially with delayed antibiotic injection.

■ True Ocular Emergencies

Ocular emergencies can be arbitrarily subdivided into 2 categories. True ocular emergencies require treatment within minutes (chemical burns, central retinal artery occlusion, acute angle-closure glaucoma). Urgent conditions require treatment within hours (various forms of ocular trauma or infections). This section describes the 3 emergency conditions most often seen in the emergency room.

Retinal Tears and Rhegmatogenous Retinal Detachments

As patients age, the central vitreous undergoes syneresis and a posterior vitreous detachment (PVD) slowly develops. The vitreous gel usually remains attached at the vitreous base, a circumferential zone that straddles the ora serrata extending about 2 mm anterior and 4 mm posterior to the ora. As the liquefied portion of the PVD moves within the globe, traction is created at the posterior vitreous base and other points of firm attachment to the retina (eg, blood vessels, margins of lattice degeneration) and can sometimes produce a retinal tear or break. A majority of retinal breaks occur in the superotemporal quadrant. Symptoms of a PVD and retinal tears include the entopic phenomena of photopsias (from mechanical traction of the retina) or multiple new floaters (possible vitreous hemorrhage or released glial and retinal pigment epithelial cells). Figure 14.8 shows a horseshoe retinal tear with associated retinal detachment.

Trauma is another potential cause of retinal breaks. While PVD-associated breaks typically occur in patients over the age of 50, ocular trauma can cause retinal tears at any age. Direct penetrating trauma that goes completely through the sclera and retina will result in a break. Blunt trauma can also cause breaks as the eye is compressed in the anteroposterior dimension and expanded in the equatorial plane. This rapid deformation results in severe traction at the vitreous base and can result in tears, dialyses, or a macular hole. Traumatic breaks are often multiple and commonly found in the superonasal and inferotemporal quadrants.

Once a tear has formed in the retina, liquefied vitreous is able to pass through to the potential subretinal space between the neurosensory retina and RPE, causing a rhegmatogenous retinal detachment (RRD). As the retina is detaching, a patient will have the sensation of a veil, curtain, or shade being pulled across his or her visual field.

After taking a careful history, testing the visual acuity, and performing a thorough pupil, adnexal, alignment, motility, confrontation visual field, and anterior segment examination, the examiner should dilate the patient's eyes. Performing accurate tonometry is important as well, given that the IOP is often relatively decreased in eyes with RRDs when compared to the fellow eye. After the eyes are dilated, use a slit lamp to examine the anterior vitreous. The presence of blood or pigment (also known as "tobacco dust" or Schaffer's sign) suggests a possible retinal break. One should then proceed with a thorough posterior segment exam via indirect ophthalmoscopy with scleral depression. This can be accomplished at the slit lamp with a 3-mirror lens or with a binocular indirect ophthalmoscope and a handheld 20 D or 28 D lens. Examination for a retinal tear or retinal detachment can be aided with the use of echography when available.

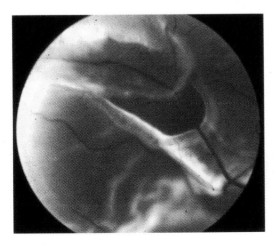

Figure 14.8   Horseshoe retinal tear with associated retina detachment. (Reprinted, with permission, from Schubert HD, Basic and Clinical Science Course, Section 12: *Retina and Vitreous.* San Francisco: American Academy of Ophthalmology, 2009–2010.)

Treatment

If after thorough examination no break or tear is found, the patient should be given specific instructions to return immediately if he or she experiences a change in symptoms, such as new photopsias, an increase in floaters, or a veil, curtain, or shadow develops. Otherwise, repeat dilated fundus examination should be performed in 3 to 4 weeks.

If a symptomatic retinal tear is found, it should be treated, especially if there is residual traction on the retina. The goal of treatment is to create a chorioretinal scar around each break to prevent liquefied vitreous from entering the subretinal space and creating a RRD. Tears can be treated either with laser demarcation or with cryotherapy. If subretinal fluid is present, the treatment area should extend beyond the fluid to an area of attached retina. If more than 1 disc diameter of fluid is present, emergent referral to a vitreoretinal specialist should be initiated. After treatment, the patient should be advised to return immediately if he or she experiences new photopsias, an increase in floaters, or a veil, curtain, or shadow develops. Otherwise, repeat dilated fundus examination should be performed at 1 week, and then again at 4 weeks. The patient should also be advised that he or she is at risk of developing a tear in the fellow eye and to return immediately if symptoms develop.

If a RRD has already occurred, it requires prompt treatment in order to prevent vision loss. A detailed discussion of retinal detachment repair is beyond the scope of this book; however, one should detail the physical examination findings as best as possible and obtain a consult from a vitreoretinal specialist as soon as possible. Depending on the location of the break(s), lens status, presence of lattice degeneration, and degree of myopia, the repair strategies may include a combination of any of the following: laser, cryotherapy, pneumatic retinopexy, scleral buckling, and pars plana vitrectomy.

Vitreous Hemorrhage

The onset of floaters and flashing lights or photopsias with associated vision loss may indicate the presence of vitreous hemorrhage, which is the most common cause of blindness in diabetic patients. Alternatively, vitreous hemorrhage may complicate a PVD in otherwise normal patients over the age of 50.

A thorough retinal examination to rule out retinal tears and detachment (as above) is indicated. If there is no view of the posterior segment, B-scan ultrasound to rule out retinal detachment is indicated. If the patient is diabetic, the likely etiology for the bleed is proliferative diabetic retinopathy. Confirmation of the presence of retinal neovascularization with clinical exam and fluorescein angiography is indicated (if the view is sufficient) and emergent panretinal laser photocoagulation should be arranged. The patient may be a candidate for pars plana vitrectomy if the hemorrhage is dense and laser therapy is not possible.

Acute Angle-Closure Glaucoma

Aqueous humor normally flows from the posterior chamber through the pupil, and then drains through the trabecular meshwork in the anterior chamber angle. Angle-closure glaucoma occurs when the iris becomes apposed to the trabecular meshwork, blocking aqueous humor drainage (Figure 14.9). Pupillary block is the most common cause of acute angle-closure glaucoma. In this condition, the flow of aqueous humor through the pupil is impeded. As a result, aqueous humor accumulates behind the iris and causes the iris to bow forward against the trabecular meshwork. Some patients are anatomically predisposed to developing pupillary block. Predisposing factors include a small, hyperopic eye and a narrow chamber angle. Pupillary block is more likely to occur when the pupil is mid-dilated. Therefore, attacks can be precipitated by topical mydriatics, systemic anticholinergics, stress, excitement (sympathetic release), or dim illumination.

Because of the acute rise in IOP, patients can present with headaches, severe eye pain, nausea, and vomiting. Ocular injection is present, and the cornea is steamy due to epithelial edema (Figure 14.10). This gives the patient the perception of rainbow-colored halos around lights and blurry or smoky vision.

On examination, patients show high IOP and ciliary flush (violaceous hue surrounding the limbus). The pupil is mid-dilated and sluggish. The anterior chamber is shallow, and aqueous flare and cells might be present. The anterior chamber angle is closed on gonioscopy, and the fellow eye almost always has a narrow angle. Corneal epithelial edema can impede the view of the anterior chamber and preclude gonioscopy or treatment by laser iridotomy. If this occurs, medical treatment to lower the IOP and topical glycerin to reduce the epithelial edema might be necessary to permit examination of the anterior chamber in detail. The corneal edema secondary to high IOP manifests as diffuse epithelial edema without stromal thickening, because the high pressure compresses the stroma, unlike edema associated with endothelial cell dysfunction (ie, Fuchs dystrophy).

Treatment

Medical treatment is used initially to break the acute attack, paving the way for definitive surgical treatment. Stepwise medical treatment consists of the following:

1. Attempt to terminate the attack by compressing the central cornea (after corneal anesthesia) with a muscle hook or Zeiss gonioprism. This might be helpful in cases of recent onset.
2. Instill a topical beta-blocker (eg, 1 drop of timolol 0.5%).

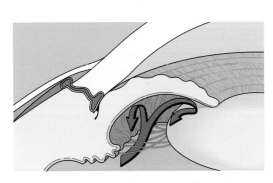

Figure 14.9 In acute angle-closure glaucoma, the iris root occludes the trabecular meshwork, impeding the flow of aqueous humor.

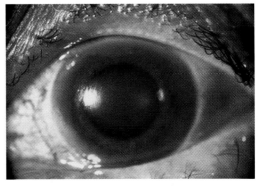

Figure 14.10 Acute angle-closure glaucoma produces corneal edema and a red eye.

3. In phakic patients, instill pilocarpine 1% to 2% q15 minutes × 3; only in pseudophakic or aphakic pupillary block, instill topical mydriatic and cycloplegic drops (eg, phenylephrine 2.5% or tropicamide 1%) q15 minutes × 3.
4. Instill topical corticosteroid drops (prednisolone acetate 1%).
5. Administer systemic carbonic anhydrase inhibitors (eg, acetazolamide 250 mg po × 2 or IV).
6. Administer systemic osmotic agents (eg, isosorbide 50 to 100 mg po over crushed ice, to be drunk slowly; or intravenous mannitol). Avoid these medications in patients with congestive heart failure or renal failure.
7. Administer systemic analgesics (eg, acetaminophen).
8. Apply topical glycerin, which can temporarily reduce corneal edema and swelling, allowing adequate view for examination and laser iridotomy. Topically applied glycerin is painful because of its hypertonicity, so topical anesthetic drops should be given first.

Definitive treatment, performed when the acute attack is broken, consists of laser iridotomy or, if not possible or not available, surgical iridectomy. The fellow eye should be treated prophylactically in the near future since it is at high risk for developing acute angle closure as well.

Ocular Chemical Burn

Chemical burns of the eye are among the few true ocular emergencies. Begin eye irrigation immediately, even before completing the history or measuring the vision.

Acid burns cause denaturation of tissue proteins, which then act as a barrier to prevent further diffusion of acid. For this reason, they are generally less devastating than alkali burns, but they can still be very severe. Alkali burns do not cause denaturation of tissue proteins. Therefore, caustic alkaline chemicals tend to penetrate deeper than acid burns and tend to be generally more destructive to ocular tissues. They can cause corneal melting, blanching of the conjunctiva, severe corneal and conjunctival scarring, and intraocular complications such as uveitis and secondary glaucoma (Figure 14.11).

Clinical findings in mild burns of either type include conjunctival hyperemia, chemosis, and corneal epithelial erosions and mild haziness. Mild stromal edema and anterior chamber reaction can also be present. More severe cases show corneal opacification and limbal ischemia.

Figure 14.11 Alkali burn.

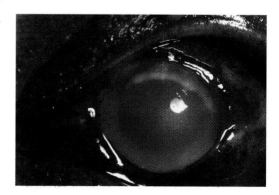

Treatment

The most important step in the treatment of acute chemical burns of any type is prompt, copious irrigation of all exposed tissues. Clinical Protocol 14.3 presents instructions for eye irrigation. After irrigation, examine the eye carefully, checking for epithelial defects, corneal melting, and other injuries. Administer topical cycloplegics, antibiotics, and corticosteroid drops, then patch the eye. Various other medications may be administered to promote collagen synthesis, inhibit the enzyme collagenase, and enhance epithelialization (eg, acetylcysteine drops 10% to 20% every 4 hours).

Central Retinal Artery Occlusion

Patients with central retinal artery occlusion present with unilateral, acute, painless, severe loss of vision. It can result from embolic episodes in patients with carotid or cardiac disease, or it can be associated with arteriolosclerosis, giant cell (temporal) arteritis, collagen vascular disease, hypercoagulation disorders, talc emboli with intravenous drug abuse, or trauma.

Affected patients show an afferent pupillary defect. Fundus examination reveals retinal arterial narrowing and blood column segmentation. The retina is white or gray except for a cherry-red spot at the fovea, which is perfused by the choroid, and except for areas supplied by a cilioretinal artery (Figure 14.12). Look for Hollenhorst plaques or other types of emboli. Over time, patients will develop inner retinal atrophy and optic atrophy. The prognosis of central retinal artery occlusion is generally poor.

Treatment

Treatment for central retinal artery occlusion should be immediate. Irreversible retinal damage is said to occur after 90 minutes, but treatment should be considered in a patient presenting within 24 hours of onset. The goals of treatment are to restore retinal blood flow and to move a potential retinal embolus distally. Emergency treatment is initiated as follows:

1. Lower intraocular pressure to improve retinal perfusion in one or more of the following ways:
   a. Massage the globe either digitally or with a fundus contact lens. In addition to lowering the intraocular pressure, this might also dislodge an embolic plaque.

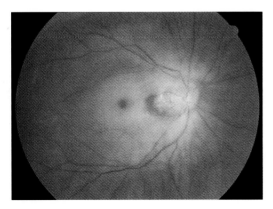

Figure 14.12 Central retinal artery occlusion. Note retinal pallor and cherry-red spot at fovea. (Photograph by Sally A. Stanley, CRA. Courtesy W.K. Kellogg Eye Center, University of Michigan.)

    b. Administer acetazolamide (500 mg IV) and/or instill topical timolol 0.5%.

    c. Consider performing anterior chamber paracentesis (Clinical Protocol 14.4).

2. Produce arterial dilation by having the patient either inhale a combination of 95% oxygen and 5% carbon dioxide (carbogen) or breathe into a paper bag. (This procedure can have complications and is no longer offered in many emergency rooms.)

3. All patients with central retinal artery occlusion should undergo a thorough medical evaluation after emergency treatment. In patients older than 55 years, erythrocyte sedimentation rate should be measured at the time of presentation to rule out giant cell arteritis. If the patient's sedimentation rate suggests temporal arteritis, give high-dose corticosteroids.

Arteritic Anterior Ischemic Optic Neuropathy

Arteritic anterior ischemic optic neuropathy (AAION) presents as painless, unilateral visual loss developing over hours to days. It occurs in patients older than 50 years of age (average age 70 years), and is more common in women. Vision loss is often accompanied by other symptoms, such as headache (most sensitive), jaw claudication (most specific), scalp tenderness, proximal muscle aches, weight loss, or fever.

Clinical exam for AAION reveals severe monocular vision loss, with over 60% of patients having visual acuity of less than 20/200 in the affected eye. An afferent pupillary defect will be present with unilateral disease, and an altitudinal visual field defect may also be observed. Funduscopic exam typically demonstrates a pale, swollen optic nerve head with flame-shaped hemorrhages along the disk margin (Figure 14.13).

If AAION is suspected, emergency laboratory evaluation with an erythrocyte sedimentation rate (ESR) and C-reactive protein (CRP) should be ordered. ESR should be considered positive if it is greater than the value obtained from the following formulas:

    Men: ESR > (Patient age)/2

    Women: ESR > (Patient age +10)/2

ESR is a nonspecific marker, however, as it can be elevated in any acute inflammatory process (ie, infection, vasculitis, malignancy). CRP can provide additional support for a diagnosis of AAION, with a specificity of 97% in patients with both a positive ESR and CRP. A definitive diagnosis is made through temporal artery biopsy, which should be performed within a week of presentation in all patients suspected of having AAION.

Treatment

Any patient who is suspected of having AAION with a positive ESR/CRP should be started on high dose corticosteroids immediately, with the goal of preventing ischemic visual loss in the contralateral eye. A typical therapeutic regimen begins with 3 to 5 days of IV methylprednisone (1g/day), followed by oral prednisone (100 mg/day) which is slowly tapered over the course of 3 to 12 months. If left

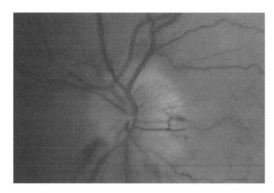

Figure 14.13 Anterior ischemic optic neuropathy. Note pale swelling of the optic disc with associated flame-shaped hemorrhages. (Reprinted, with permission, from Bradford CA, *Basic Ophthalmology*. San Francisco: American Academy of Ophthalmology, 2004.)

untreated, up to 95% of patients experience visual loss in the fellow eye within days to weeks. Therefore, corticosteroid therapy should not be delayed until temporal artery biopsy.

Pitfalls and Pointers

- Make appropriate follow-up arrangements after evaluating the patient in the emergency room.
- Make the medical records sufficiently detailed for later medicolegal and insurance purposes (see Chapter 3).
- Do not allow a patient who might require surgery to eat or drink.
- Do not use depolarizing muscular relaxants (eg, succinylcholine) in a patient with a ruptured globe.
- Embedded, hidden foreign bodies are sometimes overlooked. In cases of perforating trauma, a CT scan should be performed if there is any suspicion of a foreign body.
- Magnetic resonance imaging studies are contraindicated in patients with metallic (magnetic) foreign bodies.
- If significant head trauma exists, avoid dilating the patient's pupils for ophthalmoscopy until neurologic evaluation is completed. When you do dilate, be sure to notify other health care personnel and note the dilation on the chart.
- Traumatic hyphema in children is often associated with lethargy or somnolence; avoid confusing these symptoms with those associated with neurologic injury, and vice versa.
- Do not apply pressure (eg, ocular palpation, scleral depression) to a globe that might be ruptured or an eye that has a hyphema.
- Do not use a papoose board for restraining a child with an open or potentially ruptured globe.
- Give priority to the treatment of life-threatening conditions over the treatment of ocular trauma.
- Do not prescribe or give a patient a bottle of anesthetic eyedrops. Keep all ophthalmic medications out of reach.
- Swallowing of the contents of a bottle of atropine or pilocarpine can be fatal.

- Do not administer acetazolamide to individuals with possible or proven sickle-cell disease or trait, or patients with a sulfonamide allergy.
- First do no harm. Know your limits and don't hesitate to call for help when you need it.

Suggested Resources

Bacterial Keratitis [Preferred Practice Pattern]. San Francisco: American Academy of Ophthalmology; 2008.

Catalano RA, Belin M, eds. *Ocular Emergencies.* Philadelphia: WB Saunders; 1992.

Conjunctivitis [Preferred Practice Pattern]. San Francisco: American Academy of Ophthalmology; 2008.

Deutsch TA, Feller DB, eds. *Paton and Goldberg's Management of Ocular Injuries.* 2nd ed. Philadelphia: WB Saunders; 1985.

Kunimoto DY, Kanitkor KD, Makar M, et al. *The Wills Eye Manual: Office and Emergency Room Diagnosis and Treatment of Eye Disease.* 4th ed. Philadelphia: Lippincott, Williams & Wilkins; 2004.

Primary Angle Closure [Preferred Practice Pattern]. San Francisco: American Academy of Ophthalmology; 2005.

Posterior Vitreous Detachment, Retinal Breaks, and Lattice Degeneration [Preferred Practice Pattern]. San Francisco: American Academy of Ophthalmology; 2008.

Clinical Protocol 14.1  Applying Patches and Shields

1. Set out sterile eye pads and adhesive surgical tape. Tear the tape into 5- to 6-inch lengths.
2. Instruct the patient to close both eyes.
3. Clean the forehead and zygoma with an alcohol pad to remove the skin oils. This helps the tape stick to the skin.
4. Any of 3 techniques may be used, depending on the amount of pressure desired and what is most comfortable for the patient:
   a. 1 pad unfolded (minimal pressure)
   b. 2 pads unfolded (a bit more pressure)
   c. 2 pads, underlying one folded (still more pressure)
5. Tape the unfolded pad firmly to the forehead and zygoma (Figure 1). To prevent blinking, further bleeding, or swelling, the patch must exert some mild pressure on the lids. The patient should not be able to open the eyelid beneath the patch. The tape should not extend to the mandible or near the corner of the mouth because jaw movement could loosen the patch.
6. If the patient has any contusion or laceration of the globe or its adnexal structures, apply and tape a fenestrated aluminum (Fox) shield, instead of a patch, over the globe, to protect these tissues from further damage until healing occurs or definitive repair is performed. Rest the shield on the bony superior orbital ridge and zygoma (Figure 2). Do not patch an open globe tightly.

Clinical Protocol 14.1 *(continued)*

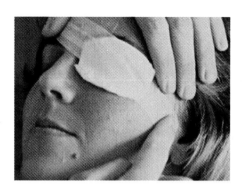
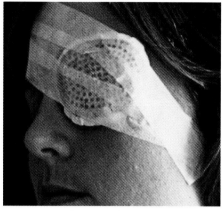

Figure 1 Positioning and taping the unfolded pad.   **Figure 2** Taping the aluminum shield over the pad.

Clinical Protocol 14.2   **Removing Corneal Foreign Bodies**

1. Apply drops of topical anesthetic solution to the affected eye.

2. While holding the patient's upper and lower lids apart with your thumb and index finger, remove a loose, nonembedded foreign body as appropriate in either of the following 2 ways:

   a. Wipe the corneal surface gently with a cotton swab moistened with saline solution or any bland ophthalmic eyedrop.

   b. Perform saline lavage, inspecting the cornea periodically, until the foreign body is no longer apparent (Clinical Protocol 14.3).

3. Remove a firmly embedded foreign body by careful extraction with a 27-gauge needle on a handle or tuberculin syringe under slit-lamp magnification. Use a flicking motion with the needle and avoid pushing the foreign body deeper into the cornea or inserting the needle any deeper into the cornea than is absolutely necessary (Figure 1).

4. If a rust ring remains, you may try to curette it with the needle or use one of the commercially available rust-ring burrs. It is not necessary to remove the entire rust ring. It is better to leave a small rust ring in the visual axis than to risk creating a dense stromal scar after the removal.

5. Treat the abrasion resulting from the foreign body as for a typical corneal abrasion.

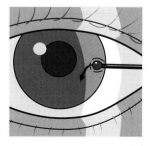

Figure 1 Extracting the foreign body.

Clinical Protocol 14.3   Irrigating the Ocular Surface

1. With the patient supine, instill drops of topical anesthetic solution into the cul-de-sac.
2. Gently keep the eyelids open either manually or with a Desmarres retractor or a lid speculum.
   a. Avoid pressure on the globe or forceful eyelid opening if you suspect a ruptured globe.
   b. Keeping the eye open with a lid speculum and administering analgesics and topical anesthetics allow effective irrigation with minimal discomfort to the patient.
   c. Inspect the ocular surface and conjunctival cul-de-sac quickly for particulate chemical substances. Remove small particles by rolling a moistened cotton-tipped applicator across the conjunctiva; remove large particles with forceps.
3. Begin irrigating the eye copiously with normal saline solution or other similarly isotonic solution.
   a. You may use a squeeze bottle or normal saline drip with plastic tubings, if available.
   b. Ask the patient to shift gaze periodically so that the entire cul-de-sac is flushed.
4. After irrigating for at least 15 or 20 minutes, using a minimum of 1 liter of fluid, reexamine the eye, especially the fornices, for particulate matter. You might need to evert the upper lid to irrigate or manually remove particulate matter that is lodged there.
5. If particulate matter is found, irrigate further after removing the particles. Continue irrigation until the pH of the conjunctival sac is neutral (ie, 7.4). Urinary pH strips are suitable for this determination.

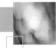

Clinical Protocol 14.4   Performing Anterior Chamber Paracentesis

1. Place the patient in the supine position.
2. Instill topical anesthetic solution (eg, proparacaine) to the eye, and hold a cotton-tipped applicator soaked with anesthetic (eg, proparacaine, tetracaine, or lidocaine) against the insertion of the medial rectus muscle.
3. Place an eyelid speculum.
4. Under the operating microscope, fixate the eye by grasping the anesthetized tendon of the medial rectus muscle.
5. Using a 30-gauge short needle on a tuberculin syringe, enter the anterior chamber at the temporal limbus with the bevel of the needle pointing up and with the needle parallel to the iris plane. Keep the tip of the needle over the midperiphery of the iris, and avoid the lens throughout the procedure.
6. Withdraw fluid from the anterior chamber until you can observe that it shallows slightly (0.1 to 0.2 cc of aqueous fluid).
7. Withdraw the needle.

15 Common Ocular Medications

This chapter presents an abbreviated overview of the most common categories of medications the beginning resident is likely to encounter.

- Anesthetic agents
- Dyes
- Anti-infective agents
- Anti-inflammatory agents
- Mydriatic/cycloplegic agents
- Glaucoma medications
- Decongestant, vasoconstrictive, and anti-allergy agents
- Lubricating agents and tear substitutes
- Corneal dehydration medications
- Agents delivered by intravitreal injection

Ocular medications are used for both ophthalmic diagnosis and treatment. They can be delivered to the eye by 4 different routes:

- As topical drops or ointments
- As thin drug-containing wafers deposited in the conjunctival sac for timed release of medication
- As injectable drugs administered directly subconjunctivally, intravitreally, sub-Tenon's capsule, or into the peribulbar or retrobulbar spaces
- As systemic medications, especially for treating serious intraocular, optic nerve, or orbital inflammations and infections

■ Anesthetic Agents

Topical anesthesia is used when performing routine procedures such as measuring intraocular pressure and removing corneal foreign bodies. Instill 1 to 2 drops in the eye for temporary anesthesia (15 to 20 minutes) to facilitate ocular examination. Common agents include tetracaine HCl 0.5% (Pontocaine), proparacaine HCl 0.5% (Alcaine, Ophthaine, Ophthetic), benoxinate 0.4% with fluorescein (Fluress), and cocaine 1% to 4%. These agents are toxic to the corneal epithelium when used habitually and should not be dispensed to the patient to take home.

■ Dyes

Certain dyes are useful for ophthalmic diagnosis. Fluorescein is a yellow-orange dye that emits a green color when exposed to a blue light. It is used topically for applanation tonometry and to diagnose corneal abrasions, punctate epithelial erosions, and other epithelial defects. The dye stains the corneal or conjunctival stroma in areas where the epithelium is absent, and it is used intravenously for fluorescein angiography.

Rose bengal is a red dye that stains devitalized epithelium and mucus. It is picked up by abnormal, but not areas of absent, epithelial cells in diseases such as keratoconjunctivitis sicca. Lissamine green is another dye that stains dead and devitalized epithelial cells; however, it is far less irritating than rose bengal.

■ Anti-Infective Agents

Medications for ocular infections comprise mainly antifungal, antibacterial, and antiviral agents. Antiprotozoal and antiparasitic agents are available but uncommonly used. The names and attributes of common antifungal, antibacterial, and antiviral medications are summarized in Tables 15.1, 15.2, and 15.3, respectively. Topical antibacterial agents should be used judiciously to avoid sensitization and emergence of resistant organisms. Agents that combine an antibiotic and anti-inflammatory agent are available, such as tobramycin plus dexamethasone (TobraDex) and sulfacetamide plus prednisolone acetate (Blephamide) but should be used with caution due to the significant side effects of corticosteroids outlined below.

Table 15.1   Antifungal Agents

Name	Preparation	Comments
Amphotericin B (Fungizone)	0.075–0.3% 1% solution or cream	Solution may be made in hospital pharmacy. May be extremely uncomfortable to the patient, but the solution is more effective than Nystatin. May be given intravitreally for fungal endophthalmitis, although toxic to the retina.
Clotrimazole	0.075–0.3% 1% solution or cream	Ophthalmic preparation not available.
Fluconazole (Diflucan)	Oral	Effective against *Candida*.
Ketoconazole (Nizoral)	Oral	Effective against *Candida*, *Cryptococcus*, *Histoplasma*.
Miconazole (Monistat)	1% intravenous solution	Intravenous solution may be used topically.
Natamycin (Natacyn)	5% suspension	Used topically for yeast and filamentary forms (corneal ulcers).
Nystatin (Mycostatin)	Ophthalmic ointment not available	The dermatologic preparation (100,000 units per gram) may be used in fungal keratitis.

Table 15.2   Topical Ophthalmic Antibacterial Agents

Antibiotic	Commercial Name	Preparation	Spectrum of Coverage
Aminoglycosides:			Enterobacteriaceae, *P aeruginosa*, *S aureus*.
Gentamicin	Genoptic, Garamycin	Ointment or solution	Fortified drops may be formulated from intravenous preparations for topical use. Widely used in serious ocular infections (eg, corneal ulcers where G-organisms are implicated). Covers many G+ staphylococci but not streptococci.
Tobramycin	Tobrex	Solution or ointment	More effective against streptococci and *Pseudomonas* than gentamicin.
Bacitracin	AK-Tracin	Ointment	G+ cocci (*Staphylococcus*, *Streptococcus*).
Bacitracin/ polymyxin B	Polysporin	Ointment	See action of each drug separately.
Chloramphenicol	Chloromycetin, Ocu-Chlor, Chloroptic	Solution or ointment	Broad-spectrum: G-bacilli (*H influenza*, *N meningitidis*), *S pneumoniae*, *Salmonella*, and anaerobes (*β fragilis*). Rare cases of aplastic anemia have been reported.
Erythromycin	Ak-Mycin, Ilotycin	Ointment	G+ organisms, chlamydiae, mycoplasmas, some atypical mycobacteria, *H ducreyi*, *C jejuni*, *N gonorrhoeae*, *Actinomyces*. Particularly good in staphylococcal conjunctivitis. Bacteriostatic.
Fluoroquinolones:			
Ciprofloxacin	Ciloxan	Solution or ointment	Broad-spectrum; anaerobes usually resistant, may not be effective against some G+ cocci (streptococci).
Gatifloxacin	Zymar	Solution	Same as Ciloxan, but improved coverage of G+ and atypical mycobacteria.
Levofloxacin	Quixin	Solution	Similar to ofloxacin.
Moxifloxacin	Vigamox	Solution	Same as Ciloxan, but improved coverage of G+ and atypical mycobacteria.
Ofloxacin	Ocuflox	Solution	Same as Ciloxan, but also covers *Chlamydia* and *Bacteroides*.
Neomycin/bacitracin/ polymyxin B	Neosporin	Ointment	Neomycin can cause contact allergies in up to 10% of users. Neomycin has broad-spectrum activity in G+ and G-organisms.
Neomycin/gramicidin/ polymyxin B	Neosporin	Drops	Polymyxin: G-enteric bacteria, *P aeruginosa*. Inactive against G+ organisms. See above regarding neomycin.
Sulfacetamide	Bleph-10, Sulf-10, Vasosulf, Sulamyd	Solution or ointment	Sulfonamides: G+ and G-organisms but not *P aeruginosa* or enterococci. Bacteriostatic.
Tetracycline	Achromycin	Solution or ointment	G+ organisms, Enterobacteriaceae, vibrios, rickettsia. Inactive for *P aeruginosa*, *Bacteroides*, and group B streptococci.
Trimethoprim/ polymyxin B	Polytrim	Solution	Trimethoprim: G+ and G-organisms but not *P aeruginosa* or enterococci.

Table 15.3   Antiviral Medications

Name of Drug	Other Names	Chemical Composition	How Administered	Mode of Action	Main Clinical Uses
Acyclovir	Zovirax	Purine analog	Ointment,, oral, parenteral (ophthalmic ointment not available in US)	Blocks viral DNA polymerase, thus selectively attacks viral replication in infected cell. Oral form (600–800 mg 5 times daily) reduces severity of skin and eye involvement. Particularly helpful in herpetic uveitis.	Herpes simplex, varicella-zoster, Epstein Barr virus, cytomegalovirus (CMV)
Famciclovir	Famvir	Purine analog	Oral	Same as ganciclovir.	Herpes simplex, varicella-zoster
Foscarnet	Foscavir	Pyrophosphate analog	Parenteral (IV)	Interferes with viral DNA polymerase and reverse transcriptase.	CMV, HSV, EBV
Ganciclovir	Cytovene	Purine analog	Oral, parenteral (IV)	Interferes with viral DNA synthesis.	CMV retinitis
Idoxuridine	IDU, Stoxil, Herplex	Thymidine analog	0.1% ophthalmic drops q1h, 0.5% ointment q4h	Inhibits thymidine incorporation into DNA.	Herpes simplex keratitis
Trifluridine	Viroptic	Thymidine analog	1% solution, usually given q2h to a maximum total of 9 drops daily	Inhibits viral DNA synthesis.	Herpes simplex keratitis; some activity against varicella-zoster virus
Vidarabine	Vira-A	Purine analog	3% ophthalmic ointment, applied q3h or 5 times daily for 6–10 days	Inhibits viral DNA synthesis	Herpes simplex keratitis
Zidovudine	Retrovir	Thymidine analog	Oral, parenteral	Interferes with RNA-directed DNA polymerase.	HIV

■ Anti-Inflammatory Agents

These drugs are used either topically or systemically to reduce ocular inflammation.

Corticosteroids

Topical corticosteroids are used for anterior segment inflammation, including refractory cases of allergic conjunctivitis, iridocyclitis, episcleritis, scleritis, and both noninfectious and infectious keratitis (once the infection has been adequately treated). Many different corticosteroid preparations are available for topical ocular use; some examples in the 3 most common categories are listed below:

- Prednisolone:
  — Prednisolone acetate suspension 0.125% (Pred Mild, Econopred)
  — Prednisolone acetate suspension 1% (AK-Tate, Econopred Plus, Pred Forte)
  — Prednisolone sodium phosphate solution 0.125% (AK-Pred, Inflamase Mild)
  — Prednisolone sodium phosphate solution 1% (AK-Pred, Inflamase Forte)
- Dexamethasone
  — Dexamethasone sodium phosphate solution 0.1% (Decadron Phosphate, AK-Dex)
  — Dexamethasone sodium phosphate ointment 0.05% (Decadron Phosphate, AK-Dex, Baldex, Maxidex)
  — Dexamethasone suspension 0.1% (Maxidex)
- Progesterone-like agents
  — Medrysone 1.0% (HMS Liquifilm)
  — Fluorometholone suspension 0.1% (FML Liquifilm)
  — Fluorometholone suspension 0.25% (FML Forte Liquifilm)
  — Fluorometholone acetate 0.1% (Flarex)
  — Fluorometholone ointment 0.1%

Some corticosteroids may also be given by subconjunctival, sub-Tenon's capsule, intravitreal, peribulbar or retrobulbar, and systemic routes. Dosage and route of administration depend on the location and severity of the inflammation. Drops or ointment may be instilled every 1, 2, or 4 hours (among other regimens), with tapering according to response. Even brief exposure to topical corticosteroids can worsen herpes simplex epithelial keratitis and fungal keratitis and can sometimes provoke severe ulceration or even perforation. In some people, corticosteroid use causes ocular hypertension or glaucoma. Loteprednol (Lotemax, Alrex) is a topical corticosteroid that has a lower risk of producing secondary intraocular pressure elevation. Long-term use of corticosteroids can cause posterior subcapsular cataracts. Other side effects include delayed wound healing, corneal melting (keratolysis), prolongation of the natural duration of the disease, mydriasis, and ptosis.

Cyclosporine (Restasis)

This is an immunomodulating drug with anti-inflammatory effects. It is available as a 0.05% ophthalmic emulsion for use twice daily for keratoconjunctivitis sicca. Cyclosporine is immunosuppressive when given systemically.

Nonsteroidal Anti-Inflammatory Drugs

The nonsteroidal anti-inflammatory drugs (NSAIDs) reduce inflammation primarily by inhibition of the cyclo-oxygenase enzyme, which is involved in prostaglandin synthesis. Topical ophthalmic preparations with widening indications have become available recently. Certain agents such as flurbiprofen (Ocufen) are used topically to reduce pupillary constriction during intraocular surgery. Ketorolac tromethamine (Acular) has been approved for treatment of ocular allergies. Diclofenac sodium (Voltaren), nepafenac (Nevanac), and bromfenac (Xibrom) are used for postoperative inflammation. Corneal melting has been described as a complication of topical NSAID use.

■ Mydriatics and Cycloplegics

Mydriasis (dilation of the pupil) is obtained either by paralyzing the iris sphincter (with parasympatholytic [cycloplegic] agents) or by stimulating the iris dilator (with sympathomimetic [mydriatic] agents). Maximal mydriasis is achieved by using a combination of both types of agents. In addition to causing mydriasis, parasympatholytic agents paralyze the ciliary muscle, which controls accommodation. Cycloplegia is useful when refracting children, whose active accommodation precludes accurate measurement of refractive errors. Cycloplegic (but not mydriatic) agents are also useful for relieving the pain of ciliary muscle spasm, which accompanies epithelial defects of the cornea, corneal inflammation, and intraocular inflammation. Dilating the pupils also helps prevent posterior synechiae in patients with anterior segment inflammation. Agents that dilate the pupil should be used with caution in patients with narrow anterior chamber angles, as they can precipitate angle-closure glaucoma. Table 15.4 lists commonly used agents and their characteristics.

Table 15.4   Mydriatics and Cycloplegics

Agent	How Available	Maximum Effect (Minutes)	Duration of Action	Comments
Phenylephrine (Neo-Synephrine) 2.5%, 10%	Solution	20	3 hours	Produces mydriasis, but no cycloplegia; avoid 10% solution. May cause angina, increased blood pressure, myocardial infraction, stroke (mainly with 10%).
Tropicamide (Mydriacyl) 0.5%, 1%	Solution	25	4–6 hours	Inadequate for cycloplegic refraction of children.
Cyclopentolate (Cyclogyl) 0.5%, 1%, 2%	Solution	30	12–24 hours	Adequate for most cycloplegic refractions. Neurotoxicity can occur, particularly in children; incoherence, visual hallucination, ataxia, slurred speech, and seizures.
Homatropine 1%, 2%, 5%	Solution	40	2–3 days	Side effects are rare.
Scopolamine (Isopto Hyoscine) 0.25%	Solution	30	4–7 days	CNS side effects; dizziness, disorientation.
Atropine 0.25%, 0.5%, 1%	Ointment or solution	30	1–2 weeks	Systemic absorption can result in flushing, fever, tachycardia, restlessness, and excited behavior.

▪ Glaucoma Medications

Glaucoma medications lower intraocular pressure to prevent optic nerve damage. Five different classes of drugs are used to treat open-angle glaucoma. In addition, hyperosmotic agents are used to lower the intraocular pressure in acute glaucoma. These 6 classes of glaucoma medications are discussed below and reviewed in Table 15.5. Agents that combine glaucoma medications from different classes are available, including timolol plus dorzolamide (Cosopt) and timolol plus brimonidine (Combigan). Benzalkonium chloride is a common preservative in most glaucoma medications. However, some glaucoma medications contain a different preservative (eg Alphagan-P) or are preservative-free (eg, Timoptic in Ocudose), which are particularly useful in glaucoma patients who are prone to benzalkonium chloride toxicity.

More Commonly Used Agents

Prostaglandin analogues

Prostaglandin analogues are the newest class of glaucoma medications. They lower intraocular pressure by increasing aqueous outflow through the uveoscleral pathway. Examples include latanoprost (Xalatan), bimatoprost (Lumigan), and travoprost (Travatan). Ocular side effects include ocular redness, iritis, increasing pigmentation of the iris and eyelid skin, eyelash growth, and cystoid macular edema.

Beta-adrenergic antagonists

Beta-adrenergic antagonists, also known as *beta-blockers*, lower intraocular pressure by reducing aqueous production in the ciliary epithelium. Timolol (Timoptic, Betimol), levobunolol (Betagan), carteolol (Ocupress), and metipranolol (Opti-Pranolol) are nonselective beta-blockers; betaxolol (Betoptic S) selectively blocks β_1 receptors. Systemic side effects include bradycardia, decreased cardiac output, exercise intolerance, bronchiolar spasm, hypotension, syncope, decreased libido, lethargy, and depression. These side effects can be additive to those associated with systemic beta-blockers that the patient might be taking for high blood pressure. Selective β_1 blockers should be less associated with bronchospasm.

Topical carbonic anhydrase inhibitors

Carbonic anhydrase inhibitors reduce aqueous production by inhibiting the enzyme carbonic anhydrase. They are sulfonamide derivatives and should be avoided in patients with sulfonamide allergies. Examples of topical carbonic anhydrase inhibitors include dorzolamide (Trusopt) and brinzolamide (Azopt). They are thought to have at least mildly adverse effects on the function of corneal endothelial cells.

Alpha-2 adrenergic agonists

Alpha-2 adrenergic agents lower intraocular pressure by reducing the production of aqueous humor and possibly by increasing uveoscleral outflow. Examples include apraclonidine (Iopidine) and brimonidine (Alphagan P). Side effects include fatigue, dry mouth, and allergic conjunctivitis.

Table 15.5   Glaucoma Medications

Name of Agent	Concentration and Dosage	Comments
Cholinergic agonists:		
Pilocarpine	0.5%–6% solution, 4% gel, also as sustained-release wafer (Ocusert)	1%–4% strengths are in widest use, instilled qid.
Carbachol	0.75%–3% solution, usually given qd-tid	Used when pilocarpine is ineffective.
Echothiophate iodide (Phospholine Iodide)	0.03%–0.25% solution, given once or twice daily or less often	Infrequently used because of its intense cholinergic effect and side effects, including salivation, nausea, vomiting, and diarrhea. Acts by indirect action as an irreversible cholinesterase inhibitor.
Adrenergic antagonists:		
Epinephrine (Epifrin, Glaucon)	0.25%, 0.5%, 1%, and 2% solution, given bid	Nonselective adrenergic agonist.
Dipivefrin (Propine)	0.1% solution given bid	Precursor to (prodrug for) epinephrine. When it enters the eye, it is cleaved to the active form of the *drug*, theoretically giving fewer local and systemic side effects
Apraclonidine (Iopidine)	0.5% and 1% solution	Commonly used for prophylaxis of post-laser IOP spike. High rate of tachyphylaxis and allergy limits its use in long-term glaucoma therapy.
Brimonidine (Alphagan P)	0.15% and 0.2% solution given bid-tid	Useful in long-term glaucoma therapy. Can cause apnea in infants.
Beta-adrenergic antagonists:		
Timolol (Timoptic, Betimol)	0.25% and 0.5% solution, given bid	A nonselective beta-blocker should be prescribed with care in patients with asthma, heart failure, and heart block. Has some corneal toxicity; also available in a once-daily-dose form (Timoptic XE).
Carteolol (Ocupress)	1% solution given bid	Comparable effects to Timolol.
Metipranolol (OptiPranolol)	0.3% solution given bid	Comparable effects to Timolol.
Betaxolol (Betoptic S)	0.25% and 0.5% solution given bid	A selective beta-blocker, should reduce the risk of pulmonary side effects, particularly in patients with reactive or restrictive airway disease.
Levobunolol (Betagan)	0.25% and 0.5% solution given bid	Comparable effects to Timolol.
Carbonic anhydrase inhibitors (CAI):		
Acetazolamide (Diamox)	125 and 250 mg tablets, sustained-release 500 mg capsule (sequel); tablets given bid to qid, capsules given once or twice daily	May also be given intravenously in 500 mg ampules.
Methazolamide (Neptazane)	25–50 mg given bid to tid	
Dichlorphenamide (Daranide)	50 mg given once daily to tid	
Dorzolamide (Trusopt)	A topical ophthalmic CAI (2% solution), given bid to tid	10% incidence of allergy.
Brinzolamide (Azopt)	A topical CAI (1% solution) given bid to tid	
Prostaglandin analogues:		
Bimatoprost (Lumigan)	0.03% solution given qHS	May cause ocular redness, increased pigmentation of the iris and eyelids, and eyelash growth
Latanoprost (Xalatan)	0.005% solution given qHS	Similar efficacy and side effects as bimatoprost.
Travoprost (Travatan)	0.004% solution given qHS	Similar efficacy and side effects as bimatoprost.

Table 15.5   Glaucoma Medications *(continued)*

Name of Agent	Concentration and Dosage	Comments
Hyperosmotic agents:		
Mannitol	20% intravenous solution given 1.5–2 g/kg intravenously	Maximum ocular hypotensive effect occurs at 1 hour and lasts 5–6 hours.
Glycerin (Glyrol, Osmoglyn)	50% solution usually given orally with water, orange juice, or flavored normal saline solution over ice, 1–1.5 g/kg	Maximum ocular hypotensive effect occurs in 1 hour and lasts 4–5 hours. Can occasionally produce nausea, vomiting, and headache.
Urea (Ureaphil)	Powder or 30% intravenous solution given 0.5–2 g/kg intravenously	

Less Commonly Used Agents

Cholinergic agonists

These agents, also known as *miotics* or *parasympathomimetics*, act by increasing outflow of aqueous humor through the trabecular meshwork. Examples include pilocarpine, carbachol, and echothiophate iodide. Ocular side effects include pupillary constriction (which can decrease vision, especially if the patient has cataract) and ciliary spasm (resulting in brow ache and a myopic shift in refraction). Young people particularly are affected by ciliary spasm.

Sympathomimetics

Sympathomimetics lower intraocular pressure by increasing conventional trabecular and uveoscleral outflow. Examples include epinephrine (Epifrin, Glaucon) and dipivefrin (Propine). Dipivefrin is a prodrug that is converted into epinephrine by esterase enzymes in the cornea. Ocular side effects include rebound hyperemia leading to a red eye, cystoid macular edema in aphakic patients, and pupillary dilation possibly triggering an acute attack of angle-closure glaucoma in patients with narrow angles. Systemic side effects are uncommon but include tachycardia, hypertension, tremor, anxiety, and premature ventricular contractions.

Systemic carbonic anhydrase inhibitors

Carbonic anhydrase inhibitors are given systemically to patients with glaucoma who do not respond sufficiently to topical medication. Examples include acetazolamide (Diamox), methazolamide (Neptazane), and dichlorphenamide (Daranide). Side effects include nausea, tingling of the fingers and toes, anorexia, peculiar taste sensations, hypokalemia, renal lithiasis, acidosis, lethargy, loss of libido, depression, and (very uncommonly) aplastic anemia.

Hyperosmotic agents

Urea, glycerin, and mannitol reduce intraocular pressure by making the plasma hypertonic to aqueous and vitreous humor, with the result that fluid is drawn from the eye into the intravascular space. These agents are used orally or intravenously to lower the intraocular pressure in cases of acute glaucoma, and they are used pre- and postoperatively in selected patients. Caution must be exercised in patients with diabetes mellitus, congestive heart failure, or kidney damage.

Decongestant, Vasoconstrictive, and Anti-Allergy Agents

Several nonprescription ophthalmic preparations (vasoconstrictors) are available to reduce ocular redness, itching, and irritation. Most contain naphazoline, tetrahydrozoline, or phenylephrine. Some of these also have an added antihistamine such as pheniramine maleate or antazoline phosphate.

Antihistamine-decongestant combinations include naphazoline HCl 0.025% plus pheniramine maleate 0.3% (Visine A, Naphcon-A, Opcon-A) and naphazoline HCl 0.05% plus antazoline phosphate 0.5% (Vasocon-A). Antihistamines (without decongestant) include levocabastine (Livostin) and emedastine (Emadine).

Mast cell stabilizers are used for allergic disorders such as vernal conjunctivitis. These include cromolyn sodium (Crolom), ketotifen fumarate (Zaditen), lodoxamide tromethamine (Alomide), and pemirolast potassium (Alamast). Combination antihistamines and mast cell stabilizers include azelastine (Optivar), epinastine (Elestat), ketotifen (Zaditor, Alaway), nedocromil (Alocril), and olopatadine (Patanol, Pataday).

Lubricating Medications and Tear Substitutes

Many formulations of artificial tears and ointments are useful in patients with dry eyes. These are available over the counter in most cases. Basic ingredients include hypotonic or isotonic buffered solution, surfactants, and viscosity agents such as methylcellulose, carboxymethylcellulose, or ethylcellulose, which prolong corneal contact time. In general, ointments and viscous solutions adhere better to the cornea and require less frequent administration, but they have the disadvantage of temporarily degrading vision. Oily medications (such as ointments) can also destabilize the tear film. Artificial tears often have preservatives (eg, benzalkonium chloride), which can cause epithelial toxicity if overused. This is especially problematic in patients with dry eyes and chronic users, but preservative-free preparations have been developed. Examples include Celluvisc, Refresh Plus, Refresh Endura, GenTeal PF, Tears Naturale Free, and Bion Tears.

Corneal Dehydration Medications

Hypertonic medications may be instilled on the eye to clear corneal edema osmotically. Patients may be placed on hypertonic sodium chloride 2% or 5% (Muro 128, Hyper-Sal, Adsorbonac). For diagnostic purposes, anhydrous glycerin (Ophthalgan) may be instilled on the cornea to clear it transiently for visualization of intraocular structures; the preparation is so hypertonic as to cause considerable pain if it is instilled without the use first of a topical anesthetic agent.

Agents Delivered by Intravitreal Injection

The delivery of medications directly into the vitreous cavity by injection (intravitreal injection) has revolutionized many aspects of clinical ophthalmology. Intravitreal injections can be performed in the office using a 27- or 30-gauge needle with an anesthetic to minimize patient discomfort and an antiseptic to minimize the risk of infection. In many cases repeated injections are necessary. Injections are performed through the pars plana in order to avoid the vascular ciliary body anteriorly and the neurosensory retina posteriorly. Care is taken to direct the needle posteriorly toward the mid-vitreous cavity to avoid trauma to the crystalline lens. Although these procedures are generally safe, intravitreal injections carry risks including endophthalmitis, sterile inflammation, retinal detachment, lens trauma, hemorrhage, increased intraocular pressure, wound leak and hypotony. Four different classes of medications are routinely given intravitreally: anti-vascular endothelial growth factor agents, anti-inflammatory agents, antibacterial and antifungal agents, and antiviral agents.

Anti-Vascular Endothelial Growth Factor Agents

Intravitreal injections are increasingly important for patients with retinal diseases. Many of these treatments are directed at inhibiting vascular endothelial growth factor (VEGF)-A. VEGF-A is a diffusible cytokine made by cells that stimulates angiogenesis and leakage of blood vessels. VEGF-A plays an important role in wet age-related macular degeneration (AMD), diabetic retinopathy, and other retinal vascular diseases. Multiple medications directed at VEGF-A inhibition may be administered intravitreally.

Pegaptanib (Macugen)

Pegaptanib is a pegylated aptamer, a single strand of nucleic acid, which selectively binds to and inactivates VEGF-A-165. It was the first of these agents to become available, gaining FDA approval in 2004. Pegaptanib has been replaced by the more efficacious agents, Avastin and Lucentis.

Ranibizumab (Lucentis)

Ranibizumab is the newest anti-VEGF-A agent, approved by the FDA in 2006 for the treatment of wet AMD. Ranibizumab is a monoclonal antibody fragment that binds to and inhibits all subtypes of VEGF-A. Ranibizumab was the first treatment for wet AMD to show an average improvement in visual acuity and therefore caused a paradigm shift in the first-line approach to treatment, from laser-based modalities toward pharmacologic agents.

Bevacizumab (Avastin)

Bevacizumab was FDA approved for intravenous use in metastatic colon cancer in 2004. Bevacizumab is a humanized monoclonal antibody that binds to and inhibits the function of VEGF-A. Bevacizumab was derived from the same murine antibody as ranibizumab and is significantly larger with less affinity for VEGF-A, but has a longer half-life inside of the eye. Bevacizumab is used in an off-label (non-FDA approved) fashion for treating a broad range of retinal vascular diseases and as a more cost-effective alternative for the treatment of wet AMD. An NIH-sponsored, multicenter, prospective trial is presently comparing the clinical efficacy of these 2 agents for wet AMD.

Anti-Inflammatory Agents

Corticosteroids are used extensively in ophthalmology. Intravitreal triamcinolone acetonide (Kenalog) and dexamethasone are often used in an off-label fashion to decrease ocular inflammation and macular edema and to treat wet AMD. The preservative-free synthetic corticosteroid Triesence (triamcinolone acetonide) was FDA approved in 2007 for visualization during vitrectomy and the treatment of certain ocular inflammatory conditions. The Retisert (fluocinolone acetonide) intravitreal implant is an FDA approved sterile device that releases fluocinolone locally to the posterior segment of the eye at a steady rate over more than 2 years.

Injecting corticosteroids into an eye carries significant risks that must be considered by the treating physician. The majority of patients will develop a cataract over the following years, and many patients will develop a high intraocular pressure requiring eye drops or surgery.

Antibacterial and Antifungal Agents

The administration of antibiotics into the vitreous cavity to treat endophthalmitis was first reported in the 1940s. It was not until the 1970s and 1980s, however, that this practice became widespread. Antibacterial agents, and less commonly antifungal agents, are now routinely given intravitreally in the setting of postoperative endophthalmitis, post-traumatic endophthalmitis and endogenous endophthalmitis. The most commonly administered intravitreal antibiotics are vancomycin (1.0 mg in 0.1 mL), ceftazidime (2.2 mg in 0.1 mL) and amikacin (0.4 mg in 0.1 mL). The most commonly used intravitreal antifungal agent is amphotericin B (usual dose is 5–10 μg) (see Table 15.1).

Antiviral Agents

Antiviral agents may be administered intravitreally as an alternative or adjunct to the systemic treatment of acute retinal necrosis (ARN), progressive outer retinal necrosis (PORN), and CMV retinitis. The most commonly employed agents are inhibitors of viral DNA polymerase, ganciclovir (200 to 2000 μg), foscarnet (1200 to 2400 μg) and cidofovir (10 to 20 μg) (see Table 15.3). Repeated intravitreal injections of ganciclovir for the management of CMV retinitis have shown no significant side effects. The advent of an intraocular sustained-release implant, which releases ganciclovir over many months, has significantly reduced the number of procedures needed to deliver the drug in some clinical settings and may be more effective than systemic anti-viral therapy alone in the treatment of CMV retinitis.

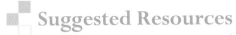

Suggested Resources

Intravitreal Injections [Clinical Statement]. San Francisco: American Academy of Ophthalmology; 2008.

Netland PA. *Glaucoma Medical Therapy. Principles and Management.* 2nd ed. New York: Oxford University Press; 2008.

O'Connor Davies PH, Hopkins GA, Pearson RM. *Ophthalmic Drugs: Diagnostic and Therapeutic Uses.* 4th ed. Boston: Butterworth-Heinemann; 1998.

Pavan-Langston D. *Manual of Ocular Diagnosis and Therapy.* 4th ed. Philadelphia: Lippincott, Williams & Wilkins; 1995.

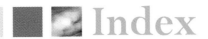 Index

Note: Medications are indexed by generic name only. Page numbers followed by "f" denote figures; "t," tables; "c," clinical protocols.

neovascularization of, 198
nodules of, 198
persistent pupillary membrane
remnants of, 198–199
sphincter, traumatic rupture of, 110
Iris bombé, 198
Iritis, 203
Irrigation of eye, 287, 292*c*
Ischemic scleritis, 186
Isopter, 114
Isopto Hyoscine. *See* Scopolamine

J

Jackson cross cylinder, 58, 59*f,* 66*f*
Jaeger notation, 28, 29*t,* 31
Jugular venous hum, 137

K

Kenalog. *See* Triamcinolone acetonide
Keratic precipitates, 196
Keratinization, 185
Keratitis
bacterial, 197*f*
dendritic, 278–280
herpes simplex, 278–280
interstitial, 193, 193*f*
microbial, 273, 273*f*
punctate epithelial, 190
Keratoconjunctivitis sicca, 181*f*
Keratometer, 11
Ketoconazole, 294*t*
Ketorolac tromethamine, 298
Kinetic perimetry, 114
Koeppe lens, 204*f*
Koeppe nodules, 198
Krimsky test, 91–92, 93*f,* 97*c*–98*c*
Krukenberg's spindle, 196

L

Lacerations
eyelid, 273
globe, 277–278
Lacrimal cannula, 129*t*
Lacrimal gland, 170–171
Lacrimal outflow measurements, 153*c*
Lacrimal probes, 129*t*
Lacrimal sac compression, 138, 153*c*
Lacrimal set, 129*t*
Lacrimal system, 134–135
Lagophthalmos, 133*t*
Lamellae, 171, 171*f*
Lancaster astigmatic clock, 65
Landolt C test, 28
Language barriers, 12
Latanoprost, 300*t*
Latent nystagmus, 95
Lattice degeneration, 256
Lattice dystrophy, 194

Lazy eye. *See* Amblyopia
Learning, 5
Legal blindness, 37
Lens (artificial)
bifocal, 75, 76*f*
compound, 52
cylindrical, 50, 51*f*
focal length of, 49
minus. *See* Minus lens
multifocal, 75, 76*f*
notation for, 54–55
plus. *See* Plus lenses
prescription for, 54–55
progressive addition, 80*c*
spherical, 49
spherocylindrical, 52
toric, 52
trifocal, 75, 76*f*
types of, 49*f*–52*f,* 49–52
variable focus, 80*c*
Lens (crystalline)
abnormalities of, 200–203
anatomy of, 199–200, 200*f*
capsule of, 199, 200*f*
cataracts of. *See* Cataracts
luxation of, 202
material from, in anterior chamber,
197
nucleus of, 199
subluxation of, 202
Lensmeter
cylinder power measurements, 79*c*
definition of, 55
eyepiece of, 78*c*–79*c*
parts of, 56*f*
prism-compensating devices in, 80*c*
sphere measurements, 79*c*
technique for using, 78*c*–79*c*
Lens power, 50*f*
Lens transposition, 54–55
Lenticular astigmatism, 36
Leukoma, 192
Levobunolol, 300*t*
Levofloxacin, 295*t*
Lid lag, 133*t*
Light-near dissociation, 106, 108
Light-perception testing, 29*t*
Light reflex (foveal), 253
Light reflex (pupillary)
pathway of, 101–103, 102*f*
testing of, 105, 111*c*
Limbal conjunctiva, 180*f,* 180–181
Linear punctate staining, 208*f*
Lisch nodules, 106
Lissamine green, 208, 294
Listening, 12
LogMAR, 27–28
Loupes, 129*t*

Lower conjunctiva, 146*c*
Low vision
classification of, 37
testing of, 32, 44*c*
Lubricating medications, 302
Luxation, of crystalline lens, 202
Lymphangiectasia, 183
Lymphedema, 183
Lymph nodes
enlargement of, 137
inspection of, 130
palpation of, 137, 137*f*

M

M, as expression of acuity, 27
Macula
anatomy of, 224, 224*f,* 225*t,* 226*f,*
252*t,* 253
drusen of, 254
Hruby lens slit-lamp biomicroscopy
of, 241
Macular dystrophy, 194
Macule, 130*t*
Madarosis, 0, 133*t,* 173*f*
Maddox rod test, 90
Magnifiers, 129*t*
Maintenance of certification, 7
Manifest refraction, 64, 73
Mannitol, 301*t*
Map-dot-fingerprint dystrophy, 190
Marcus Gunn pupil, 105, 106, 107*t*
Mast cell stabilizers, 302
Medial rectus muscle, 86, 86*f*
Medical knowledge, 3
Medical record keeping, 14
Medicare, 24
Medications
anesthetic agents, 293
antifungal, 294*t,* 304
antihistamines, 302
anti-infective, 294, 294*t*–296*t*
anti-inflammatory, 304
anti-vascular endothelial growth
factor agents, 303–304
antiviral, 296*t,* 304
cap colors for, 22–23
carbonic anhydrase inhibitors, 276,
299, 300*t,* 301
cholinergic agonists, 300*t,* 301
corneal dehydration, 302
corticosteroids, 288, 297
cycloplegics. *See* Cycloplegics
decongestants, 302
glaucoma, 299–301, 300*t*–301*t*
history-taking about, 22–23, 22–24
intravitreal administration of,
303–304
lubricating, 302